Thyroid Cancer

edited by
James A. Fagin

ENDOCRINE UPDATES

Shlomo Melmed, M.D., Series Editor

Thyroid Cancer

edited by

James A. Fagin

Division of Endocrinology & Metabolism
Department of Medicine
College of Medicine
University of Cincinnati
Cincinnati, Ohio

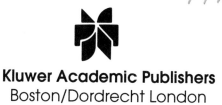

Kluwer Academic Publishers
Boston/Dordrecht London

Distributors for North, Central and South America:
Kluwer Academic Publishers
101 Philip Drive
Assinippi Park
Norwell, Massachusetts 02061 USA
Telephone (781) 871-6600
Fax (781) 871-6528
E-Mail <kluwer@wkap.com>

Distributors for all other countries:
Kluwer Academic Publishers Group
Distribution Centre
Post Office Box 322
3300 AH Dordrecht, THE NETHERLANDS
Telephone 31 78 6392 392
Fax 31 78 6546 474
E-Mail <orderdept@wkap.nl>

 Electronic Services <http://www.wkap.nl>

Library of Congress Cataloging-in-Publication Data

A C.I.P. Catalogue record for this book is available
from the Library of Congress.

Printed on acid-free paper.

Printed in the United States of America

Contents

List of Contributors

Kenneth B. Ain, M.D.
Associate Professor of Medicine
Endocrinology & Metabolism, Rm MN 520
University of Kentucky Medical Center
800 Rose St.
Lexington, KY 40536-0084

Paul Biddinger, M.D.
Associate Professor of Pathology
University of Cincinnati College of Medicine
Department of Pathology and Laboratory Medicine
Division of Surgical Pathology
231 Bethesda Avenue, ML #0529
Cincinnati, OH 45267-0529

James Brierley, M.D.
The Ontario Cancer Institute
Princess Margaret Hospital
610 University Avenue
Toronto, Ontario M5G 2M9
 Canada

A.F. Cailleux, M.D.
Institut Gustave-Roussy
39, rue Camille-Desmoulins
F-94805 Villejuif Cedex
FRANCE

Kyuran A. Choe, M.D.
Assistant Professor of Radiology
University of Cincinnati College of Medicine
Department of Radiology
231 Bethesda Avenue, ML #0742
Cincinnati, OH 45267-0742

Gilbert J. Cote, Ph.D.
Section of Endocrinology
M.D. Anderson Cancer Center, Box 15
1515 Holcombe Blvd.
Houston, TX 77030-4009

K. Michael Derwahl, M.D.
Professor
Medizinische Universitätsklinik, Bergmannsheil
Bürkle-de-la-Camp Platz 1
D-44789 Bochum
GERMANY

James A. Fagin, M.D.
Professor of Medicine
Director, Division of Endocrinology & Metabolism
University of Cincinnati College of Medicine
231 Bethesda Avenue, ML #0547
Cincinnati, OH 45267-0547

Robert Gagel, M.D.
Chief, Endocrine Section
MD Anderson Cancer Center, Box 15
1515 Holcombe Blvd.
Houston, TX 77030-4009

Hossain Gharib, M.D.
Professor of Medicine
Department of Endocrinology
Mayo Clinic
200 First Street SW
Rochester, MN 55905-0001

Yogish C. Kudva, M.D.
Division of Endocrinology
Mayo Clinic
200 First Street SW
Rochester, MN 55905

Wendy Mack, Ph.D.
Associate Professor
University of Southern California
School of Medicine
Dept. of Preventive Medicine CHP 234A
1540 Alcazar
Los Angeles, CA 90033

Harry R. Maxon, M.D.
Saenger Professor of Radiological Sciences
Director, Division of Nuclear Medicine
University of Cincinnati College of Medicine
231 Bethesda Avenue, ML 0577
Cincinnati, OH 45267-0577

Ernest Mazzaferri, M.D.
Professor and Chairman
Department of Internal Medicine
Ohio State University
215 E. Means Hall--1654 Upham Drive
Columbus, OH 43210

Yuri E. Nikiforov, M.D., Ph.D.
Instructor
University of Cincinnati College of Medicine
Department of Pathology
231 Bethesda Avenue, ML #0529
Cincinnati, OH 45267-0529

Yolanda C. Oertel, M.D.
Department of Pathology, Room 609
2300 Eye Street, N.W.
George Washington University Medical Center
Washington, DC 20037

Garry R. Peplinski, M.D.
Assistant Professor of Surgery
University of California at San Francisco
School of Medicine
Department of Surgery
513 Parnassus, S-320
San Francisco, CA 94143-0104

Susan Preston-Martin, Ph.D.
University of Southern California
Norris Cancer Center
1441 Eastlake Avenue, Room 4412-13
Los Angeles, CA 90033-0800

Jacob Robbins, M.D.
Genetics & Biochemistry Branch
NIH/NIDDK
Bldg. 10, Room 8N315
Bethesda, MD 20892-1766

Arthur B. Schneider, M.D., Ph.D.
Section Chief
Department of Endocrinology & Metabolism, M/C 640
University of Illinois at Chicago
1819 W. Polk Street
Chicago, IL 60612

Martin Schlumberger, M.D.
Professor of Oncology
Institut Gustave-Roussy
39, rue Camille-Desmoulins
F-94805 Villejuif Cedex
FRANCE

Hugo Studer, M.D.
Breichtenstrasse 13
CH-3074 Muri
SWITZERLAND

Samuel A. Wells, Jr., M.D.
Executive Director
American College of Surgeons
633 St. Clair
Chicago, IL 60611

Preface:

James A. Fagin

Thyroid cancer has been very much in the news over the past few years. Its known association with radiation exposure during childhood has manifested in a particularly cruel and unexpected way among the peoples of Belarus, Ukraine and South West Russia after the nuclear reactor accident in Chernobyl in 1986. In the United States, radioactive contamination from the atomic bomb detonations at the Nevada test site in the 1950's was reportedly widespread through the nation, and of sufficient magnitude to predict a significant excess of thyroid cancer cases. However, most patients with thyroid cancer have no known history of radiation exposure, and their pathogenesis remains uncertain.

We are now beginning to understand the genetic mechanisms of thyroid tumor initiation and progression. Genetic targets of radiation damage have been identified, as well as other defects acquired during cancer evolution. So far, the major clinical impact of molecular genetics on patient care in this field has been the identification of the gene conferring predisposition to familial medullary thyroid cancer and multiple endocrine neoplasia type II. Screening of at-risk individuals for germline mutations of the ret proto-oncogene is the most reliable test to identify carriers during early childhood, enabling prophylactic thyroidectomy.

Because of its relative rarity and favorable outcome, it has not been feasible to assess medical interventions for thyroid cancer using randomized prospective trials. The approach to diagnosis and treatment relies to a great extent on information derived from retrospective studies. Overall prognosis and survival rate have been edging upward over the past two decades. This is attributed to a wider acceptance of total thyroidectomy as the primary surgical strategy, and possibly to the use of ^{131}I therapy for remnant ablation and treatment of recurrences. The appropriate indication of radioiodine therapy remains controversial, and physicians must be familiar with staging criteria to make educated decisions. There are still major challenges ahead. Treatment of disseminated undifferentiated thyroid cancer is largely ineffective. The same can be said for invasive or metastatic medullary thyroid carcinoma. Hopefully, some of the advances in our understanding of cancer pathogenesis can be translated to new treatment schemes for advanced forms of thyroid cancer.

The contributors to this book provide comprehensive updates on epidemiology, pathogenesis, diagnosis and treatment of thyroid neoplasms. Although the material should be of particular interest to scholars in the field, we have strived to make it of practical use to physicians that treat patients with thyroid disease. I wish to acknowledge the generosity of the contributors for their support of this venture. I also want to recognize the post-doctoral fellows working in my laboratory, who have been a source of excitement and inspiration over the years. Finally, I am particularly indebted to Jeannie Wilson for her dedicated effort in preparing the final version of the chapters in a camera-ready format, which greatly accelerated our ability to publish this book in a timely fashion.

Thyroid Cancer

1 EPIDEMIOLOGY OF THYROID CANCER

Wendy J. Mack
Susan Preston-Martin
University of Southern California
Los Angeles, CA

DESCRIPTIVE EPIDEMIOLOGY

Cancer of the thyroid is a relatively rare cancer accounting for approximately 1% of all cancers in the United States (1). While the absolute incidence rates and breakdown by histologic subtypes show a marked international variation, international comparisons also show striking similarities in the age distribution and female excess of this cancer site.

Histology

Thyroid cancer is comprised of four primary histologic types. Papillary and follicular cancers arise from the thyroid follicular cells, occur primarily in young to middle-aged women, and are well differentiated. The two tumors are characterized histologically by different nuclear morphology and mode of spreading (1). Anaplastic cancers, which also arise from follicular cells, are undifferentiated, occur primarily in the elderly, and are associated with a much poorer prognosis. Medullary cancers arise from the calcitonin-secreting parafollicular cells.

While papillary and follicular cancers are the most common histologic types of thyroid cancer, the distribution of thyroid cancer by histology varies across the world. Excesses of follicular and anaplastic thyroid cancers appear to occur in iodine-deficient areas, and rates of papillary thyroid cancer have been reported to be higher in iodine-rich areas (2). Among all thyroid cancer cases diagnosed between 1973 to 1991 and identified in the United States SEER (Surveillance, Epidemiology, and End Results) registry, the distribution by histology was 76% papillary, 17% follicular, 3% medullary, and 2% anaplastic, with the remainder categorized as "other" (3). The histologic distribution is similar in Japan (4) and Hawaii (5). In Sweden between 1958-1981, the histologic distribution was 47%

papillary, 28% follicular, 4% medullary, and 17% anaplastic (6). In Switzerland between 1974-1987, the histologic distribution was 53% papillary, 27% follicular, 2% medullary, and 5% anaplastic (7). The relatively higher proportions of follicular thyroid cancers in Sweden and Switzerland likely reflect the fact that both of these countries contain iodine-deficient areas.

International Comparisons

Age-adjusted annual incidence rates of thyroid cancer vary around the world and across ethnic groups, from a low of around 0.5 per 100,000 to a high of around 25 per 100,000 (Figure 1) (8). Among United States whites, the average age-adjusted incidence rate is 2.2 per 100,000 in males, and 5.8 per 100,000 in females (Figure 1). Lower incidence rates are observed in African-American populations, in certain Asian populations (India, China), and in the United Kingdom. Populations with relatively high incidence rates are Iceland (6.2 per 100,000 in males and 8.3 per 100,000 in females), the Philippines (3.5 per 100,000 in Manila males and 8.6 per 100,000 in Manila females), Filipino immigrant populations in areas such as Los Angeles and Hawaii, and various other ethnic groups in Hawaii (Figure 1).

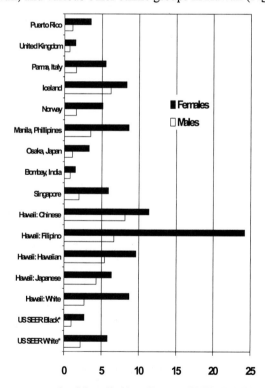

Figure 1: Age-adjusted incidence rates (per 100,000) of thyroid cancer, 1983-1987 (8).
* SEER = Surveillance, Epidemiology, and End Results cancer registry
** State of Hawaii cancer registry contributes data to U.S. SEER registry

Age

Cancer incidence data from 1972-1995, obtained from the Los Angeles County population-based Cancer Surveillance Program (CSP), were used to plot age-specific rates of thyroid cancer in the Caucasian population (Figure 2). Rates are quite low for both sexes in childhood. In females, rates increase from age 15-40. After this, rates plateau in women while male rates continue to rise through ages 75-79 when male and female rates are similar.

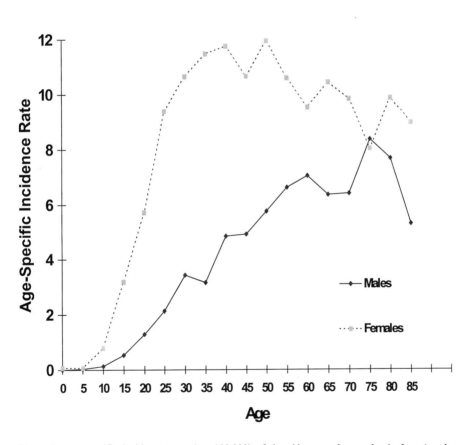

Figure 2: Age-specific incidence rates (per 100,000) of thyroid cancer by gender in Los Angeles County, 1972-1995.

Gender

Throughout the world, age-adjusted incidence rates for thyroid cancer show a 2- to 3-fold excess among females relative to males (Figure 1). This female excess is apparent not only in geographically diverse areas, but is also evident across ethnic groups residing in the same area.

The female:male ratio varies by age and histology. Age-specific incidence data from Los Angeles County (Figure 2) show that the female:male rate ratio is highest from ages 15-40, ranging from 3.1 to 6.0. The female excess remains approximately double from age 40-55 and declines thereafter. Among almost 12,000 thyroid cancer cases diagnosed among whites between 1973-1987 and identified in the United States SEER registry, the female:male ratio was 2.6 for papillary cancer, 2.2 for follicular cancer, 2.0 for medullary cancer, and 1.0 for anaplastic cancer (1).

Ethnicity

Figure 3 displays age-adjusted incidence rates (AAIRs, per 100,000) for thyroid cancer in Los Angeles County by ethnicity. In both males and females, rates are lowest in African-Americans, and are roughly equivalent in Non-Hispanic and Hispanic whites. Consistent with international data (Figure 1), Filipinos show the highest incidence rates in Los Angeles County. Other Asian groups in general show thyroid cancer rates that are slightly lower than those among whites. This is in contrast to data from the United States SEER cancer registries, which show, relative to non-Hispanic whites, higher rates in Chinese-Americans, Japanese-Americans, and Filipino-Americans (9). The SEER analysis also reported lower thyroid cancer incidence rates in African-Americans and Puerto Rico Hispanics and higher rates in all Hawaiian ethnic groups (9).

Migration

In Hawaii, incidence rates are elevated for all non-white ethnic groups in comparison to rates from their countries of origin and in comparison to rates from the same ethnic groups in other countries of migration (Figure 1). This suggests that environmental factors specific to Hawaii may be important factors contributing to the incidence of thyroid cancer (5).

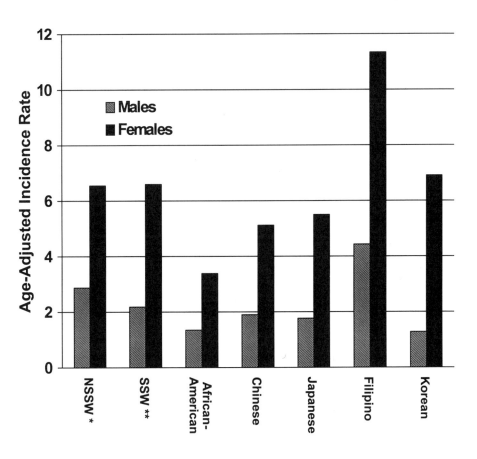

Figure 3: Age-adjusted incidence rates (per 100,000) of thyroid cancer by ethnicity, Los Angeles County, 1972-1995.
* NSSW = Non-Spanish surnamed white
** SSW = Spanish-surnamed white

Data from cancer registries in Hawaii, San Francisco Bay, and Washington State, were used to compare thyroid cancer incidence rates among U.S-born whites, U.S.-born Asians, and foreign-born Asians (10). Differences in thyroid cancer incidence rates according to birthplace were most striking in Filipino men and women. In comparison to U.S.-born whites, Filipino men and women born in the Philippines had higher rates of thyroid cancer. In contrast, the rates in U.S.-born Filipinos were not significantly higher than rates of U.S.-born whites. Papillary thyroid cancer rates in Japanese-born women, but not men, were higher than U.S.-born whites, and the rates in U.S.-born Japanese women were significantly lower than U.S.-born whites. In both U.S.- and foreign-born Japanese women, the rates of follicular cancer were lower than U.S.-born whites. Rates of papillary thyroid cancer were elevated in both U.S-born and foreign-born Chinese men.

Secular trends

Increases in the incidence of thyroid cancer have been observed all over the world (6, 11-14). It has been hypothesized that the increases observed in the United States may be due to the use of radiation therapy for treatment of benign conditions of the head and neck (11,15). These medical practices were not widely used in Europe, however (13,14).

In Connecticut between 1935-1975, there was a 5-fold increase in thyroid cancer rates, which was largely attributed to increases in papillary and follicular cancers (11). When analyzed by birth cohort, increases in the incidence of papillary cancer in females were seen with each birth cohort born from 1910 to 1960, after which decreases in incidence were observed. This pattern was attributed to use of radiation therapy to treat benign childhood conditions of the head and neck, which was widely practiced in the United States from the 1920's through 1950's. An extended analysis from 1935-1992 of data from the same Connecticut Tumor Registry was consistent with the previous study (15). Increases in thyroid cancer incidence in this analysis were almost completely due to increases in papillary cancer, which has continued to increase throughout the study period. Follicular cancer showed small increases between 1940 through the early 1980's, and plateaued after this. There was a strong effect of birth cohort on the trends in incidence; in males and females, thyroid cancer rates increased continuously for cohorts born prior to 1950 and either decreased or leveled off for cohorts born after 1950. The observed increases in incidence up to 1992 in this study contrasts with an earlier analysis of incidence data from United States SEER cancer registries (1973-1981) which suggested a leveling off of thyroid cancer rates in the 1970's (9).

In England and Wales, increases in thyroid cancer rates were observed from 1962-1984 in both sexes among persons under age 45 (13). A sharp rise in incidence was observed in women born in 1952-1955. The same pattern was not observed in males. Similar patterns were observed in Sweden from 1958-1981 (6). In Sweden, the observed increases in thyroid cancer were also primarily due to increases in papillary cancer, were larger in women (average annual increases in papillary cancer rates of 4.9% in women and 2.1% in men), and were observed in birth cohorts from 1919 on. The increases could not be completely attributed to changes in diagnostic practices and histologic classification.

In Norway, thyroid cancer rates increased in the 1970's and began to decrease in the early 1980's (12, 14). The trend of decreasing thyroid cancer incidence in the 1980's was most evident in women and in papillary cancers. Analysis of birth cohort showed increases in incidence by cohort starting approximately after 1900 and leveling off in 1950 birth cohorts (14). In addition, a weaker time period effect was observed with higher rates in the period 1965-1984.

It is certain that a portion of the secular trend can be explained by the introduction of more sophisticated diagnostic procedures, such as fine-needle biopsy and radioisotope thyroid scans (6). Trends in the completeness of ascertainment of cancer cases must also be considered as a possible explanation for secular trends in cancer incidence. However, these factors cannot explain why much of the increases in incidence have occurred in papillary cancer. Changes in medical technology and case ascertainment would be expected to influence incidence rates of all histologic types. Changes in diagnostic classification would also influence incidence rates. In this respect, revised histological classification criteria in the 1970's likely resulted in the re-classification of certain follicular cancers as papillary cancer (6). However, these changes in histologic classification would not explain increases in incidence of papillary cancer observed prior to this period. A better explanation, at least for observed secular trends in the United States, is the administration of radiation treatment for benign childhood conditions practiced from the 1920's to 1950's. Analyses showing that increases in thyroid cancer incidence are limited to birth cohorts born prior to 1950 support this notion (15).

Survival

Survival rates for thyroid cancer exceed all other cancers except for nonmelanoma skin cancer (3). Survival varies markedly by histology. In a follow-up of 15,698 thyroid cancer cases diagnosed between 1973 and 1991 as part of the Surveillance, Epidemiology and End Results (SEER) program, a network of population-based cancer registries in the United States, the overall 10-year survival rate was 58% (3). Survival varied strongly by histology. While the 10-year survival rate for papillary (98%), follicular (92%), and even medullary (80%) thyroid cancers are quite good, the relative 10-year survival rate for anaplastic thyroid cancer is poor (13%). Several demographic factors are associated with survival; lower survival rates are observed with increasing age, more poorly differentiated tumors at diagnosis, and a more advanced tumor stage at diagnosis (3). Papillary thyroid cancer diagnosed at a distant stage was still associated with a remarkably good 10-year survival rate (82%), compared to tumors of similar staging in follicular (45%), medullary (31%) and anaplastic (6%) cancers. Although survival did not vary markedly by gender, females had distinctly higher 10-year survival rates for medullary thyroid cancer (87% in females and 68% in males). For follicular and medullary thyroid cancers,

African-Americans have lower survival rates than any other ethnic group, even after adjusting for tumor stage at diagnosis (3). The reasons for this higher mortality in African-Americans are not clear.

Analytic Epidemiology -- Risk Factors

Radiation

Exposure to ionizing radiation is by far the most well established risk factor for thyroid cancer. The excess risk has been consistently demonstrated in cohorts of persons exposed to therapeutic radiation for a variety of medical conditions. While the literature regarding exposure to I^{131} and risk of thyroid cancer is less clear, elevations in risk at high doses is evident. Despite the strong relationship with radiation exposures, only a small proportion of thyroid cancer cases can be attributed to high dose radiation exposures because of the low prevalence of such exposures in the general population. What remains to be determined is the thyroid cancer risk associated with lower radiation doses characteristic of diagnostic radiography, since these are the doses that are highly prevalent in industrialized nations. Because radiation-induced thyroid cancer is extensively covered in Chapter 2, it will not be reviewed in detail here. We focus instead on other factors that might relate to the large proportion of thyroid cancers that cannot be attributed to high dose radiation exposure, and that might help explain the female predominance of this disease.

Other Risk Factors

The search for risk factors other than radiation for thyroid cancer has been stimulated by the hypothesis that chronic elevation of serum TSH and other alterations in the hormonal environment may be important etiologic factors in thyroid carcinogenesis (16). TSH induces thyroid growth, and chronic elevations in TSH produced through a variety of mechanisms yield thyroid hyperplasia and thyroid tumors in laboratory animals (17).

Benign thyroid disease

The occurrence of certain thyroid conditions, in particular conditions that are associated with thyroid hyperplasia, is a well-established risk factor for thyroid cancer. The consistency of the associations among a number of studies conducted throughout the world is striking (including the United States, Sweden, Switzerland, Italy, and Shanghai, China). It is interesting to note that these thyroid conditions, like thyroid cancer, are more prevalent in females than males. This may partially explain the high female:male ratio of thyroid cancer incidence. Like thyroid cancer, it is not known why benign thyroid diseases are more common in females than males. It is possible that excesses in TSH, possibly related to reproductive and hormonal events, may also be important in the pathogenesis of benign thyroid disease.

A prior history of goiter has been shown to be a risk factor in epidemiological studies (18-25) with odds ratios (ORs) ranging from 2.4 to 8.2 when assessed over all histologic subtypes. Although goiter was a risk factor for all histologic subtypes of thyroid cancer among females in Washington State, the association with follicular thyroid cancer (OR = 17.0) was much stronger than for other subtypes (18). This finding is consistent with descriptive data, which reports higher rates of follicular thyroid cancer in geographical areas characterized by endemic goiter (2). However, in a study conducted among Italian males and females, elevated relative risks associated with goiter were of a similar magnitude for both follicular and papillary cancers (25). Only one case-control study in Sweden reported a non-significantly elevated risk associated with goiter (OR=1.5) (26).

A history of benign thyroid nodules or adenomas is another condition which shows a highly elevated relative risk of subsequent thyroid cancer (18, 19, 21, 23-25). Relative risks associated with this condition range from 12.0 to 33.3. In Washington State females, the relative risk was higher in papillary thyroid cancer (OR=19.8) compared to all histologic subtypes (OR = 12.0) (18). Benign nodules or adenomas may actually be precursor lesions to thyroid cancer (23). In addition, benign thyroid adenomas are associated with radiation therapy in childhood (27). This would in part explain the very high relative risks associated with these conditions.

Other thyroid conditions associated with elevated risk for thyroid cancer include thyroid enlargement as an adolescent (20, 24), thyroiditis (23, 25), a general variable of benign thyroid disease (22), and a combined variable of either goiter or benign thyroid nodules (20, 28). Hyperthyroidism has been inconsistently associated with thyroid cancer. While some studies report this condition to be a risk factor (21, 24-26, 28), others have shown no association (18, 19, 22, 23). A history of hypothyroidism has consistently shown no association with the risk of thyroid cancer (18, 19, 22, 25).

Although benign thyroid disease is relatively infrequent in most populations, the highly elevated relative risks for thyroid cancer associated with these conditions lead to appreciable estimates of attributable risk. The occurrence of any hyperplastic thyroid disease (including thyroid enlargement as an adolescent, goiter, and benign nodules or adenomas) accounted for approximately 20% of thyroid cancers in Los Angeles County females (20) and 10% of thyroid cancers in Shanghai females (24). A history of thyroid disease (including the hyperplastic conditions plus hyperthyroid disease, thyroiditis, and hypothyroid disease) was associated with attributable risk estimates of 13% in Italy (21), 34% in Switzerland (23), and 19% in Northern Italy (25).

While part of the relationship of hyperplastic thyroid conditions with thyroid cancer is likely due to increased medical surveillance among persons with thyroid disease, the fact that hypothyroid disease is not related to thyroid cancer reduces this possibility. The fact that benign thyroid adenomas may be precursor conditions to thyroid cancer (23) makes it difficult to interpret these associations in etiologic terms.

Reproductive factors

Spurred by the striking elevations in thyroid cancer incidence in women of reproductive age relative to males, a host of epidemiologic studies have examined a variety of reproductive variables as possible risk factors.

Menarche. While TSH does not vary over the menstrual cycle (29), thyroid volume has been shown to vary up to 50% throughout the menstrual cycle (30). A cohort study of over 63,000 Norwegian women showed a decreased risk for papillary thyroid cancer and an increased risk for follicular thyroid cancer with later age at menarche (31). In Connecticut, a case-control study (which did not evaluate risk by histology) found a non-significant increasing trend in thyroid cancer risk with later age at menarche, apparent only in women who were diagnosed before the age of 35 (19). In Italy, an elevation in risk with menarche after age 11 was found, with no apparent trend by increasing age at menarche (32); this study also found increased risk with the report of irregular menstrual patterns. Most studies have found no association with age at menarche (20, 22, 24, 33, 34) or whether a woman had ever menstruated regularly (20, 33).

Parity. Because the female:male excess in thyroid cancer incidence peaks in the reproductive years, it has been hypothesized that hormonal changes related to pregnancy might be relevant etiologic factors. Among healthy pregnant women, TSH levels show a gradual rise throughout pregnancy (35-37). A progressive increase in thyroid volume occurs throughout pregnancy, with an average 18-30% increase from initial evaluation in early pregnancy to delivery (37, 38). Serum hCG, with marked elevations occurring in early pregnancy, may directly stimulate the thyroid through its TSH-like activity (37, 39, 40). The precise nature and mechanisms of this thyroid stimulatory activity are not clear.

A number of epidemiologic studies have shown a relatively modest increase in the risk of thyroid cancer associated with parity. Several studies have found no increase in risk in parous compared to non-parous women or any trend in risk with numbers of pregnancies (22, 31, 41, 42). In contrast, other studies have found a positive trend in thyroid cancer risk with increasing numbers of pregnancies and/or live births (19, 20, 28, 32-34, 43). One study reported this positive trend to be limited to women older than age 50 at diagnosis (44), while others have reported the association only in women less than 35 at diagnosis (19) or premenopausal women (32). Still others have found an increased risk associated with at least one pregnancy, but no trend in risk with number of pregnancies (24, 26, 45). In one study, the association with at least one pregnancy was stronger for follicular than papillary thyroid cancer (45). Multiple pregnancies increased the risk for papillary thyroid cancer associated with diagnostic radiography (34) and for thyroid cancer associated with therapeutic radiation to the head or neck (19). Such findings might result from elevated levels of TSH during pregnancy promoting cellular proliferation and replication of radiation-induced mutations.

Higher risks have been noted with shorter time since pregnancy (44), and the effect of a recent pregnancy was found to be even stronger in follicular, compared to papillary, thyroid cancer (43). In general, age at first birth has not been found to be related to thyroid cancer risk (19, 20, 28, 33, 41, 43, 44). One Italian case-control study did find a strong trend of increasing risk for thyroid cancer with older age at first (and last) birth (32). In contrast, a case-control study from Sweden found decreasing risk of papillary thyroid cancer with older age at first pregnancy (34).

Several studies have noted an increase in risk of thyroid cancer in women who had miscarriages, particularly in the first pregnancy (19, 20, 22, 24, 33). Only one study has failed to support this finding (41). A case-control study found a higher prevalence of miscarriage prior to the index pregnancy in the mothers of thyroid cancer cases as compared to control mothers (46). Infertility has also been associated with an elevated thyroid cancer risk (22).

Underlying thyroid disorders are responsible for dysfunctional menstrual cycles, anovulation, infertility, and miscarriages (47). Pregnant women with mild thyroid abnormalities (including past thyroid disorder, goiter, benign nodules, and autoimmune thyroid disorders) had a higher frequency of spontaneous abortions ((48). A small percentage of these women also had abnormally elevated TSH levels at delivery. Pregnant women with a past history of a thyroid disorder, goiter, or thyroid nodules had elevated serum thyroglobulin levels throughout gestation; this may indicate an oversensitivity to stimulatory factors influencing the thyroid during pregnancy. In pregnant women with thyroid nodules, there was an increase in the number and size of nodules at delivery. About one third of the women with goiter showed an increase in thyroid size at delivery, which was related to hormonal stimulation of the thyroid (48).

Menopause. Natural menopause has been related to the risk of thyroid cancer in only two case-control studies conducted in China (24) and Sweden (33). In the few studies that have examined the type of menopause experienced, the occurrence of a surgical menopause has shown a highly elevated risk for thyroid cancer (22, 24, 33, 42). This finding was not replicated in one case-control study (19). The age at menopause, either natural or surgical, has shown no clear relationship to thyroid cancer.

Exogenous hormones

In animal studies, thyroid tumors induced by N-methyl-N-nitrosourea and a low iodine diet were more frequent in female than male rats (49). Thyroid weight and serum TSH was also higher in female than in male rats. Relative to gonadectomized rats not given estrogen, the administration of estrogen increased thyroid weight, TSH, and the incidence of thyroid tumors in castrated and ovarectomized rats. While this animal study suggests that exogenous estrogen may promote thyroid tumors, the epidemiologic data is less compelling.

Oral contraceptives. TSH levels are slightly higher in women on oral contraceptives as compared to women on normal menstrual cycles (29), and it is hypothesized that estrogen may have an inhibitory effect on the thyroid. Several epidemiologic studies have found no association between thyroid cancer and prior use of oral contraceptives (22, 26, 33, 42). However, case-control studies conducted in Shanghai women aged 54 or less (24), in Connecticut women below age 35 (19), in women in Washington state (45), in Los Angeles women aged 40 and under (20), and in Italian women (32) have found slightly to moderately elevated risk associated with any use of oral contraceptives (with odds ratios ranging around 1.5 to 2.4). The Connecticut study found a nonsignificantly elevated risk with use of oral contraceptives that was confined to women diagnosed before age 35 (19). Risk associated with oral contraceptive use was not elevated in women diagnosed at age 35 or older, or among the total sample. In Washington state, risk was slightly elevated over all histologies and among papillary cancers, but was significantly elevated (odds ratio = 3.6) among follicular cancers (45). In all studies, there was no clear trend with duration of use.

Hormone replacement. Few epidemiologic studies have examined the risk of thyroid cancer in relation to postmenopausal hormone use. Most of these studies have found no association between the incidence of thyroid cancer in females and use of hormone replacement therapy (19, 22, 32, 42). In a Swedish cohort of over 22,000 women who had received prescriptions for hormone replacement therapy, there was no excess of thyroid cancer compared to incidence rates in the general Swedish female population after an average 13 years of follow-up (50). A case-control study in Washington state found a small increase in risk (odds ratio=1.4) for any use of noncontraceptive estrogens (45). The association was strengthened (odds ratio=1.9) and became statistically significant when the analyses were confined to papillary thyroid cancer; however there was no clear trend in risk by duration of use of noncontraceptive estrogens. A non-significantly elevated risk associated with postmenopausal hormone use was found in a Swiss case-control study (33).

Other hormones. Only a few studies have studied hormones used for reasons other than birth control or hormone replacement. Connecticut women who used estrogens for gynecologic problems had an increased risk of thyroid cancer (19). While the use of fertility drugs was found to elevate thyroid cancer risk in Hawaiian women (22), no association with fertility drugs was apparent among women in Connecticut (19). The use of lactation suppressants moderately elevated risk in two case-control studies (19, 45). In one of these studies, the elevated risk was apparent only among women less than age 35 (19). The second study reported a significant trend of increasing risk with the number of pregnancies in which lactation suppressants were used (45). No associations with thyroid cancer risk were found for use of DES (19).

Dietary factors

The exploration of diet in the etiology of thyroid cancer was initially motivated by the potential role of iodine-rich seafoods and goitrogenic vegetables. Both iodine excess and iodine deficiency may lead to elevations in TSH (51). For example, endemic goiter has been observed in association with excess dietary iodine, and low levels of dietary iodine result in decreased levels of thyroid hormones and a subsequent rise in TSH (51). Dietary goitrogens can inhibit thyroid uptake of iodine resulting also in an elevation of TSH (51). While epidemiologic studies regarding diet have now been reported from a variety of geographic areas, the inconsistency of the findings is striking. Inconsistencies in testing dietary hypotheses may involve: (1) the difficulty in measuring diet, particularly retrospectively, (2) variation in methods of dietary assessment across studies, (3) the large geographical variation in the iodine content of foods (meat and dairy products may or may not contain relatively large amounts of iodine depending on whether the animal ate iodine-rich foods; for example, in Utah following nuclear testing, grazing land became iodine-rich from fallout, and milk from backyard cows and goats became extraordinarily high in iodine), and (4) the variation in thyroid cancer histology and foods eaten across studies (since the association with diet may vary by histology).

Seafood and other fish. It has been hypothesized that consumption of high levels of iodine-rich seafoods will increase the risk of thyroid cancer. Epidemiologic studies to date have shown inconsistent findings in relation to this hypothesis. A case-control study in Norway (a country with a relatively high incidence of thyroid cancer) supported this hypothesis by showing increased risk for regular consumers of cod liver oil, fish liver, or fish sandwich-spread as well as for persons reporting to eat more fish dinners per week (52). The higher incidence of thyroid cancer in coastal versus inland regions of Norway may reflect this reported association with increased consumption of seafood. These findings were supported by a case-control study in Connecticut showing elevated risks with frequent (at least 3 times a week) consumption of shellfish, saltwater fish, and freshwater fish (19); the elevated risk with shellfish was evident in follicular, but not papillary thyroid cancer. In contrast, a case-control study from Sweden and Norway found no increase in risk associated with the consumption of saltwater fish or shellfish; this study did find a decreased risk with greater consumption of freshwater fish (53). In Hawaii, there was a suggestion of elevated risk with high levels of seafood intake; however the dose-response trends by frequency of consumption were not statistically significant (22). This same study found higher average levels of dietary iodine in female cases versus controls. This same pattern of elevated risk (particularly with saltwater fish) without a clear dose-response trend was observed in a case-control study among Shanghai women (24). Yet another case-control study from Norway suggested that the elevated risk associated with seafood may be due to the high content of longchain fatty acids rather than iodine (54). While this association was inferred from serum levels of longchain fatty acids (measured after diagnosis), it is unfortunate that a retrospective diet was not obtained in this study to determine whether seafood was indeed associated with increased risk in this study sample. One case-control study from Italy actually found a pattern of decreased risk with higher consumption of fish (although the type of fish, fresh or saltwater, was not detailed) (21). Decreased risk with higher consumption of all fish and shellfish was found in a Swedish case-control study (34), while others have found no relationship with fish and shellfish (26).

Fruits and vegetables. Epidemiological studies of vegetable consumption have tended to focus on cruciferous vegetables (such as cauliflower and broccoli) because they contain thioglucosides, which can form goitrogens (19). By blocking iodine uptake and synthesis of thyroid hormones, goitrogens can cause the pituitary gland to increase secretion of TSH. In animal studies, goitrogens in large quantities have been shown to cause thyroid cancer (19). However, it is unlikely that these effects are seen in most populations because the levels of dietary goitrogens normally consumed are too low; in the rare populations where dietary goitrogens are a major part of the diet and the population resides in an iodine-deficient area, elevated levels of TSH and abnormal thyroid states have been observed (51, 55). In this respect, it is interesting that one case-control study suggested that the consumption of cruciferous vegetables may increase the risk of thyroid cancer only among persons who had resided in areas of endemic goiter (53).

Far more case-control studies have found a decreased risk associated with cruciferous vegetables (19, 34) and green vegetables (21, 56). It has been hypothesized that the decreased risk may be due to the indoles, isothiocyanates and phenols contained in vegetables (19). Most epidemiological studies of diet have not examined risk according to residence in iodine-rich versus iodine-poor areas.

In general, consumption of fruit has not been associated with the risk of thyroid cancer (56). Elevated risk was found for higher consumption of fruit in a case-control study from Norway (53), while an Italian case-control study found decreased risk (21).

Dairy products. Dairy products can be a major source of dietary iodine if the animal source was fed iodine-supplemented foods (51). Butter and cheese, but not yogurt and milk, were found to increase the risk of thyroid cancer in case-control studies in Sweden and Norway (53) and Italy (21). Further analyses in the Swedish study (53) showed the effect of milk products to be limited to subjects who had lived in areas of endemic goiter.

Iodine supplementation. Incidence rates of papillary thyroid cancer tend to be higher in iodine-rich areas than in iodine-deficient areas, while the opposite pattern has been reported for follicular thyroid cancer (2). Concern with iodine supplementation programs in endemic goiter areas thus relates to a possible increase in the incidence of papillary thyroid cancer. Earlier studies did report an overall increase in rates of papillary cancer of the thyroid in the 20 years following iodine supplementation (57, 58). A more detailed analysis in Sweden found a secular increase in papillary thyroid cancer following iodine supplementation in endemic goiter areas; however the increase was no different in iodine-deficient versus iodine-rich areas, suggesting that the increase was not related to iodine supplementation (2). A decreased risk of thyroid cancer associated with use of iodized salt was evident in Norway, but not Sweden in one case-control study (53).

Caffeinated beverages. A protective association with increasing coffee consumption was noted in a Greek case-control study (59) and in a recent case-control study from Japan (28). This association was not seen in Sweden and Norway (53) or Italy (21).

Dietary and Serum Micronutrients. A small number of epidemiological studies have evaluated specific micronutrient levels in subjects' diets in relation to thyroid cancer. Such studies have found decreased risk with dietary betacarotene and vitamins C and E (60). The association with betacarotene was apparent in both papillary and follicular thyroid cancer. This same study interestingly found an elevated risk with higher dietary intake of retinol. Serum levels of selenium have been found to be lower in thyroid cancer cases than controls (61).

Vitamin supplementation. In Sweden and Norway, a decreased risk for thyroid cancer was found for regular use of vitamins A, C and E; these associations were apparent in women only (53). In contrast, a Connecticut case-control study found non-significantly elevated risks for thyroid cancer in regular users of vitamins A and C (19). This study also found a significantly increased risk in regular users of vitamin D; this association was particularly high for medullary cancer of the thyroid. Animal studies have shown that vitamin D increases the production of calcitonin and causes hyperplasia of the parafollicular cells, from which medullary cancer arises (19).

Alcohol. Regular consumption of alcohol (including wine, beer, and hard liquor) was not related to incident thyroid cancer in several case-control studies from geographically diverse regions (19, 21, 28, 53). Earlier data from the Third National Cancer Survey had found an increased risk for thyroid cancer associated with use of wine, beer, and hard liquor (62); it had been hypothesized that alcohol might increase TSH levels.

Body Size

Body size and weight gain have been shown to increase the risk of thyroid cancer in several case-control studies. Thyroid volume increases with higher body weight (30). Elevated risk for thyroid cancer has been associated with a higher absolute weight prior to diagnosis (63, 64), a high body mass index at 18 years of age and as an adult in women, but not in men (19), weight gain (from menarche to adulthood) in Shanghai women (24), as well as a greater weight gain in mothers of thyroid cancer cases versus controls (46). Few studies have failed to find this association in women (32). In a detailed analysis of case-control data on weight and body mass index in Hawaii, weight gain from early adulthood was a significant risk factor in women, but not men (64). This study also suggested that higher absolute weight and body mass index are stronger risk factors when experienced in older adulthood compared to early adulthood, and when experienced after menopause compared to premenopause. Intriguing analyses of interactions suggested that the influence of prior use of fertility drugs was potentiated by higher weight (odds ratio for fertility use in women below median weight = 1.4; odds ratio for fertility use in women above the median weight = 17.2) (64).

Familial Aggregation and Molecular Genetics

Approximately 20-25% of medullary thyroid cancer is of a familial form that is inherited in an autosomal dominant pattern with a high, age-related penetrance (65). While no clear pattern of genetic inheritance has been demonstrated for other types of thyroid cancer or for the remaining 75% of sporadic medullary thyroid cancer, a number of case-control studies have reported an elevated relative risk associated with having a positive family history of thyroid disease (22-26, 34, 46), or thyroid cancer (19, 26, 28, 46, 66, 67). The excess risk of thyroid cancer in case families may be limited to subjects with papillary thyroid cancer (67).

An excess of all cancers among family members of thyroid cancer cases found in one case-control study (68) has not been supported by others (19, 22, 24, 67). A case-control study from Serbia found excesses of cancers of the breast, uterus, and digestive organs among first- and second-degree family members of thyroid cancer cases (68). In Sweden, mothers of thyroid cancer cases had a lower rate of breast cancer than the general population; an excess risk of cancers of the uterus and stomach were apparent only among mothers' of follicular cancer cases (67). Relative to controls, an excess of female genital cancers (sites unspecified) was found among family members of Swedish females with papillary thyroid cancer (34).

The multiple endocrine neoplasia (MEN) type 2 syndrome is an inherited autosomal dominant disorder characterized by three subtypes, all of which include medullary thyroid cancer as a primary tumor type: MEN 2A, MEN 2B, and familial medullary thyroid cancer (65). Activation mutations of the ret proto-oncogene have been found in persons exhibiting the MEN 2 syndromes as well as in sporadic medullary thyroid cancers (69). Germline mutations in specific regions of this proto-oncogene have been found in the three MEN 2 subtypes. These findings have been clinically applied to recommend genetic screening for these mutations in of MEN 2 families and prophylactic thyroidectomy in family members in whom these mutations are found (70) (see Chapter 4). Somatic mutations in another region have been found in some persons with sporadic medullary thyroid cancer (69), and rearrangements of the gene have been noted in papillary thyroid cancer (71). The specific genetic rearrangements found in papillary cancer were particularly apparent among children diagnosed with thyroid cancer who resided in areas contaminated by the Chernobyl nuclear accident (72, 73). Both mutations and rearrangements of this gene lead to oncogenic activity.

Mutations of the ras oncogene have been associated with follicular thyroid cancer, and mutations of the p53 tumor suppressor gene are highly prevalent in undifferentiated (anaplastic) thyroid cancer, but not in the differentiated thyroid cancers (74). Activating mutations in the trk, Gs alpha, and TSH-receptor genes have also been associated with thyroid nodules and cancers (75, 76) (see Chapter 3).

Occupational and chemical exposures

Relatively few studies have investigated the role of occupational or specific chemical exposures in relation to thyroid cancer. Cohort studies are hampered by the low incidence rates of thyroid cancer. Mortality studies are even more problematic because of the high survival rates of the primary subtypes, papillary and follicular thyroid cancers. Although mortality studies do not generally specify histology-specific deaths, it is likely that relatively more deaths are due to anaplastic than other thyroid cancer subtypes. Generalizations from mortality studies to all thyroid cancers should thus be made with extreme caution.

Using a linkage between the Swedish cancer registry and occupation reported on the population census, elevated risk of incident thyroid cancer was found for X-ray operators and laboratory assistants, pharmacists, textile workers (males only), canning and preserving industry workers, petroleum refinery workers (males only), stenographers and typists (males only), buyers and dealers (females only), and drivers (males only) (77). Horticultural workers, painters in the construction industry, and unskilled manual laborers were at significantly decreased risk for thyroid cancer.

A case-control study of papillary thyroid cancer in females found elevated risks in women who had ever worked as dentists or dental assistants, teachers, shoemakers, or warehouse workers (78). In addition, women who reported to have ever been occupationally exposed to chemicals in general, x-rays, or video display terminals were at increased risk for papillary cancer of the thyroid. A related case-control study, which contributed a portion of its data to the previous study, reported non-significantly elevated risk among cleaners, lineman, shoemakers, x-ray work, butchers, electrical workers, and dental nurses (79).

Elevated risk of thyroid cancer has been associated with several occupations involving exposure to x-rays, including x-ray operators and laboratory assistants (77, 79), dentists or dental assistants (78), and medical diagnostic x-ray workers (80). In China, excesses in thyroid cancer risk in medical x-ray workers occurred among persons employed prior to 1960, when radiation exposures in this country were relatively high (80). Two studies which failed to support these findings both tested a general variable of occupational exposure to radiation, rather than specific occupations (19, 22).

Female textile workers in North Carolina were found to have elevated risk of thyroid cancer mortality (81). Although no specific agent was hypothesized, an elevated risk for incident thyroid cancer was also reported in Swedish male textile workers (77).

Elevated risks of thyroid cancers were found for male farm laborers (22). Two additional case-control studies did not support this finding in Italian females (32) or among Swedish males and females (79).

A history of occupational exposure to specific chemicals showed no elevated risk associated with herbicides or insecticides (79). However, elevated risks (with very small numbers of exposed subjects) were found for occupational exposure to chlorophenols and creosote. In a cohort study of almost 19,000 production workers and sprayers exposed to chlorphenoxy herbicides and chlorophenols, an elevated risk of thyroid cancer mortality (with 4 observed deaths) was found (82). Both types of compounds may be contaminated with TCDD (dioxin) during production. Following the accidental contamination of an Italian residential community with TCDD, a non-significant 4.6-fold elevation in thyroid cancer incidence was found (2 incident cases) (83).

In a mortality study of dry cleaning workers, a non-significant three-fold elevation in thyroid cancer mortality was found (3 deaths) (84). Dry cleaning workers are potentially exposed to a variety of organic solvents, most notably perchloroethylene. A Spanish community with highly elevated airborne levels of organochlorinated compounds, in particular hexachlorobenzene (HCB), noted an almost 7-fold increase in risk of thyroid cancer in males (2 incident cases); the excess was not seen in females (85). The different association by gender may have been explained by the occupational as well as residential exposure; both male cases had been employed in the neighboring organochlorinated-compounds factory, while the female case had not. Animal experiments have linked feeding of HCB with thyroid cancer.

Residence

A history of residence in areas characterized by endemic goiter has been consistently shown to be a risk factor for thyroid cancer. In Switzerland (23) and Sweden (53), thyroid cancer risk was doubled in persons with a history of residence in endemic goiter areas. Similar findings in an Italian case-control study showed an approximate doubling in risk for persons living at least 20 years and in those living in childhood in endemic goiter areas (21). These findings were evident for both papillary and follicular thyroid cancers. Subjects who had lived in endemic goiter areas reported a history of goiter or thyroid nodules twice as often as persons never residing in these areas; adjustment for these thyroid diseases reduced the association between thyroid cancer and residence (21). A later case-control study in Italy showed a positive trend with the duration of residence in endemic goiter areas which was evident in both papillary and follicular cancers (25). This positive association was most apparent in females and in persons diagnosed prior to age 50. Residence of more than 5 years in a seaside community was estimated to reduce the thyroid cancer risk by half in Sweden (34).

Other medical conditions and use of medications

Breast cancer. A relationship between thyroid and breast cancer has been noted. Reports on these associations are inconsistent. Based on the positive findings in these and other data, it has been hypothesized that cancers of the thyroid and breast share some common etiologic factors. In particular, the female excess of both cancers have led investigators to suspect that hormonal and reproductive factors may be important in the etiology of both cancers.

Data from the Connecticut Tumor Registry showed a significant excess (relative to the general population) of thyroid cancers following a diagnosis of breast cancer (standardized incidence ratio (SIR) = 1.68) and of breast cancers following a diagnosis of thyroid cancer (SIR = 1.89) (86). The excesses of these second primary cancers were even higher in women diagnosed before age 40. A similar study conducted in Sweden did not confirm the excess of breast cancers following a diagnosis of thyroid cancer (87). One case-control study of thyroid cancer found an elevated thyroid cancer risk in women with a prior breast cancer (63). Another case-control study failed to confirm this finding, but did find a slightly elevated risk for thyroid cancer in women who had reported a prior breast surgery (19).

Thyroid disease, including thyroid enlargement, has been found to be more prevalent in women with breast cancer and benign breast disease compared to women without breast disease (88). TSH levels were also found to be higher in women with breast cancer compared to women with benign breast disease and women free of breast disease (88). A case-control study of breast cancer found that more cases than controls had been treated for hyperthyroidism (89). A history of other thyroid conditions, including hypothyroidism and nodules, goiter, or thyroid cancer, did not increase a woman's risk of breast cancer (89). Another case-control study of breast cancer found no association with a history of hyperthyroidism or other benign thyroid conditions (90). In a cohort of women treated for hyperthyroidism, no excess risk of breast cancer was noted on a subsequent average follow-up of 18 years (91). Among Japanese women, serum levels of FT_3 and FT_4 were significantly lower in breast cancer cases versus controls; TSH levels were not significantly different between the two groups (92).

Other Medical Conditions and Medications. Other than benign thyroid conditions and breast disease, the extent to which other medical conditions and medications are associated with thyroid cancer has been infrequently studied. One case-control study found a decreased risk associated with a history of asthma or allergies, and a slightly increased risk with a history of cardiovascular disease (26). The same study found thyroid cancer risk was elevated in persons with a history of use of beta-blockers, while a history of cortisone use was associated with a decreased risk for thyroid cancer. A multivariate model showed that the use of cortisone was an independent protective factor for thyroid cancer. Another case-control study similarly found a nonsignificantly decreased risk for thyroid cancer among women with a history of steroid use (19). Possible mechanisms for a protective association with steroids have not been proposed. Other conditions and medications shown not to be associated with thyroid cancer in this study included tonsillectomy, adenoidectomy, and use of diuretics and antihypertensive medications. The use of antihistamines, antibiotics, and steroids all showed nonsignificantly decreased risk for thyroid cancer (19).

Smoking

Epidemiological studies examining cigarette smoking have fairly consistently shown a (usually nonsignificant) decrease in the risk of thyroid cancer among women (22, 26, 28, 42). This result was not observed in men (22). In one case-control study, the decrease in risk was related to an earlier age at initiation of smoking (42). Potential mechanisms of this slight reduction in risk include: (1) a possible reduction of TSH levels in smokers (93, 94), (2) a smoking-related reduction in serum estrogen in women taking oral estrogens (95, 96) that is not observed in women not taking oral estrogens (97), (3) a small smoking-related reduction in serum estrogen during pregnancy (98), and (4) the association of smoking with a lower body weight in women (since higher body weight is a risk factor for thyroid cancer) (42). Reported associations with smoking have usually not adjusted for body weight or weight gain. Somewhat paradoxically, a higher prevalence of goiter in smokers relative to non-smokers (99) and nodular goiter in heavy smokers compared to moderate smokers and non-smokers (100) has been noted.

Summary

Exposure to high dose radiation (particularly in childhood) and a history of benign hyperplastic thyroid conditions are the two well-established risk factors for thyroid cancer. It would be of interest in the future to prospectively follow cohorts of subjects with these thyroid conditions with sequential ultrasonography to track changes in thyroid volume and structure which might provide some insight as to when and how these conditions progress to thyroid neoplasia. Weight gain or higher body weight also is fairly consistently found to be a risk factor for thyroid cancer, particularly in women. The mechanisms of this association are unclear. While there is evidence that diet plays a role in the etiology of thyroid cancer, the epidemiologic data are often conflicting. It appears that the histologic subtype of thyroid cancer as well as geographical characteristics of iodine sufficiency may be important considerations in determining dietary effects. Future research in this area should pay close attention to these factors. While much of the recent epidemiologic research has focussed on exposures which might explain the female excess of thyroid cancer occurring in reproductive years, only modest effects, if any, are seen for reproductive and hormonal factors. Nonetheless, the role of hormones, particularly TSH and estrogen, remains an important area of future research. Larger studies analyzed by histologic subtype are warranted; such an approach will require a longer period of case ascertainment and the use of many cancer registries to obtain sufficient numbers of subjects. It also appears likely that only a portion of women experience excessive thyroid stimulation and growth in pregnancy. While there is no simple way in a retrospective case-control study to identify these women, it would be very interesting to know if these women are more likely than others to develop thyroid cancer and to identify factors (genetic or environmental) which may predispose a woman to excessive thyroid response. Finally, the recent surge in research into the molecular genetics of thyroid tumors shows clear differences by histologic subtype and offers intriguing evidence of specific mutations associated with radiation. Future research thus promises some insight into mechanisms of effect of known exposures and offers promise for screening high-risk individuals.

Acknowledgements.

This work was supported by NIH RO3CA71409. Cancer incidence data for Los Angeles County were collected with support from grant CA17054 and contract NO1-CN-25403 from the National Institutes of Health and subcontracts 050(1987-95)-8709 from the California Department of Health Services as part of its statewide cancer reporting program.

References

1.   Correa P, Chen VW. Endocrine gland cancer. Cancer 1995; 75:338-352.
2.   Pettersson B, Coleman MP, Ron E, Adami H-O. Iodine supplementation in Sweden and regional trends in thyroid cancer incidence by histopathologic type. Int J Cancer 1996; 65:13-19.
3.   Gilliland FD, Hunt WC, Morris DM, Key CR. Prognostic factors for thyroid carcinoma: a population-based study of 15,698 cases from the Surveillance, Epidemiology and End Results (SEER) Program 1973-1991. Cancer 1997; 79:564-573.
4.   Koike A, Naruse T. Incidence of thyroid cancer in Japan. Seminars in Surgical Oncology 1991; 7:107-111.
5.   Goodman MT, Yoshizawa CN, Kolonel LN. Descriptive epidemiology of thyroid cancer in Hawaii. Cancer 1988; 61:1272-1281.
6.   Pettersson B, Adami H-O, Wilander E, Coleman MP. Trends in thyroid cancer incidence in Sweden, 1958-1981, by histopathologic type. Int J Cancer 1991; 48:28-33.
7.   Levi F, Franceschi S, Te V-C, Negri E, LaVecchia C. Descriptive epidemiology of thyroid cancer in the Swiss Canton of Vaud. J Cancer Res Clin Oncol 1990; 116:639-647.
8.   Parkin DM, Muir CS, Whelan SL, Gao YT, Ferlay J, Powell J (ed). Cancer Incidence in Five Continents. International Agency for Research on Cancer, Lyon, vol 6, 1992.
9.   Spitz MR, Sider JG, Katz RL, Pollack ES, Newell GR. Ethnic patterns of thyroid cancer incidence in the United States, 1973-1981. Int J Cancer 1988; 42:549-553.
10. Rossing MA, Schwartz SM, Weiss NS. Thyroid cancer incidence in Asian migrants to the United States and their descendants. Cancer Causes and Control 1995; 6:439-444.
11. Pottern LM, Stone BJ, Day NE, Pickle LW, Fraumeni J, J.F. Thyroid cancer in Connecticut, 1935-1975: an analysis by cell type. Am J Epidemiol 1980; 112:764-774.
12. Glattre E, Akslen LA, Thoresen SO, Haldoren T. Geographic patterns and trends in the incidence of thyroid cancer in Norway 1970-1986. Cancer Detection and Prevention 1990; 14:625-631.

13.   dos Santos Silva I, Swerdlow AJ. Thyroid cancer epidemiology in England and Wales: time trends and geographical distribution. Br J Cancer 1993; 67:330-340.

14.   Akslen LA, Haldorsen T, Thoresen SO, Glattre E. Incidence pattern of thyroid cancer in Norway: influence of birth cohort and time period. Int J Cancer 1993; 53:183-187.

15.   Zheng T, Holford TR, Chen Y, Ma JZ, FLannery J, Liu W. Time trend and age-period-cohort effect on incidence of thyroid cancer in Connecticut, 1935-1992. Int J Cancer 1996; 67:504-509.

16.   Henderson BE, Ross RK, Pike MC, Casagrande JT. Endogenous hormones as a major factor in human cancer. Cancer Res 1982; 42:3232-3239.

17.   Williams ED. TSH and thyroid cancer. Horm Metab Res 1990; 23:72-75.

18.   McTiernan AM, Weiss NS, Daling JR. Incidence of thyroid cancer in women in relation to previous exposure to radiation therapy and history of thyroid disease. J Natl Cancer Inst 1984; 73:575-581.

19.   Ron E, Kleinerman RA, Boice JD, Jr., LiVolsi VA, Flannery JT, Fraumeni JF, Jr. A population-based case-control study of thyroid cancer. J Natl Cancer Inst 1987; 79:1-12.

20.   Preston-Martin S, Bernstein L, Pike MC, Maldonado AA, Henderson BE. Thyroid cancer among young women related to prior thyroid disease and pregnancy history. Br J Cancer 1987; 55:191-195.

21.   Franceschi S, Fassina A, Talamini R, Mazzolini A, Vianello S, Bidoli E, Serraino D, LaVecchia C. Risk factors for thyroid cancer in Northern Italy. International Journal of Epidemiology 1989; 18:578-584.

22.   Kolonel LN, Hankin JH, Wilkens LR, Fukunaga FH, Hinds MW. An epidemiologic study of thyroid cancer in Hawaii. Cancer Causes and Control 1990; 1:223-234.

23.   Levi F, Franceschi S, LaVecchia C, Negri E, Gulie C, Duruz G, Scazziga B. Previous thyroid disease and risk of thyroid cancer in Switzerland. European Journal of Cancer 1991; 27:85-88.

24.   Preston-Martin S, Jin F, Duda MJ, Mack WJ. A case-control study of thyroid cancer in women under age 55 in Shanghai (People's Republic of China). Cancer Causes and Control 1993; 4:431-440.

25.   D'Avanzo B, LaVecchia C, Franceschi S, Negri E, Talamini R. History of thyroid diseases and subsequent thyroid cancer risk. Cancer Epidemiology, Biomarkers, and Prevention 1995; 4:193-199.

26.   Hallquist A, Hardell L, Degerman A, Boquist L. Thyroid cancer: reproductive factors, previous diseases, drug intake, family history and diet. A case-control study. European Journal of Cancer Prevention 1994; 3:481-488.

27.   Shore RE, Hildreth N, Dvoretsky PH, Pasternack B, Andresen E. Benign thyroid adenomas among persons x-irradiated in infancy for enlarged thymus glands. Radiation Research 1993; 134:217-223.

28.   Takezaki T, Hirose K, Inoue M, Hamajima N, Kuroishi T, Nakamura S, Koshikawa T, Matsuura H, Tajima K. Risk factors of thyroid cancer among women in Tokai, Japan. J Epidemiol 1996; 6:140-147.

29.   Weeke J, Hansen AP. Serum TSH and serum T3 levels during normal menstrual cycles and during cycles on oral contraceptives. Acta Endocrinol 1975; 79:431-438.

30.   Hegedues L. Thyroid size determined by ultrasound. Influence of physiological factors and non-thyroidal disease. Danish Medical Bulletin 1990; 37:249-263.

31.   Akslen LA, Nilssen S, Kvale G. Reproductive factors and risk of thyroid cancer. A prospective study of 63,090 women from Norway. Br J Cancer 1992; 65:772-774.

32.   Franceschi S, Fassina A, Talamini R, Mazzolini A, Vianello S, Bidoli E, Cizza G, LaVecchia C. The influence of reproductive and hormonal factors on thyroid cancer in women. Rev Epidem et Sante Publ 1990; 38:27-34.

33.   Levi F, Franceschi S, Gulie C, Negri E, LaVecchia C. Female thyroid cancer: the role of reproductive and hormonal factors in Switzerland. Oncology 1993; 50:309-315.

34.   Wingren G, Hatschek T, Axelson O. Determinants of papillary cancer of the thyroid. Am J Epidemiol 1993; 138:482-491.

35.   Malkasian GD, Mayberry WE. Serum total and free thyroxine and thyrotropin in normal and pregnant women, neonates, and women receiving progestogens. Am J Obstet Gynecol 1970; 108:1234-1238.

36.   Rastogi GK, Sawhney RC, Sinha MK, Thomas Z, Devi PK. Serum and urinary levels of thyroid hormones in normal pregnancy. Obstet Gynecol 1974; 44:176-180.

37.   Glinoer D, De Nayer P, Bourdoux P, Lemone M, Robyn C, Van Steirteghem A, Kintheart J, Lejeune B. Regulation of maternal thyroid during pregnancy. J Clin Endocrinol Metab 1990;

71:276-287.
38. Burrow GN. Thyroid function and hyperfunction during gestation. Endocrine Reviews 1993;
     14:194-202.
39. Kennedy RL, Darne J. The role of hCG in regulation of the thyroid gland in normal and
     abnormal pregnancy. Obstet Gynecol 1991; 78:298-307.
40. Mann K, Hoermann R. Thyroid stimulation by placental factors. J Endocrinol Invest 1993;
     16:378-384.
41. LaVecchia C, Negri E, Franceschi S, Parazzini F. Long-term impact of reproductive factors on
     cancer risk. Int J Cancer 1993; 53:215-219.
42. Galanti MR, Hansson L, Lund E, Bergstrom R, Grimelius L, Stalsberg H, Carlsen E, Baron JA,
     Persson I, Ekbom A. Reproductive history and cigarette smoking as risk factors for thyroid
     cancer in women: a population-based case-control study. Cancer Epidemiology, Biomarkers and
     Prevention 1996; 5:425-431.
43. Kravdal O, Glattre E, Haldorsen T. Positive correlation between parity and incidence of thyroid
     cancer: new evidence based on complete Norwegian birth cohorts. Int J Cancer 1991; 49:831-
     836.
44. Galanti MR, Lambe M, Ekbom A, Sparen P, Pettersson B. Parity and risk of thyroid cancer: a
     nested case-control study of a nationwide Swedish cohort. Cancer Causes and Control 1995;
     6:37-44.
45. McTiernan AM, Weiss NS, Daling JR. Incidence of thyroid cancer in women in relation to
     reproductive and hormonal factors. Am J Epidemiol 1984; 120:423-435.
46. Paoff K, Preston-Martin S, Mack WJ, Monroe K. A case-control study of maternal risk factors
     for thyroid cancer in young women (California, United States). Cancer Causes and Control 1995;
     6:389-397.
47. Chiovato L, Lapi P, Fiore E, Tonacchera M, Pinchera A. Thyroid autoimmunity and female
     gender. J Endocrinol Invest 1993; 16:384-391.
48. Glinoer D, Soto MF, Bourdoux P, Lejeune B, Delange F, Lemone M, Kintheart J, Robijn C,
     Grun J-P, De Nayer P. Pregnancy in patients with mild thyroid abnormalities: maternal and
     neonatal repercussions. J Clin Endocrinol Metab 1991; 73:421-427.
49. Mori M, Naito M, Watanabe H, Takeichi N, Dohi K, Ito A. Effects of sex difference,
     gonadectomy, and estrogen on N-methyl-n-nitrosurea induced rat thyroid tumors. Cancer Res
     1990; 50:7662-7667.
50. Persson I, Yuen J, Bergkvist L, Schairer C. Cancer incidence and mortality in women receiving
     estrogen and estrogen-progestin replacement therapy--long-term follow-up of a Swedish cohort.
     Int J Cancer 1996; 67:327-332.
51. Franceschi S, Talamini R, Fassinia A, Bidoli E. Diet and epithelial cancer of the thyroid gland.
     Tumori 1990; 76:331-338.
52. Glattre E, Haldorsen T, Berg JP, Stensvold I, Solvoll K. Norwegian case-control study testing the
     hypothesis that seafood increases the risk of thyroid cancer. Cancer Causes and Control 1993;
     4:11-16.
53. Galanti MR, Hansson L, Bergstrom R, Wolk A, Hjartaker A, Lund E, Grimelius L, Ekbom A.
     Diet and the risk of papillary and follicular thyroid carcinoma: a population-based case-control
     study in Sweden and Norway. Cancer Causes and Control 1997; 8:205-214.
54. Berg JP, Glattre E, Haldorsen T, Hostmark AT, Bay IG, Johansen AF, Jellum E. Longchain
     serum fatty acids and risk of thyroid cancer: a population-based case-control study in Norway.
     Cancer Causes and Control 1994; 5:433-439.
55. McLaren EH, Alexander WD. Goitrogens. Clin Endocrinol Metab 1979; 8:129-144.
56. Negri E, LaVecchia C, Franceschi S, D'Avanzo B, Parazzini F. Vegetable and fruit consumption
     and cancer risk. Int J Cancer 1991; 48:350-354.
57. Heitz P, Moser H, Staub J. A study of 573 thyroid tumours and 161 autopsy cases observed over
     a 31 year period. Cancer 1976; 37:2329-2337.
58. Harach RH, Escalante D, Onativia A, Outes J, Day S. Thyroid carcinoma and thyroiditis in an
     endemic goiter region before and after iodine prophylaxis. Acta Endocrinol 1985; 108:55-60.
59. Linos A, Linos DA, Vgotza N, Souvatzoglou A, Koutras DA. Does coffee consumption protect
     against thyroid disease? Acta Chir Scand 1989; 155:317-320.
60. D'Avanzo B, Ron E, La Vecchia C, Franceschi S, Negri E, Ziegler R. Selected micronutrient
     intake and thyroid carcinoma risk. Cancer 1997; 79:2186-2192.
61. Glattre E, Thomassen Y, Thoresen SO, Haldorsen T, Lund-Larsen PG, Theodorsen L, Aaseth J.
     Prediagnostic serum selenium in a case-control study of thyroid cancer. International Journal of

Epidemiology 1989; 18:45-49.

62. Williams RR. Breast and thyroid cancer and malignant melanoma promoted by alcohol-induced pituitary secretion of prolactin, TSH, and MSH. Lancet 1976; I:996-999.

63. McTiernan A, Weiss NS, Daling JR. Incidence of thyroid cancer in women in relation to known or suspected risk factors for breast cancer. Cancer Res 1987; 47:292-295.

64. Goodman MT, Kolonel LN, Wilkens LR. The association of body size, reproductive factors and thyroid cancer. Br J Cancer 1992; 66:1180-1184.

65. Marsh DJ, Mulligan LM, Eng C. RET proto-oncogene mutations in multiple endocrine neoplasia type 2 and medullary thyroid carcinoma. Hormone Research 1997; 47:168-178.

66. Goldgar DE, Easton DF, Cannon-Albright LA, Skolnick MH. Systematic population-based assessment of cancer risk in first-degree relatives of cancer probands. J Natl Cancer Inst 1994; 86:1600-1608.

67. Galanti MR, Ekbom A, Grimelius L, Yuen J. Parental cancer and risk of papillary and follicular thyroid carcinoma. Br J Cancer 1997; 75:451-456.

68. Vlajinac HD, Adanja BJ, Zivaljevic VR, Jankovic RR, Dzodic RR, Jovanovic DD. Malignant tumors in families of thyroid cancer patients. Acta Oncologica 1997; 36:477-481.

69. Eng C, Mulligan LM. Mutations of the RET proto-oncogene in the multiple endocrine neoplasia type 2 syndromes, related sporadic tumors, and hirschsprung disease. Human Mutation 1997; 9:97-109.

70. Skinner MA, Wells J, S.A. Medullary carcinoma of the thyroid gland and the MEN 2 syndromes. Seminars in Pediatric Surgery 1997; 6:134-140.

71. Kusafuka T, Puri P. The RET proto-oncogene: a challenge to our understanding of disease pathogenesis. Pediatric Surgery International 1997; 12:11-18.

72. Takahashi M. Oncogenic activation of the ret protooncogene in thyroid cancer. Critical Reviews in Oncogenesis 1995; 6:35-46.

73. Williams ED, Pacini F, Pinchera A. Thyroid cancer following Chernobyl. Journal of Endocrinological Investigation 1995; 18:144-146.

74. Komminoth P. The RET proto-oncogene in medullary and papillary thyroid carcinoma. Molecular features, pathophysiology and clinical implications. Virchows Archiv 1997; 431:1-9.

75. Derwahl M. Molecular aspects of the pathogenesis of nodular goiters, thyroid nodules and adenomas. Experimental and Clinical Endocrinology and Diabetes 1996; 104 (Supp):32-35.

76. Wynford-Thomas D. Origin and progression of thyroid epithelial tumors: cellular and molecular mechanisms. Hormone Research 1997; 47:145-157.

77. Carstensen JM, Wingren G, Hatschek T, Fredriksson M, Noorlind-Brage H, Axelson O. Occupational risks of thyroid cancer: data from the Swedish Cancer-Environment Register, 1961-1979. Am J Ind Med 1990; 18:535-540.

78. Wingren G, Hallquist A, Degerman A, Hardell L. Occupation and female papillary cancer of the thyroid. Journal of Occupational and Environmental Medicine 1995; 37:294-297.

79. Hallquist A, Hardell L, Degerman A, Boquist L. Occupational exposures and thyroid cancer: results of a case-control study. European Journal of Cancer Prevention 1993; 2:345-349.

80. Wang J-X, Boice J, J.D., Li B-X, Zhang J-Y, Fraumeni J, J.F. Cancer among medical diagnostic x-ray workers in China. J Natl Cancer Inst 1988; 80:344-350.

81. Delzell E, Grufferman S. Cancer and other causes of death among female textile workers, 1976-78. J Natl Cancer Inst 1983; 71:735-740.

82. Saracci R, Kogevinas M, Bertazzi P-A, DeMesquita BHB, Coggon D, Green LM, Kauppinen T, L'Abbe KA, Littorin M, Lynge E, Mathews JD, Neuberger M, Osman J, Pearce N, Winkelmann R. Cancer mortality in workers exposed to chlorophenoxy herbicides and chlorophenols. Lancet 1991; 338:1027-1032.

83. Pesatori AC, Consonni D, Tironi A, Zocchetti C, Fini A, Bertazzi PA. Cancer in a young population in a dioxin-contaminated area. International Journal of Epidemiology 1993; 22:1010-1013.

84. Blair A, Stewart PA, Tolbert PE, Grauman D, Moran FX, Vaught J, Rayner J. Cancer and other causes of death among a cohort of dry cleaners. British Journal of Industrial Medicine 1990; 47:162-168.

85. Grimalt JO, Sunyer J, Moreno V, Amaral OC, Sala M, Rosell A, Anto JM, Albaiges J. Risk excess of soft-tissue sarcoma and thyroid cancer in a community exposed to airborne organochlorinated compound mixtures with a high hexachlorobenzene content. Int J Cancer 1994; 56:200-203.

86. Ron E, Curtis R, Hoffman DA, Flannery JT. Multiple primary breast and thyroid cancer. Br J

Cancer 1984; 49:87-92.
87. Hall P, Holm LE, Lundell G. Second primary tumors following thyroid cancer. A Swedish record-linkage study. Acta Oncologica 1990; 29:869-873.
88. Adamopoulos DA, Vassilaros S, Kapolla N, Papadiamantis J, Georgiakodis F, Michalakis A. Thyroid disease in patients with benign and malignant mastopathy. Cancer 1986; 57:125-128.
89. Moseson M, Koenig KL, Shore RE, Pasternack BS. The influence of medical conditions associated with hormones on the risk of breast cancer. International Journal of Epidemiology 1993; 22:1000-1009.
90. Talamini R, Franceschi S, Favero A, Negri E, LaVecchia C. Selected medical conditions and risk of breast cancer. Br J Cancer 1997; 75:1699-1703.
91. Hoffman DA, McConahey WM. Thyroid disease and breast cancer. Lancet 1981; 1:730
92. Takatani O, Okumoto T, Kosano H, Nishida M, Hiraide H, Tamakuma S. Relationship between the levels of serum thyroid hormones or estrogen status and the risk of breast cancer genesis in Japanese women. Cancer Res 1989; 49:3109-3112.
93. Eden S, Jagenburg R, Lindstedt G, Lundberg PA, Mellstrom D. Thyroregulatory changes associated with smoking in 70-year-old men. Clinical Endocrinology 1984; 21:605-610.
94. Fisher CL, Mannino DM, Herman WH, Frumkin H. Cigarette smoking and thyroid hormone levels in males. International Journal of Epidemiology 1997; 26:972-977.
95. Jensen J, Christiansen C, Rodbro P. Cigarette smoking, serum estrogens, and bone loss during hormone-replacement therapy early after menopause. N Engl J Med 1985; 313:973-975.
96. Cassidenti DL, Vijod AG, Vijod MA, Stanczyk FZ, Lobo RA. Short-term effects of smoking on the pharmocokinetic profiles of micronized estradiol in postmenopausal women. Am J Obstet Gynecol 1990; 163:1953-1960.
97. Cassidenti DL, Pike MC, Vijod AG, Stanczyk FZ, Lobo RA. A reevaluation of estrogen status in postmenopausal women who smoke. Am J Obstet Gynecol 1992; 166:1444-1448.
98. Petridou E, Panagiotopoulou K, Katsouyanni K, Spanos E, Trichopoulos D. Tobacco smoking, pregnancy estrogens, and birth weight. Epidemiology 1990; 1:247-250.
99. Christensen SB, Ericsson UB, Janzon L, Tibblin S, Melander A. Influence of cigarette smoking on goiter formation, thyroglobulin, and thyroid hormone levels in women. J Clin Endocrinol Metab 1984; 58:615-618.
100. Lio S, Napolitano G, Marinuzzi G, Monaco F. Role of smoking in goiter morphology and thyrotropin response to TRH in untreated goitrous women. J Endocrinol Invest 1989; 12:93-97.

2 IONIZING RADIATION AND THYROID CANCER

Arthur B. Schneider
University of Illinois, Chicago

Jacob Robbins
NIH/NIDDK, Bethesda, MD

The relationship between radiation and thyroid cancer is so well established that one might forget that a great deal remains to be learned, especially about how this association arises. One way to illustrate this point is to draw an analogy with a traditional hormonal system such as the effects of TSH on the thyroid gland (Table 1). The analogy emphasizes the need to characterize all of the steps from the stimulus to the final effect, particularly the intermediate steps where much work is now focused. The purpose of this chapter is to outline the current understanding of the pathway leading from radiation to thyroid cancer.

The discussion of each topic will focus on clinically relevant issues. For example, the discussion of the types and characteristics of radiation should help a physician obtain an accurate radiation history so that a patient's thyroid cancer risk can be estimated. Previous clinical studies will be reviewed in the context of what their findings reveal about the risks of different types of radiation exposure and how they illustrate the role of epidemiology in understanding radiation-related thyroid cancer. The effects of radiation on thyroid cancer-related genes will be mentioned only briefly, as they are discussed in a separate article in this book (Chapter 3).

Basic concepts

Physical properties of radiation

Ionizing radiation refers to radiation with sufficient energy to dislodge electrons from atoms (1). X-rays and gamma rays (these are characterized either as waves with a specific wave length or as particles called photons) are forms of ionizing radiation. In tissues ionizing radiation produces chemically reactive products. Ultraviolet radiation has lower energy and is not ionizing. It can cause cancer, but by different mechanisms and not below the surface of the body. Therefore, in the clinical setting, the distinction is an important one and one that may be made by an accurate history. Often, for ultraviolet treatment, a purple light will be recalled, the condition would have been a superficial dermatological one, and the treatment would have been administered without other people leaving the immediate area.

Table 1. Analogy between areas of study for radiation-induced thyroid cancer and a representative hormone response system.

	TSH Thyroxine production	Radiation Thyroid cancer
Stimulus	TSH: Varies by molecular characteristics, particularly carbo-hydrate composition	Ionizing radiation: Varies by type and energy
Receptor	TSH receptor: Conformational activation of receptor	Site of initial lesion: Solvent (H_2O) or macromolecules (DNA modifications and breaks)
Signal transduction	cAMP, phospholipids, calcium, etc.: Multiple, potentially interacting pathways	DNA repair mechanisms: Multiple enzymes, some related to radiation sensitivity
Effects on genes	Gene promotors: Increased transcription of genes involved in synthetic pathways	Structural genetic changes: Increased or decreased activity of oncogenes, tumor suppressors, and growth factors
Functional effect	Increased thyroid hormone production and other effects on thyroid cells	Cancer and benign neoplasms, goiter, and possibly immune thyroid disease

By one of several energy-dependent mechanisms ionizing radiation interacts with matter to produce charged particles (1). Also, charged particles (electron, protons, and alpha particles) can be generated directly for clinical use by using accelerators and radioactive isotopes . Neutrons, although not charged, can convert some of its energy into ionizing radiation by interacting with atomic nuclei.

Radiation is also classified according to the frequency of energy transfer events along its path. This is called linear energy transfer (LET). This classification takes into account the frequency, but not the magnitude, of energy loss along the path. X-rays, gamma rays and beta particles (electrons) lose energy relatively infrequently and are referred to as low LET radiation. For alpha particles, which lose energy frequently, LET is high. High LET radiation is more carcinogenic than low LET radiation, in part because the distance between energy releases may be close to the distance between the strands of DNA. However, the energy of high LET radiation is dissipated rapidly in superficial tissues.

Given the different kinds of radiation and their different reactions with biological tissues, it is not surprising that biological effectiveness of each varies (2). In other words, a given amount of radiation, measured using the physical unit Gray (formerly rad, 1 gray = 100 rads, 1 cGy = 1 rad), produces different biological effects. To take this into account, the concept of relative biological equivalent (RBE) was introduced. This is a factor that normalizes the biological effectiveness of different kinds of radiation, with the RBE for low LET radiation defined as 1.0. The product of grays and RBE is measured in sieverts (formerly rem). For X-rays, 1 Gray = 1 Sievert. Neutrons have a high RBE. The dose-response relationships for tumors in atomic bomb survivors was revised recently to take into account the newly estimated contribution of neutrons to the radiation exposure (2). As discussed below, the carcinogenic potential (RBE) of iodine isotopes has not been established.

External radiation

Types. In the medical setting, external radiation is delivered by teletherapy (conventional beam treatment) or brachytherapy (the placement of a radioactive source next to the surface of the body). Teletherapy is delivered using orthovoltage, megavoltage, cobalt-60 and electron-generating machines. Brachytherapy uses radium, radon or other sources. The former sources generated alpha particles, electrons and photons in which case the applicator itself absorbed virtually all of the alpha particles and most of the electrons (3,4).

Uses and biological effects. In the past, teletherapy was used to treat a wide variety of benign conditions in the head and neck area. These conditions included 1) the "enlarged" thymus gland thought to be associated with "crib death", 2) the "enlarged" tonsils and adenoids that were otherwise treated by routine tonsillectomy, 3) tinea capitis by removal of all scalp hair, 4) cystic acne and a variety of other dermatological conditions, 5) bronchitis, 6) cervical lymph node enlargement, and others. In general, the thyroid doses from these treatments were in the 10-100 cGy range (5-7). For some dermatological conditions Grenz ray treatment was used. This is teletherapy using radiation that is largely absorbed at the surface of the body (8). Teletherapy continues to be used to treat malignant conditions. In this instance, the thyroid dose may be large enough to result in thyroid insufficiency and hypothyroidism (9).

Brachytherapy was used to treat hemangiomas and other skin conditions. The placement of the source determined how much radiation was absorbed by the thyroid gland. When the source was place in the region of the gland, the thyroid dose was in the same range as teletherapy for benign conditions (3). Probably the most wide-spread use of brachytherapy was the placement of a radium-tipped rod into the posterior pharynx to shrink the lymphoidal tissue in that region and surrounding the outlets of the eustachian tubes. It has been estimated that 0.5-2.0 million such treatments were administered in the United States (10). The distance from the radiation source to the thyroid resulted in a low dose, about 3 cGy in a 6 year old child (4).

Carcinogenesis studies in model systems. Model systems have had only limited use in the study of the effects of external radiation on the thyroid. This arises In part from the convenience of using iodine isotopes for such studies (see below) and in part because many clinical questions are hard to extrapolate to model systems.

In one model system 1680 beagle dogs from 8 days gestation to 365 days old, in groups of 120, were irradiated. Two-day neonatal dogs that received 17 cGy or 85 cGy of whole-body irradiation and 70-day old dogs that received 83 cGy of whole-body irradiation developed thyroid neoplasms more frequently than the others (11). Beagle dogs are prone to develop spontaneous thyroiditis-associated hypothyroidism. Irradiation reduced the frequency of hypothyroidism. More thyroid neoplasms occurred in hypothyroid dogs, but hypothyroid dogs were not more susceptible to the carcinogenic effects of radiation. An age-dependent relationship for thyroid radiation susceptibility was present and similar to what is seen in humans.

In other model systems thyroid cells in tissue culture are irradiated. *In vitro* irradiation of a human thyroid cancer-derived cell line resulted in activation of the *ret* gene by chromosomal rearrangement, an activation that occurs in many radiation-related and unrelated human thyroid cancers (12). Similar rearrangements occurred after irradiation of a human fibrosarcoma cell line. This is notable because *ret* rearrangements in humans are strictly limited to papillary thyroid cancers.

Irradiation of freshly dispersed rat thyroid cells increases the frequency with which they form cancers when they are reinjected into recipient rats. Using this system, Domann et al. determined that increasing the TSH level in the recipient rats did not change the number of cancers formed, but did change the rapidity with which they developed (13). In a related system, Mizuno et al. (14) irradiated human fetal thyroid tissue that had been transplanted into SCID mice and studied oncogene activation. They found radiation activation of the *ret* and *bcr* oncogenes, but only the former persisted for up to 2 months after the radiation.

Internal radiation from iodine isotopes

The special relationship between iodine and the thyroid is a key factor in the gland's vulnerability to internal ionizing radiation. Iodine is a low abundance element in the environment and the thyroid gland possesses a mechanism for its concentration. In the normal human thyroid iodide transport can give an intracellular iodide concentration 30 - 40 fold that in the blood. Normally, however, the iodide is rapidly organified and the homeostatic mechanism under which the thyroid gland operates provides for a large store of hormone within the thyroid follicles in the form of thyroglobulin. As a result, the rate at which iodine leaves the gland is extremely slow, with a half time of about 90 days. The ultimate concentration of iodine in the gland far exceeds that in the environment.

Another significant factor, especially in the young, is that cow's milk is a major dietary source of iodine. Cows grazing on contaminated pastures concentrate any iodine radioisotopes into their mammary glands and milk. The radioiodine in consumed milk then accumulates in the thyroid gland. Additionally, if there is a low abundance of stable iodine in the environment, this leads to increases in iodine uptake and thyroid gland size. These changes affect the radioiodine concentration within the gland in opposing directions.

Types and uses. Of the more than 20 known radioiodines, five are of major interest in the context of this discussion (Table 2). I-123 and I-131, as the iodide ion, are currently used clinically, the latter for diagnosis and therapy. Another isotope used clinically to visualize the thyroid gland is Tc-99m in the form of pertechnetate. Pertechnetate ion is trapped by the thyrocyte but is not organified. I-125 and I-132 were used clinically in the past, the former for therapy and the latter to measure trapping, but they did not have very wide use. I-125 and I-131 are the major radioiodines that are used in laboratory work.

Table 2. Radioisotopes having potential health effects on the thyroid gland

Isotope	Half life	Emission energy[*]	
		Beta	Gamma
I-123	13 h	none	Moderate
I-125	60 d	none	Low[+]
I-131	8 d	high	Moderate
I-132	2.3 h	high	High
I-133	21 h	high	Moderate
Te-132	78 h	moderate	Moderate
Tc-99m	6 h	none	Moderate

[*]Average emission energies are defined as follows: low = <0.1 MeV, moderate = 0.1-0.4 MeV, high = >0.4 MeV. All of the isotopes give rise to low LET (linear energy transfer) radiation.
[+]Mainly x-rays from electron capture.

I-131, I-132 and I-133 are the main sources of environmental contamination because they are produced in nuclear reactors, nuclear processing facilities, and as a result of nuclear explosions. An important precursor of I-132 in nuclear accidents is Te-132 (tellurium) because it is equally volatile and has a much longer half life than its daughter isotope. Other potentially damaging radioiodine contaminants are ignored because the half life is short (I-135, t ½ = 6.7 h) or the abundance is very low (I-125, I-129). I-129, however, is useful in monitoring radioiodine contamination of the environment because it has an extremely long half life and can be assayed by neutron activation.

Biological effects. Damage to the thyroid from internal radiation is dependent on intracellular absorption of the emitted energy and the resulting ionization. Most of the damage is caused by beta irradiation, although a portion of the gamma irradiation is absorbed. In the human thyroid, for example, only about 10% of the damage from I-131 is from the gamma rays. The average path length of the I-131 beta particles is 2 to 3 mm whereas the diameter of an adult thyroid follicle is about 0.3 mm and the thickness of its epithelial lining is about 15 μm. As a result, the beta energy is deposited in adjacent follicles and the damage is more uniform than the distribution of the isotope itself. In experiments with rodents, especially mice, the thyroid is so small that about 30% of the beta irradiation is not absorbed within the gland, but in the human thyroid at least 90% is absorbed, even in an infant (15). In the early fetal thyroid, however, less beta energy is deposited in the gland (16).

Since the radiation dose to the thyroid is a function of the isotope's concentration in the gland, it depends on its size and the uptake. The other determinants are the half life of the isotope and its residence time in the gland, which depends on both the physical half life and the rate of thyroid iodine secretion or biological half life. The residence time, or the effective half-life, also governs the rate at which the radiation energy is delivered. Thus, irradiation from an internal slowly decaying isotope may be less damaging than the same amount of radiation delivered acutely by external radiation, since the former allows more time for DNA repair.

Summaries of these aspects of radiation dosimetry from internal thyroid radiation, and a guide to the relevant literature, can be found in several references (2,15-17).

Carcinogenesis studies in model systems. I-131 is useful in radiation therapy of thyrotoxicosis and thyroid cancer because the radiation within the gland or the tumor can be so high that it is possible to destroy the thyroid cells without damaging extrathyroidal tissues. Thus the radiation dose received from I-131 or other radioiodines can range from insignificant to lethal. Somewhere between these extremes is the range in which the damage can induce neoplasia. This has been explored in experimental animals, especially in rodents, with various iodine isotopes, and the results have been collected in the NCRP Report No.80 (17). An important goal of these experiments has been to compare the carcinogenicity of internal and external irradiation. Early experiments indicated that I-131 was less carcinogenic than x-ray by a factor of ½ to 1/25, as might be expected from the difference in the rate of radiation delivery . They also indicated that I-132 was more carcinogenic than I-131 and similar to x-ray . In a more recent experiment with rats, however, the carcinogenic radiation effect from I-131 was no different than from x-ray (18), although it was about half as effective as x-ray in inducing benign neoplasms. Unlike in humans, the malignant lesions were follicular rather than papillary carcinoma, presumably a species difference. This experiment has led many to assume that the risk from I-131 and x-ray are comparable, but the experience with human carcinogenesis (see below) makes this conclusion unlikely. The conclusion of NCRP Report No.80 from the combined animal experiments is that, at radiation doses above 10 Gy (1000 rad), I-131 is 1/10 as carcinogenic as x-ray, but that at doses from 1 to 10 Gy I-131 has about the same carcinogenicity as x-ray , although a relative effectiveness as low as 1/3 could not be excluded. For production of adenomas, I-131 was about 40% as effective as x-ray at 10 Gy, but similar at lower doses.

Radiation Effects on the Genome

Radiation-induced mutations may occur in germline DNA where, in theory, heritable mutations could occur and in somatic DNA, where tumors may arise. Radiation carcinogenesis involves somatic mutations in cancer-related genes. Evidence for radiation-induced mutations in germline DNA comes from minisatelllite analysis. Comparison of minisatellites in children in the Chernobyl area to their radiation-exposed parents show changes compatible with germline mutations (19,20). However, inherited, disease-producing mutations induced by irradiation have not been shown in humans as yet (21).

Damage and Repair. Even though radiation can affect all components of a cell, it is generally accepted that its cell killing and carcinogenic effects are mediated by DNA damage. In part this is due to the fact that DNA contains unique information, so that damage in a single location, e.g., a key gene, can affect the properties of the entire cell. Some of the DNA damage results from the direct effects of the radiation-produced scattered electrons. The majority of the damage results from reactions with free radical species generated by the radiation-induced ionization of cellular water (2).

A great deal of effort has been placed in trying to determine the nature of the DNA damage that leads to cancer. There are two main questions: 1) what sort of DNA damage is most important and 2) are the main effects directly on cancer related genes, on genes that maintain the integrity of the genome, or on both? Neither of these questions is completely resolved.

DNA damage following radiation includes single-strand breaks, changed bases, double-strand breaks and other forms of multiple, closely spaced damaged sites. Several *in vitro* model systems have been used to study the frequency of these different forms of damage following radiation. Unfortunately, due to the unique characteristics of each system, varying results have been obtained. The prevailing view is that DNA double strand breaks (caused by multiple, closely spaced DNA damaging events) are the initial and most important lesions (22). It is also accepted that some double strand breaks are converted into the chromosome breaks that are seen following radiation exposure, although the mechanism for this has not been elucidated. In part, this conclusion comes from the observation that restriction enzyme-induced double strand breaks can be converted into chromosomal breaks (23). Two systems for the repair of double strand breaks exist, homologous recombination and nonhomologous end joining. The latter is active in immunoglobulin gene recombination, is dominant in mammalian cells, and has been reviewed recently (24).

Two results of chromosome breaks are chromosomal rearrangements including translocations and inversions and loss of chromosomal material resulting in loss of heterozygosity (25). The *ret* gene is activated by chromosomal rearrangements in papillary thyroid cancer. Therefore the findings of frequent *ret* gene translocations in the Chernobyl cases is consistent with a direct radiation effect. Radiation also produces smaller genetic changes including base substitutions. Evidence so far indicates that these may play some, but not a predominant role in radiation-associated thyroid cancer (26,27).

The translocation of the *ret* gene following radiation suggests a straightforward model of carcinogenesis; that is, that radiation activates a gene that causes cancer (28,29). However, carcinogenesis often involves the accumulation of multiple mutations. Recognizing that it would be unlikely that radiation and subsequent random events would be enough to allow a single cell to accumulate these multiple mutations, an alternative hypothesis has been proposed. In this alternative view, the initial step in radiation carcinogenesis is an event that produces instability in the genome, increasing the chances of subsequent mutations (30). Whether instability plays a part in radiation-induced thyroid cancer and whether *ret* activation leads to instability is not known.

Modifiers. In addition to the type of radiation, discussed above, the dose and rate of exposure may modify the carcinogenic effects of radiation, especially if carcinogenesis requires two closely juxtaposed damaging events on the two strands of DNA (31). For high LET radiation, closely spaced ionizations occur along a single track, so the effects are expected to be linearly related to dose. For low LET radiation this is more complex. If two events arising from two separate tracks are needed, then the probability that two decays would occur close enough to each other would increase as an exponential function of the dose. However, low LET radiation may produce closely spaced ionizations at the end of its track. If these were dominant, then the carcinogenic effect would be linear. In either case, at high doses, the effects of cell killing become increasing important and should result in a flattening of the dose-response relationship.

The dose rate may also modify the carcinogenic effect of radiation. Since radiation initiates a complex set of cellular responses, the reparative component of these responses may function more effectively when dealing with a low dose rate. For thyroid cancer, it is possible that the difference in carcinogenic effects of external and internal radiation may be due to the different dose rates for these two types of radiation. However, in epidemiological studies confined to external radiation, it has not been possible to show a significant dose rate effect. Also, the epidemiological studies have not been able to demonstrate a quadratic component at low doses, although there is evidence of flattening of the risk at higher doses (5).

Since radiation carcinogenesis is thought to be a multistep process, it is reasonable to expect that additional factors, called promotors, are involved. In order to extrapolate the results of one clinical study to another, it is important to characterize these factors. However, the identification of these promotors is difficult. Some, such as the age at exposure, have been clearly confirmed. Others, such as sex, reproductive factors, and diet, require further investigation (32). Of special interest are genetic factors (33). While variations in radiation susceptibility on a genetic basis is likely, ataxia telangiectasia is an example, the importance of genetic factors remains to be determined. The identification of factors that influence the dose-response relationship for thyroid cancer by epidemiological methods is discussed below.

Oncogenes. The role of oncogenes in the pathogenesis of thyroid cancer is reviewed elsewhere in this volume (Chapter 3). Several important questions related to radiation carcinogenesis will be clarified by ongoing studies, as mentioned in the section "Future Research" below.

Epidemiological study methodology

Modeling and estimation of cancer risks. By establishing a strong association between radiation exposure and thyroid cancer, the first goal of epidemiological studies has been achieved. The second goal is to to provide a quantitative description of the association. In order to achieve this, it is necessary to determine which model is most appropriate and gives the best fit to the data. Any model must take into account the background rate; i.e., the rate in the absence of radiation exposure. In one type of model, the effect of radiation is to add additional cases of thyroid cancer to the background in proportion to the dose of radiation. In another type of model, the effect of radiation is to multiply the background rate. The former is an additive risk model and the latter is an excess relative risk (ERR) model. In both models an effect of radiation can be a linear function of dose, the simplest form, or can have an exponential component or other complex components. For thyroid cancer and external radiation, a linear ERR model fits the data well, although other models cannot be excluded with certainty (5).

Studying covariates. One of the strengths of epidemiological studies is the ability to evaluate the effects of multiple factors (covariates) that influence the measured outcome (thyroid cancer). The first part of an epidemiological study is to determine which covariates affect the background rate. In a study of thyroid cancer, sex is one such factor since women have many more thyroid cancers than men. If a study were conducted where the proportion of women was higher in an irradiated group compared to a control group or where women received a different dose than men, these differences would need to be taken into account before concluding that radiation is associated with thyroid cancer. Host effects and environmental influences on the background rate of thyroid cancer have been reviewed elsewhere (7).

Another question that involves covariates, but a distinctly separate one, is whether there are any factors that affect susceptibility to the effects of radiation. In other words, the second part of an epidemiological study is to determine whether there are factors that change the slope, or possibly the shape, of the dose-response curve. The most clearly established susceptibility factor for external radiation is age at the time of radiation exposure. The younger the age, the greater the risk for developing radiation-related thyroid cancer (5). It has been proposed that at an early age the thyroid contains more dividing, and therefore more susceptible cells. As yet, direct proof of this hypothesis has not been provided.

The factor with the largest effect on the background rate of thyroid cancer is sex, but it is not clear whether sex affects radiation susceptibility. In a relative risk model the dose-response relationship is somewhat steeper for women than for men, but the difference is not statistically significant (5). However, in a relative risk model, the radiation effect multiplies the background rate. Therefore, since the background rate is higher for women, even if they are not more susceptible, they will develop more cases of radiation-related thyroid cancer. Whether preexisting or coexisting thyroid disease, dietary iodine insufficiency or excess, reproductive history, family history, or other factors modify the effects of radiation remain to be seen.

Populations studied

External radiation

Medical X-ray.

Therapeutic radiation for benign conditions. The practice of treating benign conditions with x-ray reached its peak in the 1940's and 1950's, and persisted mostly in dermatological practice in the 1970's. First recognized in 1950 (34), the relationship between such exposure and thyroid cancer has been studied extensively (7,35-38).

The most thorough evaluation of the epidemiological aspects of this relationship was performed by pooling the data from seven large studies (citations to the individual studies are found in the reference) (5). Four of the studies followed patients whose childhood radiation treatment had been directed to the thymus, tonsils, and scalp, the latter as a part of the treatment of tinea capitis. The average thyroid doses in these studies, in cGy, were 136 (thymus), 24 (tonsils), 59(tonsils) and 9 (scalp). Treatments were given either in one session or in a few sessions spaced over days. An important observation was that the risk estimates from each of the studies included in the parallel analysis were similar to each other. This supports the validity of combining the data and provides convincing confirmation of the relationship between radiation exposure and thyroid cancer. The following comments highlight the conclusions from the pooled analysis, rather than describing each of the studies individually.

Three conclusions relate to the shape of the dose-response curve. First, the effects of radiation were seen at thyroid doses as low as 10 cGy. There was no evidence for a threshold dose below which the effect disappeared. Second, a relative risk model fit the data well. The fit did not improve with the inclusion of additional exponential terms. An additive risk model was not entirely excluded, but the analysis favored the relative risk description of the data. Third, the risk did not decline significantly at the highest doses included, although there appeared to be some flattening of the curve.

Additional conclusions concern identification of factors that affect radiation sensitivity. Age at the time of exposure was extremely important, with younger age associated with higher risk. The effect was seen at the youngest ages and tapered rapidly toward 15 years. In fact, the analysis was unable to detect any increased risk for people exposed after age 15. Althoug there was a tendency for the effect of radiation to be greater in women than in men, but, as mentioned above, the difference was not statistically significant.

The studies were not designed to address the question of latency, since the risk was not recognized initially and periodic examinations were not performed. Some early cases of thyroid cancer were observed about 5 years after exposure, but the marked increase began at about 10 years. More important were the observations on the duration of the risk, given that radiation treatments for almost all benign conditions have been abandoned. This analysis had to take into account the increase in the background rate of thyroid cancer as people get older. This was done by determining the effect of time on the dose-response relationship. At the longest times of observations, several decades after the initial exposure, a significant dose effect on thyroid cancer was still seen, but it appeared that the risk had reached a plateau and was beginning to decline. The continuing risk is of particular concern because radiation-related cases occurring at advanced ages may have the same aggressive tendencies as thyroid cancer occurring in older people in general.

Further conclusions about thyroid cancer and external radiation come from analysis of data from the Chicago (Michael Reese Hospital) cohort. First, screening for thyroid cancer in an exposed population can increase the rate of thyroid cancer by nearly 10-fold (39). The risk estimates, however, were the same before and after the initiation of screening (6). From this observation it is concluded that radiation is associated with thyroid cancers of all sizes, those large enough to be found by routine clinical care and those too small to be found by routine means, but large enough to be seen by thyroid imaging.

The suggestions of one of the authors (ABS) of this review for the management of people exposed to childhood radiation treatments, and the management of nodules and cancer in the setting of a history of radiation, have been summarized elsewhere (35-37,40,41). In part, these suggestions are based on the following observations: In an irradiated patient a thyroid nodule is more likely to be a thyroid cancer than if there has been no radiation exposure. Thyroid cancer occurring in an irradiated patient is frequently multicentric and associated with lymph node metastases (42). Taking these and other presenting features, particularly size, into account, the clinical behavior of these cancers is the same as that reported for thyroid cancers in patients not exposed to radiation.

The extent of clinical examination for a radiation-exposed person depends on an estimate of the risk factors mentioned throughout this review. For those with high risk factors, screening with thyroid imaging, currently ultrasonagraphy, is indicated. Additional attention to the possibilities of salivary gland neoplasms, neural neoplasms including vestibular schwannomas and hyperparathyroidism is indicated. The evaluation of thyroid nodules should be the same as for nodules in patients withoout radiation exposure, but is often more difficulty when more than one nodule is present. Thyroid cancer should be treated as in patients without radiation exposure.

Therapeutic radiation for malignant conditions. There are two categories of therapeutic radiation treatments to be considered. In the first, the primary cancer and the radiation field are remote from the thyroid; however, because of the large doses employed the thyroid is exposed to some extent. An example of this is found in the study of radiation treatment for cervical cancer (43) that was included in the pooled analysis of Ron et al (5). Although there are few data, it is to be expected that the risks from this type of exposure is equivalent to that from comparable thyroid doses resulting from treatment for benign head and neck conditions.

When the thyroid is close to, or in the field of radiation therapy for a malignancy, both hypothyroidism and thyroid cancer need to be considered. Hypothyroidism is much more frequent than thyroid cancer and the evidence associating it with high dose radiation exposure is convincing, as recently reviewed (9). For thyroid cancer, the association has been more difficult to establish. Inpart, this may be because therapeutic radiation is used most often in adults where the thyroid is less sensitive to its effects. In one study of about 1800 patients with Hodgkin's disease, treated at a mean age of 26 years with radiation at Stanford University and followed for an average of 9.9 years, 46 developed thyroid nodules and 6 were found to have thyroid cancer (44). Compared to the expected number derived from the Connecticut tumor registry, the relative risk was 15.6. However, the increased medical attention due to the original diagnosis may have contributed to increased ascertainment of the thyroid cancers. In another study, 9170 patients who survived at least two years after a childhood cancer were followed for an average of 5.5 years (45). The number of observed cases of thyroid cancer was 23, 53-times higher than the expected number based on the Connecticut registry. The association was supported by the finding of a dose-response relationship, mainly due to an increase in the relative risk estimates for exposures at doses >200 cGy compared to < 200 cGy.

Diagnostic radiation. The most comprehensive studies of diagnostic x-rays and thyroid cancer were performed in Sweden. In one report, the pooled data from two case-control studies suggested that an association was present (46). These pooled data were obtained from questionnaires mailed to 186 female cases of papillary thyroid cancer and twice as many controls. A statistically significant trend of thyroid cancer with estimated thyroid dose was found. In comparison to those with no thyroid exposure from diagnostic x-rays, those with the highest estimated dose, >0.1 cGy, had an odds ratio for thyroid cancer of 2.6. More than 10 dental x-rays also were associated with an elevated odds ratio. However, elevated odds ratios were found for some diagnostic x-rays remote from the thyroid gland, e.g. the kidneys, and the authors recognize that their findings could be affected by recall bias.

In a larger study, of 484 cases of papillary and follicular thyroid cancer and an equal number of controls, medical records were searched extensively to find exposure to diagnostic x-ray (47). The total number of diagnostic x-ray procedures found in this way was 3,853 for the cases and 4,039 for the controls. No association between the number of x-rays, the number of x-rays near the thyroid, or the estimated thyroid dose and thyroid cancer was found. This was also true when only x-rays performed during childhood, when the thyroid is most sensitive, were considered in the analysis.

Atomic bomb survivors. In the studies of atomic bomb survivors, thyroid cancer was the first solid tumor for which an excess number of cases was recognized for thyroid cancer. The thyroid doses were derived from whole body radiation from direct exposure to X-rays and neutrons. The bombs exploded so far above the ground that most volatile components, including the radioiodine isotopes, were dispersed. None of the studies take into account any internal exposure to radioactive iodine. The most recent studies were published in 1994 (48) and the data were included in the pooled analysis of Ron, et al (5). These studies use the dose estimates that were revised in 1986. They take into account individual exposures to X-rays and neutrons and use an RBE of 10 for neutrons. Using 0.01 Sievert as the cutoff, there were 41,234 exposed and 38,738 unexposed people included. The average thyroid dose was equivalent to 27 cGy. Follow-up information was obtained from the Hiroshima and Nagasaki tumor registries.

The findings conform to the results of the pooled analysis, in particular showing the magnitude of the age at exposure effect (ERR=9.5 for age at exposure <10 years versus no excess risk for age >20 years). In this regard the study is especially important because, due to the nature of the exposure, all age groups were represented. The follow-up studies of the atomic bomb survivors include all malignancies, thus permitting a comparison of the sensitivity of various organs to radiation. In an excess relative risk model, the risk for thyroid cancer is among the highest for all solid malignancies (48).

Physical examinations and thyroid ultrasound imaging was used during 1984-1987 in a study of 2856 survivors in Nagasaki (49). Ninety solid nodules >5 mm were detected. They occurred with a significant dose-response relationship. A relatively large number of thyroid cysts, 110 of them, were also found. Since more sensitive ultrasound machines have shown that most cysts have a solid component, reanalysis of the population with these higher resolution machines could give different results. No dose-response relationship was found for thyroid cancer. An interesting finding was that autoimmune hypothyroidism increased at low doses of exposure and then declined at higher doses. The significance of this observation and whether it will be confirmed by continued studies in this and other populations remains to be seen.

Occupational exposure. Several studies have suggested a relationship between occupational exposure to radiation and thyroid nodules and thyroid cancer. The largest of these studies compared 27,011 diagnostic x-ray workers in China to 25,782 non-exposed medical workers (50). Doses were not estimated; rather duration and type of occupation were used as indicators of exposure. Follow-up information was obtained by interview whenever possible and by other means in other cases. In x-ray workers with more than 10 years of employment there were 7 cases of thyroid cancer compared to 3.3 expected cases. The relative risk was 2.1 with a lower confidence limit just above 1.0.

In a much smaller study in Italy, but one that used thyroid ultrasound for evaluation, 50 medical workers working with radiation were compared to 200 medical workers without exposure (51). It was estimated that the exposed workers had an average cumulative thyroid dose of 67 mSv (7 cGy). Nodules were defined as lesions >5 mm seen by two independent ultrasonographers. In the exposed group there were 19 (38%) nodules compared to 32 (16%) in the control group. After stratification by age, this difference was significant.

In the Swedish case-control studies of diagnostic x-ray exposure and thyroid cancer mentioned above (46), a significantly elevated odds ratio was found for dentists and dental assistants. However, the data should be evaluated cautiously. Surprisingly, teachers also had a statistically significant elevated odds ratio, although not as large as for the dental workers. Also, in addition to the problem of recall bias noted above, the study was not designed specifically to evaluate occupational exposure and there were few cases in each group.

Natural background radiation. Background levels of radiation vary geographically due to elevation or to the proximity of radiation-containing mineral deposits. So far, there is no evidence that the lifetime exposure to this radiation is related to thyroid cancer. The most comprehensive study of this was carried out in southern China comparing 50-65 year old women living in adjacent areas that were similar except for differing levels of background radiation (52). About 1,000 women from each area were examined by history, physical examination and laboratory testing. People living in this area were extremely stable, with most coming from families that lived in the same region for many generations. Therefore, lifetime doses from the background sources could be calculated accurately and were, on the average, 12-16 cGy and 4-6 cGy in the two areas. The prevalence of all nodular disease was 9.5% and 9.3% in the high and low background areas, respectively, and the prevalence of single nodules was 7.4% and 6.6% in the same areas. The study was large enough to be sure that the effect of the lifetime dose was smaller than predicted for the same dose of external radiation administered acutely to children. One explanation is that prolonged exposure allows time for DNA repair. However, another equally plausible explanation, proposed by the authors, is that most of the exposure came during the adult years of life when the thyroid is less sensitive to radiation.

Internal radiation from iodine isotopes

Medical. The use of radioiodine in the medical setting is extensive and well accepted. The thyroid gland receives radiation exposure when iodine isotopes are used as diagnostic agents, for the treatment of hyperthyroidism, and for the treatment of differentiated thyroid cancer.

Diagnostic uses of radioiodine isotopes. The isotope that was used first for functional and imaging studies of the thyroid was I-131. In Sweden, where the most significant follow-up studies have been carried out, the mean thyroid dose estimate in 34,104 people who had diagnostic tests with I-131 during 1950-1969 was 110 cGy (53). Interestingly, and of importance in the subsequent evaluation of radiation effects, patients who were referred for nodular thyroid disease received higher doses than other patients. At a specific institution in Sweden, the Karolinska Hospital, the mean dose for a cohort of 1,005 people who were part of a follow-up screening program was 54 cGy (54). Diagnostic thyroid uptake and imaging studies are now performed with I-123 or Tc-99m-pertechnetate. Thyroid doses from the former are 1.3-5.2 cGy, and 0.26-0.65 cGy from the latter (55). These doses are so small that, even if the carcinogenic potential of internal 123-I and 99mTc was equal to that of external radiation, only an extremely large study could detect an effect.

In the larger study of 34,104 people, the Swedish tumor registry was used to ascertain cases of thyroid cancer during follow-up (53). A small increase in the number of cases was found (67 thyroid cancers reported versus 50 expect), but the excess was confined entirely to people who had suspected thyroid tumors as the reason for their diagnostic exposure to I-131. No increase was seen in people who had diagnostic procedures with I-131 for other reasons and no dose-response relationship was present. The authors concluded that the small excess was due to the original thyroid condition and not to radiation exposure.

The findings were amplified by a study that included physical examination of a subset of the Swedish patients (1005 women) and matched controls (54). The average length of follow-up was 26 years and the average age at exposure was 26 years. The prevalence of thyroid nodules in the two groups was nearly identical (10.6% versus 11.7%); however, among the exposed women there was a small, but statistically significant dose-response relationship. The authors speculate that the original indication for the diagnostic testing with I-131 may account for this observation.

In summary, the study of thyroid cancer follow diagnostic I-131 exposure is complicated by the nature of the indication for the original testing and the absence of a substantial number of exposed children, but the effect is either smaller than the one from external radiation or completely absent.

Benign conditions treated with I-131. Given the wide utilization of I-131 to treat hyperthyroidism and the prevalence of thyroid cancer, especially in a setting where there would be increased clinical attention to the thyroid, it is not surprising that cases reports linking the two have appeared. In the I-131 treatment of Graves' disease the thyroid is exposed to both radiation and thyroid stimulating immunoglobulins. However, two large and carefully conducted epidemiological studies, one in the U.S. and the other in Sweden, have failed to detect any increase in thyroid cancer following I-131 therapy of hyperthyroidism.

In the U.S. study, about 22,000 patients treated with I-131 were compared to about 12,000 patients treated surgically (56). Treatment was performed between 1946 and 1964 and follow-up ended in 1968. The average length of follow-up for the I-131-treated patients was 8 years. The frequency of thyroid cancer during follow-up was not different for the two groups. Five cases of anaplastic thyroid cancer occurred, all in the I-131-treated patients. An important strength of this study is that both groups started with hyperthyroidism and both groups would have had similar clinical attention to their thyroid glands during follow-up. Limitations are that the follow-up was relatively short, the effects of age at exposure were not studied, and the possibility of increased anaplastic thyroid cancer was not resolved.

In the Swedish study, about 11,000 patients treated with I-131 between 1950 and 1975 for hyperthyroidism were studied. Follow-up was for an average of 15 years and the average dose was >10,000 cGy. Two approaches were taken; matching to the Swedish Cancer registry (57) and matching to the Swedish Cause-of-Death Register (58,59). Compared to the expected number of cases for the general population, there was no increase in the number of cases of thyroid cancer or in mortality from thyroid cancer in the I-131-treated patients. Despite the radiation exposure, there was no evidence for increased cases of leukemia, but there was some evidence for increased occurrence of, and mortality from stomach cancer. Mortality in general was higher in patients treated with I-131, but the hyperthyroidism, rather than the radiation exposure was felt to be the likely explanation.

Thyroid cancer treated with I-131. In patients who already have thyroid cancer, two questions arise about the radiation exposure from I-131 used in their therapy. First, since carcinogenesis is thought to be a multistep process, could radiation exposure of residual thyroid cancer tissue enhance its progression to a more aggressively malignant form? In brief, there is no evidence supporting this possibility. Second, is there a possibility that other malignancies will arise as a result of I-131 treatment. Several studies have addressed this question by looking at second cancers following thyroid cancer (please see also Chapter 12).

One problem in studying this question has been that each epidemiological study finds potential associations because the patients at risk are subgrouped (e.g., into males and females) and multiple endpoints are evaluated. In fact, no uniform findings have emerged as yet . Earlier reports suggested that leukemia might be associated with I-131 thyroid cancer treatment (reviewed in (60)), but none of the more recent studies have confirmed this (61-64). In London, England, 285 thyroid cancer patients treated with I-131 were followed by periodic examinations for an average of 11.2 years. In comparison to the general population, small, but significant excesses of bladder cancer (3 observed cases vs 0.5 expected) and breast cancer (6 observed vs 2.53 expected) were seen (65). In Sweden, 834 thyroid cancer patients treated with I-131 were followed using the cancer registry and comparison to the general population (63). A 43% excess of cancer (confidence interval, 17% - 75%) was detected, predominantly ascribable to salivary, genital, kidney and adrenal cancer in women. However, since the excess did not change over time, the authors suggest that the I-131 exposure is an unlikely explanation. Salivary tumors also emerged in a study from Italy in which 730 patients treated with I-131 were followed (62). However, this was based on only 3 observed cases and the means of ascertainment were not clear. The overall rate of cancer was not increased in this study. In Japan a study was conducted of 3321 thyroid cancer patients operated on in one clinic, the majority with additional I-131 therapy, with an average follow-up of 13 years (64). Cancer mortality at all sites, the central nervous system and the respiratory organs were significantly elevated (by 60% for all sites) compared to the general population. However, in an analysis limited to papillary thyroid cancer, no differences in these three categories were found comparing I-131-treated patients (N=2307) with those who did not receive I-131 (N=355). Clearly, more data are needed to evaluate more definitively the potential carcinogenic effects of I-131 on non-thyroid tissues.

Nuclear weapons installations and detonations.

Marshall Islands. The first convincing evidence that radioiodine is capable of inducing thyroid cancer in humans came from follow-up studies on Marshall Islanders who were exposed to fallout from an above ground nuclear weapons test (66-68). The explosion on a tower on Bikini in 1954 unexpectedly contaminated two inhabited islands, Rongelap and Utitrik. About 100 miles downwind and 4-6 hours later, Rongelap was covered by a grossly particulate, ash-like deposit. The nature of this fallout was very different from the high altitude fallout contaminating the continental United States during the nuclear weapons testing in Nevada, and not at all like the high altitude explosions over Hiroshima and Nagasaki that resulted in acute gamma and neutron radiation but little if any particulate deposit on those cities. The fallout on Utirik arrived after 22 hours and was invisible. A series of reviews of this event has been published recently in Health Physics (vol 73(1), 1997).

By the time of the Bikini accident, the thyroid gland was becoming known as an organ sensitive to external radiation-induced neoplasia (see above), but the first thyroid tumors were not detected on Rongelap until 9 yrs later, after the residents had recovered from alopecia, skin burns, and bone marrow depression. Thyroid tumors continued to accumulate during the ensuing 25 years until 20 of the 24 residents who were in utero, or were younger than 10 yrs, at the time of the accident had developed thyroid nodules (17 cases), complete thyroid ablation (2 cases) or evidence of thyroid insufficiency unrelated to surgery (7 cases) (69). In addition, 3 of 12 residents who were 10-18 yrs old when exposed and 3 of the 31 adults developed thyroid nodules. Of the 23 with thyroid nodules, 5 had papillary carcinoma, and 3 of these were younger than 18 yrs when exposed to the fallout. On Sifo (Ailingnae Atoll), where Rongelap residents were working and where the fallout was less severe than on neighboring Rongelap, 5 of 19 individuals developed thyroid nodules but none were malignant. Two of the affected residents were <10 yrs when exposed. On Utirik, 23 of 167 residents developed thyroid nodules, 4 of whom had papillary carcinoma. Only 8 of those with nodules, and one of those with cancer, were adults at the time of the accident.

The ages at which the nine cancers developed on these three contaminated islands were during adulthood in all but one, but the number exceeded that expected in an unexposed Marshallese population by a factor of 4.5. The total of 51 residents with nodules exceeded the expected incidence by a factor of 3 (66,70). All but 4 of those with benign nodules, which were characteristically multiple, were classified as having "adenomatous nodules", the 4 others having a follicular adenoma. In addition, there were 4 individuals with occult papillary cancers that were not included in the analysis, and one case in which there was a divided opinion among the pathologists between follicular carcinoma and atypical adenoma.

Until the accident at Chernobyl, the Marshall Islands experience presented the best opportunity to evaluate the carcinogenic risk of radioiodine in humans, and it appeared to be comparable to that from external radiation (66). Several complicating factors, however, made it difficult to calculate an accurate risk coefficient, especially if one wishes to know the risk that can be attributed to I-131. The small exposed population, a total of 253 on the three islands, was one factor, but even more important was the mixture of the types of radiation. The contribution from external radiation on Rongelap, estimated at 190 cGy, is in a range that can cause thyroid cancer in children (70). On Utirik, however, the external radiation dose was only 11 cGy. On all three islands there appeared to be a substantial contribution to internal radiation by iodine radioisotopes with short half lives that emit high energy beta particles (70,71). The internal radiation dose was reconstructed from a single pooled urine measurement performed about two weeks after the accident and from various measured and derived quantities related to the time of fallout arrival, the particle size and composition of the fallout, and dietary and living patterns. Unlike the fallout experience around Chernobyl and in the continental United States, there is no milk production in the Marshall Islands. The calculations indicated that I-131 accounted for a small fraction of the internal radiation dose, about 13% in Rongelap adults and 21% in Utirik adults (72). Thus the similarity of the carcinogenic risk from internal radiation in the Marshall Islands (approximately $2/10^6$ person years/cGy) and external x-ray irradiation (66,73) should be attributed to the short half-life radioiodines, not to I-131. Furthermore, it should be recognized that the dose received on Rongelap was high enough to cause severe radiation damage to thyroid cells, and this could affect their ability to undergo neoplasia. It should also be noted that the prevalence of benign thyroid nodules in the exposed Marshall Islanders exceeds the prevalence of cancer by a factor of about five, which is higher than experienced with external radiation.

Screening of the Marshall Islanders for thyroid nodules still continues (74) and it has been extended to other regions of the archipelago (75,76). It is uncertain, however, whether the lower contamination levels on the other atolls is associated with thyroid cancer induction. Evidence suggesting that this might be the case was obtained by screening the population of 14 atolls previously thought to be uncontaminated (2,76). The prevalence of a solitary nodule with diameter at least 1 cm varied from 0.9 to 10.6% and tended to increase with proximity to Bikini. The prevalence of malignant nodules, however, was not determined. The more recent and more extensive data (75) is consistent with this interpretation but, although a higher prevalence of nodules was detected (16.2% by palpation, 15.7% by ultrasound only), the correlation with distance from Bikini was marginally significant. In the latter study, 10 cases of papillary cancer were discovered in a cohort of 1322 individuals. Although this prevalence is higher than observed in other Pacific island populations (77), which range from 5 to 25 cancers/10^3 females, the influence of intensive screening of the Marshallese may be a factor. There also is continuing investigation of thyroid dosimetry (78,79) which should help to clarify some of the remaining questions.

Nevada test site. A large number of above ground nuclear weapons tests were performed at the Nevada Test Site in the 1950s, mainly during 1952, 1953, 1955 and 1957. In response to Congressional directive, the National Cancer Institute has recently published the results of an extensive dose reconstruction project that estimates the thyroid radiation dose range received from I-131 by residents in each of the counties of the continental United States (16). The implications for the future health of those who received these exposures are now being addressed by committees of the National Academy of Sciences. At present, the best indication of what these effects might be can be derived from surveys that were carried out in the immediate downwind region in Utah and Nevada (80-83) in two counties that had among the highest average radiation doses to the thyroid, estimated at 30 cGy and higher in young children (16). The reconstructed cumulative doses, from I-131 plus I-133, in the individuals screened in Utah, Nevada and Arizona ranged from 0 to 4.6 Gy (81,84). The greatest contribution to the dose (73%) was from milk ingestion. Inhalation, which should include more of the I-133, accounted for only 3%, and 13% was from external radiation. The highest exposure was in Washington County, Utah (mean $\pm$ SD = 17 $\pm$ 27 cGy, median = 7.2 cGy). In comparison, the average lifetime thyroid dose to the US population born on Oct. 1, 1951 ranged from 0.3 cGy in Los Angeles, to 5.0 cGy in New York City, and 10 cGy in Salt Lake City (16).

Several thousand school age children were examined during 1965 to 1968 and about 70% of this cohort were reexamined 20 years later. In the first survey (80,82), 12 thyroid nodules (with no other thyroid pathology) and no cancers were found among 1378 exposed children, 6 nodules and 2 cancers in 1313 "unexposed" children who moved into those counties at a later time, and 10 nodules and no cancers in 2140 unexposed children in Arizona. In the latest survey (81), 34 non-neoplastic thyroid nodules and 19 neoplasms, 8 of them malignant, were detected in the three counties. The malignant tumors were papillary carcinomas and the adenomas were 8 follicular, 1 Hurthle cell, 1 fetal and 1 papillary. Analysis revealed a significant association with reconstructed thyroid dose for total neoplasms, but not for benign or malignant neoplasms separately or for non-neoplastic nodules. As reviewed by Boice et al (85), there are several concerns in this analysis, including the small sample size, a higher referral rate for thyroid examination in Utah than in Arizona, and the failure to find an association between dose and the more numerous non-neoplastic nodules, as was observed in the Marshall Islands.

Hanford. The Hanford Nuclear facility in Washington state was established in 1943 to produce nuclear materials for atomic weapons. In 1985 and 1986 previously secret documents were released, revealing that large quantities of radioactive isotopes had been released into the environment during the functioning of the facility. Legislation was passed requiring a study with two components: dose reconstruction and thyroid health effects.

It is estimated that 740,000 Ci of I-131 were released from the plant into the atmosphere during its operations (86). The releases occurred after a period of storage on the site, so isotopes of iodine with shorter half lives were mostly gone by the time of release. In contrast, releases from a nuclear explosion or a production plant accident include short-lived iodine isotopes. The dose reconstruction effort confirmed the importance of the milk pathway for thyroid exposure and also quantitated exposure by direct transport through the atmosphere and by indirect transport through the ground water route. With respect to thyroid exposure, the latter routes were not major contributors.

As a result of the dose reconstruction project it is now possible to estimate individual doses based on factors including, most importantly, a person's age during the period of maximum releases and the source of the milk that was consumed. The best estimate for the maximally exposed person, i.e., a person who was young during the releases and obtaining milk from a backyard cow, is 230 cGy. The study of health effects was completed in late 1997 and is currently being analyzed and prepared for publication. No preliminary indication of the findings has been released.

Mayak. The facility in the former Soviet Union analogous to Hanford, the Mayak nuclear production facility, was located in a closed city in Siberia (Ozyorsk), near the major city Chelyabinsk. Preliminary data indicate that the releases of I-131 during operations were large. It has been estimated that the effective equivalent dose accumulated by 1990 for people born in 1952 and 1953 was about 40 centisieverts (87). Assuming that the authors calculated total body exposure, the thyroid dose would be about 20-fold higher. An effort is underway to determine whether the radioactive releases from this facility can be related to thyroid neoplasms. A potential advantage of this study is that, as a closed city, people would not have had the opportunity to move about during the period of releases and it may be easier to trace the milk supply during that time. A possible disadvantage is that it may be more difficult to determine the amounts and types of isotopes released. Also, accidents in long-term nuclear waste storage facilities in the region contributed additional radiation exposure (88).

Other. Nuclear testing in the Soviet Union began in 1949 and was carried out in the Semipalatinsk area. The exposure from the first test alone was dramatic. The explosion occurred close to the ground and at a time of day when most inhabitants were outdoors tending to their fields. Thyroid doses have been estimated as 300 cSv (equivalent to 300 cGy) and 5-10-fold higher for children (89). This was the first of a large series of tests in the area. Only preliminary data on thyroid disease in the residents have been reported (in Russian) so far.

Other nations that later undertook nuclear weapons production programs presumably would have done so with the precautions that the U.S. and Soviet Union eventually adopted. However, in October, 1957 at the British facility located at Sellafield for the production of plutonium, a fire occurred in one of the plutonium producing piles. As a result about 20,000 Ci of I-131 and other isotopes were released into the environment (90). The dose to the thyroid was minimized by control of milk supplies and thyroid glands were monitored. The largest dose to a child's thyroid was estimated to be 16 cGy.

The full extent of thyroid doses received as a result of the worldwide nuclear weapons enterprise remains to be determined.

Nuclear reactor accidents.

Chernobyl. Despite the fact that approximately 400 nuclear power plants are operating currently worldwide, three fourths of them in the United States and Western Europe (91), there has been only one accident of sufficient magnitude to pose a substantial risk of causing thyroid cancer (92). This happened in one of the four reactors at Chernobyl in northern Ukraine on 26 April 1986. The Chernobyl accident released 32 to 46 MCi of I-131 (93) and has been followed by a dramatic increase in childhood thyroid cancer (94).

The accident at Chernobyl exemplifies the potential complexity of such an event, and it will require an intensive effort over a prolonged period to correctly evaluate the extent of the health effects. Interestingly, compared to other environmental disasters of comparable magnitude, there were only 31 deaths (from the acute radiation syndrome) and these involved only plant workers and firefighters. A possible increase in leukemia in the several hundred thousand cleanup workers has not yet been detected, and aside from the enormous psychosocial aftermath, thyroid cancer has until now been the major resulting illness.

Release of volatile radionuclides from the reactor core occurred rapidly on the first day, decreased from the second to the sixth day, then increased again until the tenth day when it abruptly decreased almost to zero (91). In addition to I-131, the initial release included 68 MCi of I-133 and 27 MCi of Te-132 which decays to I-132 (cf Table 2) (93). Although the fallout covered a significant portion of Europe (91), the major contamination was in southern Belarus, northern Ukraine and southwestern Russian Federation, at that time all part of the USSR, where an area covering about 150,000 sq.km was contaminated with at least 1 Ci of Cs-137 per sq.km.

An increase in thyroid cancer in children in Belarus and Ukraine began in 1990, after an interval of only 4 years (95-98). Despite initial concern that the early onset and increased incidence might have been the result of ascertainment bias from intensive screening, subsequent observations made this possibility untenable (94,99). Many of the early tumors were not discovered by routine screening and were relatively large, invasive, and accompanied by spread to cervical lymph nodes. Their prevalence far exceeded that of childhood thyroid cancer in any other region in the world. Furthermore, the number of cancers decreased dramatically in children who were born after 1986 (100); i.e., those who were neither in utero nor already born at the time of the accident. The concentration of cases in the most highly contaminated regions of Belarus and Ukraine clearly associates them with the Chernobyl accident but does not prove that radiation, in particular radioiodine, is the cause. A case-control study in Belarus, however, has revealed a strong relationship between thyroid cancer and thyroid radiation dose (101). Although the thyroid dosimetry used in that analysis must be regarded as preliminary, it was chosen to allow the least biased comparison between cases and controls. Further epidemiological and dose reconstruction studies now underway or planned are expected to provide a better estimate of the carcinogenic risk (102).

The radiation dose to the thyroid in the aftermath of Chernobyl could have been reduced significantly if KI had been given to the children throughout the period of exposure to the fallout. Unfortunately, this appears not to have been done on an adequate scale (94). In Poland, however, KI was administered to more than 10 million individuals, including newborn children and pregnant women, and it was shown that this can be done in a large population with no serious ill effects (103).

Continuing accrual of thyroid cancer in the exposed children into adult life is anticipated (104,105), but the cases thus far recognized as accident-associated have all occurred during childhood. The very large number, about 1000 as of 1997, and the otherwise low incidence of childhood thyroid cancer, has provided an opportunity to assess the pathology, biochemistry, and clinical behavior of radiation-induced thyroid cancer. Because prior experience with thyroid cancer at young ages is rather limited, it is important to differentiate between the properties that might be related to radiation as opposed to the age of onset . The finding of papillary cancer that behaves aggressively, often with extraglandular invasion and with lymph node metastases in virtually every case, and that recurs very frequently after initial removal, as was seen in the children around Chernobyl (106), is typical of thyroid cancer occurring at an early age. The cancers that followed exposure to radiation, however, whether external (107) or internal at Chernobyl (100,108,109), tend to have the following characteristics: they occur at younger ages, the ratio of males to females is higher, the pathological type of papillary carcinoma is more frequently the "solid/follicular variant", and they are more likely to be associated with benign nodular disease. Recent studies, suggest that radiation-associated tumors may also show the following genetic differences: more frequent K-*ras* mutations (not yet seen in Chernobyl cases), more frequent *p53* mutations, and more *ret*- PTC3 translocations compared to *ret*-PTC1 or 2 (reviewed in (109)). Please see Chapter 3 for further discussion.

Insufficient data has been collected to determine the ultimate prognosis in the Chernobyl thyroid cancers, but there is no reason to expect that it will be different from that seen in cases not caused by radiation. The cancer related mortality rate, therefore, may be about 2 to 3% in the childhood cases (107) and overall, including cancers beginning in adults, about 10%. Other questions to be answered by future investigation are the risk of adults developing thyroid cancer as compared to children, the influence of the mild iodine deficiency in the region on the carcinogenesis, the possible occurrence of radiation-induced hypothyroidism, and the risk of developing benign thyroid nodules, autoimmune thyroiditis, and perhaps parathyroid adenomas.

Three-Mile Island. While the accident on March 28, 1979 at the Three-mile Island received a great deal of publicity, only about 20 curies of I-131 were released into the environment (110). Although the potential for a major release of radioisotopes existed, this did not come about due to the containment design of the plant and the fact that the anticipated explosion did not occur. No detectable increase in thyroid cancer is to be expected at this level of contamination (110). The collective dose to the population of 2 million within a 50 mile radius of 3-Mile Island has been estimated at 33 person-Sv, and the average dose to an individual at < 2 μSv (< 2 mrem).

Protection methods

For external radiation the most effective protection methods are the design of radiation fields that avoid the thyroid and physical shielding of the thyroid. If exposure of the thyroid is unavoidable, then subsequent monitoring of the thyroid is indicated. For high dose exposure, serial measurements of TSH and early intervention with thyroid hormone replacement is indicated. This is to avoid the theoretically additive effects of radiation and hypothyroidism. The monitoring of irradiated individuals has been reviewed elsewhere (9,36,37,40,111).

When I-131 enters the environment, the most effective protection methods are avoidance of contaminated milk and other foods and the use of iodide prophylaxis. It has been estimated that the dose of I-131 received by children in Poland after the Chernobyl accident was reduced approximately in half by these two measures (103). The American Thyroid Association has recommended that iodine be available for this purpose (112). However, administrative considerations have intervened and the recommendation has yet to be implemented in the United States.(113). A review of iodide prophylaxis, including its effectiveness, potential side effects, and mechanism of action has been published recently (114).

Future research

Clinical issues

Its long course and generally favorable outcome has made it difficult to resolve several clinical questions, not only for radiation-related thyroid cancer, but for thyroid cancer in general. This has been true so far because, with few exceptions, only well-differentiated papillary thyroid cancer and its variants have been implicated as effects of radiation. However, two important questions about prognosis need to be addressed in ongoing studies. The first is whether more aggressive well differentiated thyroid cancers and undifferentiated thyroid cancer will occur in irradiated people as they become older. This possibility needs to be considered because the effects of radiation are very long lasting and the background rate of more aggressive thyroid cancers increases with age. The second is whether the thyroid cancers occurring in children in the Chernobyl area are more aggressive than other thyroid cancers in children. This possibility arises because there appears to be an increase in certain histological variants, particularly the solid variant of papillary thyroid cancer, and because the oncogene activation pattern may be different than in other childhood thyroid cancers.

As this review emphasizes throughout, resolution of the question of the carcinogenic potency of I-131 is extremely important. In the medical setting, the studies   from Sweden on its diagnostic and therapeutic use are reassuring. However, ongoing studies are needed to determine if there are any subtle effects that have not been recognized as yet. In the area of environmental exposure to I-131, the extent of exposure, particularly resulting from military nuclear weapons programs throughout the world, is becoming clearer with time. It remains to be determined how to recognize individuals and populations at particular risk. How should modifying factors such as other radioactive isotopes in the exposure, dietary factors, age factors, etc. be taken into account? For those determined to be at high risk, it is necessary to determine how they and their physicians should respond. The issue of screening needs to reevaluated in the light of advances in the imaging of the thyroid. On the one hand screening for thyroid neoplasms by palpation is not sensitive. On the other hand, screening by thyroid imaging may be considered too sensitive, revealing many findings that are of no clinical significance (41).

Pathogenesis

It is to be expected that new insights about the pathogenesis of radiation-related thyroid cancer will come from work at the genetic level in two areas. One is in the role of radiation-induced somatic mutations and the other is in the role of hereditary and other radiation susceptibility factors.

With respect to the somatic mutations found in radiation-related thyroid cancer, one question stands out: Is there a specific or preferential pattern of oncogene activation in radiation-related cases? This has been referred to as a "radiation signature". Support for this possibility comes from a study of lung cancer occurring after radiotherapy for Hodgkin's disease (115). The pattern of single base mutations in the *p53* gene of the radiation-related cases was different from *p53* mutations in other cases. In the childhood cases of thyroid cancer in the Chernobyl area, it appears that translocations of *ret* are more common and the pattern of the translocations may be different than in other cases (109). A specific pattern could help identify cases that are related to radiation, a distinct advantage in epidemiological studies. Also, a specific pattern could be correlated to clinical behavior and lead to better clinical management.

One reason to suspect that there are inherited susceptibility factors comes from the patterns of radiation-related tumors that have been observed. The number of individuals with multiple radiation-related tumors and the concordance of thyroid neoplasms found in irradiated siblings is higher than can be explained by chance or known risk factors (33,116,117). There are rare genetic conditions that already have been associated with radiation susceptibility, most notably ataxia telangiectasia. Even heterozygotes for this condition, according to a study that has yet to be corroborated, may be at increased risk for radiation-related breast cancer (118). Recently, it has been recognized that the breast cancer susceptibility genes BRCA1 and BRCA2 interact with proteins involved in one of the DNA repair systems, raising the as yet untested possibility that mutations in these genes may result in increased radiation susceptibility in humans (119,120). While radiation susceptibility is likely to be multifactorial, it is likely that there are substantial genetic components and it is likely that the identity of the genes related to susceptibility will be discovered in the future.

Acknowledgement

Some of the work described in this review was supported, in part, by grant CA 21518 (to ABS) from the National Cancer Institute.

References

1.   Rauth AM. "Radiation Carcinogenesis," In: Tannock IF, Hill RP, eds. *The Basic Science of Oncology.* 2nd edition. New York: McGraw-Hill Inc, 1992; 119-135.

2.   National Research Council. *Health Effects of Exposure to Low Levels of Ionizing Radiation (BEIR V)*, Washington, D.C. National Academy Press, 1990.

3.   Lundell M. Estimates of absorbed dose in different organs in children treated with radium for skin hemangiomas. Radiat Res 1994; 140:327-333.

4.   Stovall M. Nasopharyngeal brachytherapy for lymphoid hyperplasia: Review of dosimetry. Otolaryngol Head Neck Surg 1996; 115:395-398.

5.   Ron E, Lubin JH, Shore RE, Mabuchi K, Modan B, Pottern LM, Schneider AB, Tucker MA, Boice JD, Jr. Thyroid cancer after exposure to external radiation: A pooled analysis of seven studies. Radiat Res 1995; 141:259-277.

6.   Schneider AB, Ron E, Lubin J, Stovall M, Gierlowski TC. Dose-response relationships for radiation-induced thyroid cancer and thyroid nodules: Evidence for the prolonged effects of radiation on the thyroid. J Clin Endocrinol Metab 1993; 77:362-369.

7.   Ron E. "Thyroid Cancer," In: Schottenfeld D, Fraumeni Jr JF, eds. *Cancer Epidemiology and Prevention.* 2nd edition. New York: Oxford University Press, 1996; 1000-1021.

8.   National Research Council. *A Review of the Use of Ionizing Radiation for the Treatment of Benign Diseases*, Rockville, MD: U.S. Dept. of Health, Education, and Welfare (FDA), 1977.

9.   Schneider AB. "Cancer Therapy and Endocrine Disease: Radiation-induced Thyroid Tumours," In: Sheaves R, Jenkins PJ, Wass JA, eds. *Clinical Endocrine Oncology.* Oxford: Blackwell Science, 1997; 514-517.

10.   Mellinger-Birdsong AK. Estimates of numbers of civilians treated with nasopharyngeal radium irradiation in the United States. Otolaryngol Head Neck Surg 1996; 115:429-432.

11.   Benjamin SA, Saunders WJ, Lee AC, Angleton GM, Stephens LC, Mallinckrodt CH. Non-neoplastic and neoplastic thyroid disease in beagles irradiated during prenatal and postnatal development. Radiat Res 1997; 147:422-430.

12.   Ito T, Seyama T, Iwamoto KS, Hayashi T, Mizuno T, Tsuyama N, Dohi K, Nakamura N, Akiyama M. In vitro irradiatioin is able to cause ret oncogene rearrangement. Cancer Res 1993; 53:2940-2943.

13.   Domann FE, Freitas MA, Gould MN, Clifton KH. Quantifying the frequency of radiogenic thyroid cancer per clonogenic cell *in vivo*. Radiat Res 1994; 137:330-337.

14.   Mizuno T, Kyoizumi S, Suzuki T, Iwamoto KS, Seyama T. Continued expression of a tissue specific activated oncogene in the early steps of radiation-induced human thyroid carcinogenesis. Oncogene 1997; 15:1455-1460.

15.   Dumont JE, Malone JF, Van Herle AJ. *Irradiation and Thyroid Disease: Dosimetric, Clinical and Carcinogenic Aspects. Report EUR 6713ER*, Luxembourg: Comminsion of the European Communities, 1980.

16.   National Cancer Institute. *Estimate Exposures and thyroid Doses received by the American People from I-131 in Fallout Following Nevada Atmospheric Nuclear Bomb Tests*, Bethesda, MD: National Institutes of Health, 1997.

17.   National Council on Radiation Protection and Measurement. *Induction of Thyroid Cancer by Ionizing Radiation. NCRP Report No. 80*, Bethesda, MD: National Council on Radiation Protection and Measurement, 1985.

18.   Lee W, Chiacchierini RP, Shleien B, Telles NC. Thyroid tumors following ^{131}I or localized X irradiation to the thyroid and pituitary glands in rats. Radiat Res 1982; 92:307-319.

19.   Dubrova YE, Nesterov VN, Krouchinsky NG, Ostapenko VA, Neumann R, Neil DL, Jeffreys AJ. Human minisatellite mutation rate after the Chernobyl accident. Nature 1996; 380:683-686.

20.   Dubrova YE, Nesterov VN, Krouchinsky NG, Ostapenko VA, Vergnaud G, Giraudeau F, Buard J, Jeffreys AJ. Further evidence for elevated human minisatellite mutation rate in Belarus eight years after the Chernobyl accident. Mutat Res-Fundam Mol Mech Mut 1997; 381:267-278.

21. Sankaranarayanan K. Ionizing radiation, genetic risk estimation and molecular biology: Impact and inferences. Trends Genet 1993; 9:79-84.
22. Ward JF. Radiation mutagenesis: The initial DNA lesions responsible. Radiat Res 1995; 142:362-368.
23. Bryant PE. DNA damage, repair and chromosomal damage. Int J Radiat Biol 1997; 71:675-680.
24. Chu G. Double Strand Break Repair. J Biol Chem 1997; 272:24097-24100.
25. Moynahan ME, Jasin M. Loss of heterozygosity induced by a chromosomal double-strand break. Proc Nat Acad Sci Usa 1997; 94:8988-8993.
26. Fogelfeld L, Bauer TK, Schneider AB, Swartz JE, Zitman R. p53 gene mutations in radiation-induced thyroid cancer. J Clin Endocrinol Metab 1996; 81:3039-3044.
27. Nikiforov YE, Nikiforova MN, Gnepp DR, Fagin JA. Prevalence of mutations of ras and p53 in benign and malignant thyroid tumors from children exposed to radiation after the Chernobyl nuclear accident. Oncogene 1996; 13:687-693.
28. Jhiang SM, Sagartz JE, Tong Q, Parker-Thornburg J, Capen CC, Cho JY, Xing SH, Ledent C. Targeted expression of the ret/PTC1 oncogene induces papillary thyroid carcinomas. Endocrinology 1996; 137:375-378.
29. Santoro M, Chiappetta G, Cerrato A, Salvatore D, Zhang L, Manzo G, Picone A, Portella G, Santelli G, Vecchio G, Fusco A. Development of thyroid papillary carcinomas secondary to tissue-specific expression of the RET/PTC1 oncogene in transgenic mice. Oncogene 1996; 12:1821-1826.
30. Morgan WF, Day JP, Kaplan MI, McGhee EM, Limoli CL. Genomic instability induced by ionizing radiation. Radiat Res 1996; 146:247-258.
31. Hall EJ. "Principles of carcinogenesis: Physical," In: DeVita VT, Hellman S, Rosenberg SA, eds. *Cancer: Principles and Practice of Oncology.* 4th edition. Philadelphia: J. B. Lippincott, 1993; 213-227.
32. Wong FL, Ron E, Gierlowski T, Schneider AB. Benign thyroid tumors: General risk factors and their effects on radiation risk estimation. Am J Epidemiol 1996; 144:728-733.
33. Perkel V, Gail MH, Lubin J, Pee D, Weinstein R, Shore-Freedman E, Schneider AB. 1988. Radiation-Induced Thyroid Neoplasm: Evidence for Familial Susceptibility Factors. J Clin Endocrinol Metab 66:1316-1322.
34. Duffy BJ, Fitzgerald P. Thyroid Cancer in Childhood and Adolescence: A Report on Twenty-Eight Cases. Cancer 1950; 10:1018-1032.
35. Sarne DH, Schneider AB. Evaluation and management of patients exposed to childhood head and neck irradiation. Endocrinologist 1995; 5:304-307.
36. Schneider AB, Ron E. "Thyroid diseases: Tumors: Carcinoma of Follicular Epithelium: Pathogenesis." In: Braverman LE, Utiger R, eds. *Werner and Ingbar's The Thyroid.* 7th edition. Philadelphia: Lippincott-Raven, 1996; 902-909.
37. Schneider AB, Ron E. "Radiation and Thyroid Cancer: Lessons from 46 Years of Study," In: Braverman LE, ed. *Contmporary Endocrinology: Diseases of the Thyroid.* Totowa, NJ: Humana Press, Inc. 197; 265-286.
38. Shore RE. Issues and Epidemiological Evidence Regarding Radiation-Induced Thyroid Cancer. Radiat Res 1992; 131:98-111.
39. Ron E, Lubin JH, Schneider A. Thyroid Cancer Incidence. Nature 1992; 360:113.
40. Sarne DH, Schneider AB. External radiation and thyroid neoplasia. Endocrinol Metab Clin North Am 1996; 25:181-195.
41. Schneider AB, Bekerman C, Leland J, Rosengarten J, Hyun H, Collins B, Shore-Freedman E, Gierlowski TC. Thyroid nodules in the follow-up of irradiated individuals: Comparison of thyroid ultrasound with scanning and palpation. J Clin Endocrinol Metab 1997; 82:4020-4027.
42. Schneider AB, Recant W, Pinsky S, Ryo UY, Bekerman C, Shore-Freedman E. Radiation-induced thyroid carcinoma: Clinical course and results of therapy in 296 patients. Ann Intern Med 1986; 105:405-412.
43. Boice JD, Jr., Engholm G, Kleinerman RA, Blettner M, Stovall M, Lisco H, Moloney WC, Austin DF, Bosch A, Cookfair DL, et al. Radiation dose and second cancer risk in patients treated for cancer of the cervix. Radiat Res 1988; 116:3-55.
44. Hancock SL, Cox RS, Mcdougall IR. Thyroid diseases after treatment of Hodgkin's disease. N Engl J Med 1991; 325:599-605.
45. Tucker MA, Jones PH, Boice JD, Jr., Robison LL, Stone BJ, Stovall M, Jenkin RD, Lubin JH, Baum ES, Siegel SE, Meadows AT, Hoover RN, Fraumeni JF, Jr. Therapeutic radiation at a young age is linked to secondary thyroid cancer. The Late Effects Study Group. Cancer Res 1991;

51:2885-2888.

46. Wingren G, Hallquist A, Hardell L. Diagnostic X-ray exposure and female papillary thyroid cancer: a pooled analysis of two Swedish studies. Eur J Cancer Prev 1997; 6:550-556.

47. Inskip PD, Ekbom A, Galanti MR, Grimelius L, Boice JD, Jr. Medical diagnostic x rays and thyroid cancer. J Natl Cancer Inst 1995; 87:1613-1621.

48. Thompson DE, Mabuchi K, Ron E, Soda M, Tokunaga M, Ochikubo S, Sugimoto S, Ikeda T, Terasaki M, Izumi S, Preston DL. Cancer incidence in atomic bomb survivors. Part II: Solid tumors, 1958-1987. Radiat Res 1994; 137:S17-S67.

49. Nagataki S, Shibata Y, Inoue S, Yokoyama N, Izumi M, Shimaoka K. Thyroid diseases among atomic bomb survivors in Nagasaki. JAMA 1994; 272:364-370.

50. Wang JX, Boice JD, Jr., Li BX, Zhang JY, Fraumeni J. Cancer Among Medical Diagnostic X-Ray Workers In China. J Natl Cancer Inst 1988; 80:344-350.

51. Antonelli A, Silvano G, Bianchi F, Gambuzza C, Tana L, Salvioni G, Baldi V, Gasperini L, Baschieri L. Risk of thyroid nodules in subjects occupationally exposed to radiation: A cross sectional study. Occup Environ Medicine 1995; 52:500-504.

52. Wang Z, Boice JD, Jr., Wei L, Beebe G, Zha Y, Kaplan M, Tao Z, Maxon H, III, Zhang S, Schneider AB, Tan B, Wesseler T, Chen D, Ershow A, Kleinerman R, Littlefield LG, Preston D. Thyroid Nodularity and Chromosome Aberrations Among Women in Areas of High Background Radiation in China. J Natl Cancer Inst 1990; 82:478-185.

53. Hall P, Mattsson A, Boice JD, Jr. Thyroid cancer after diagnostic administration of iodine-131. Radiat Res 1996; 145:86-92.

54. Hall P, Furst CJ, Mattsson A, Holm LE, Boice JD, Jr., Inskip PD. Thyroid nodularity after diagnostic administration of iodine-131. Radiat Res 1996; 146:673-682.

55. Cavalieri RR, Mcdougall IR. "In Vivo Isotopic Tests and Imaging," In: Braverman LE, Utiger R, eds. *Werner and Ingbar's The Thyroid.* 7th edition. Philadelphia: Lippincott-Raven, 1996; 352-376.

56. Dobyns BM, Sheline GE, Workman JB, Tompkins EA, McConahey WM, Becker DV. Malignant and benign neoplasms of the thyroid in patients treated for hyperthyroidism: A report of the Cooperative Thyrotoxicosis Therapy Study. J Clin Endocrinol Metab 1974; 38:976-998.

57. Holm LE, Hall P, Wiklund K, Lundell G, Berg G, Bjelkengren G, Cederquist E, Ericsson UB, Hallquist A, Larsson LG, Lidberg M, Lindberg S, Tennvall J, Wicklund H, Boice JD, Jr. Cancer risk after iodine-131 therapy for hyperthyroidism. J Natl Cancer Inst 1991; 83:1072-1077.

58. Hall P, Berg G, Bjelkengren G, Boice JD, Jr., Ericsson UB, Hallquist A, Lidberg M, Lundell G, Tennvall J, Wiklund K, Holm LE. Cancer mortality after iodine-131 therapy for hyperthyroidism. Int J Cancer 1992; 50:886-890.

59. Hall P, Lundell G, Holm LE. Mortality in patients treated for hyperthyroidism with iodine-131. Acta Endocrinol 1993; 128:230-234.

60. Maxon HR, Smith HS. Radioiodine-131 in the diagnosis and treatment of metastatic well differentiated thyroid cancer. Endocrinol Metab Clin N Amer 1990; 19:685-718.

61. Akslen LA, Glattre E. 1992. Second malignancies in thyroid cancer patients - a population-based survey of 3658 cases from norway. Eur J Cancer 28:491-495

62. Dottorini ME, Lomuscio G, Mazzucchelli L, Vignati A, Colombo L. Assessment of female fertility and carcinogenesis after iodine-131 therapy for differentiated thyroid carcinoma. J Nucl Med 1995; 36:21-27.

63. Hall P, Holm LE, Lundell G, Bjelkengren G, Larsson LG, Lindberg S, Tennvall J, Wick. Cancer risks in thyroid cancer patients. Br J Cancer 1991; 64:159-163.

64. Ishikawa K, Noguchi S, Tanaka K, Fukuda A, Hirohata T. Second primary neoplasms in thyroid cancer patients. Jpn J Cancer Res 1996; 87:232-239.

65. Edmonds CJ, Smith T. The long-term hazards of the treatment of thyroid cancer with radioiodine. Br J Radiol 1986; 59:45-51.

66. Robbins J, Adams WH. "Radiation Effects in the Marshall Islands," In: Nagataki S, ed. *Radiation and the Thyroid.* Amsterdam: Excerpta Medica, 1989; 11-24.

67. Conard RA. "Late Radiation Effects in Marshall Islanders Exposed to Fallout 28 Years Ago," In: Boice JD, Jr., Fraumeni JR, eds. *Radiation Carcinogenesis: Epidemiology and Biological Significance.* New York: Raven Press, 1984; 57-71.

68. Conard RA, Paglia DE, Larsen PR, Sutow WW, Dobyns BM, Robbins J, Krotosky WA, Field JB, Rall JE, Wolff J. *Review of Medical Findings in a Marshallese Population Twenty-six Years After Accidental Exposure to Radioactive Fallout.* Brookhaven National Laboratory Report BNL 51261, Springfield, VA: National Technical Information Service, 1980.

69. Larsen PR, Conard RA, Knudson AG, Robbins J, Wolff J, Rall JE, Nicoloff J, Dobyns BM. Thyroid hypofunction after exposure to fallout from a hydrogen bomb explosion. JAMA 1982; 247:1571-1575.

70. Lessard E, Miltenberger R, Conard RA, Musolino S, Naidu J, Moorthy A, Schopfer C. *Thyroid Absorbed Dose for People at Rongelap, Utrik, and Sifo on March 1, 1954. Brookhaven National Laboratory Report BNL 51882*, Springfield, VA: National Technical Information Service, 1985.

71. Lessard E, Miltenberger RP, Cohn SH, Musolino SV, Conard RA. Protracted exposure to fallout: The Rongelap and Uterik experience. Health Phys 1984; 46:511-527.

72. Adams WH, Harper JA, Rittmaster RS, Heotis P, Scott WA. *Medical Status of Marshallese Accidentally Exposed to 1954 BRAVO Fallout Radiation: January 1980 through December 1983. Brookhaven National Laboratory Report BNL 51761*, Springfield, VA: National Technical Information Service, 1982.

73. Adams WH, Engle RJ, Harper JA, Heotis P, Scott WA. *Medical Status of Marshallese Accidentally Exposed to 1954 BRAVO Fallout Radiation: January 1983 through December 1984. Brookhaven National Laboratory Publication 51958*, Springfield, VA: National Technical Information Service, 1984.

74. Howard JE, Vaswani A, Heotis P. Thyroid disease among the Rongelap and Utirik population - An update. Health Phys 1997; 73:190-198.

75. Takahashi T, Trott KR, Fujimori K, Simon SL, Ohtomo H, Nakashima N, Takaya K, Kimura N, Satomi S, Schoemaker MJ. An investigation into the prevalence of thyroid disease on Kwajalein atoll, Marshall Islands. Health Phys 1997; 73:199-213.

76. Hamilton TE, van Belle G, LoGerfo JP. Thyroid neoplasia in Marshall Islanders exposed to nuclear fallout. JAMA 1987; 258:629-635.

77. Blot WJ, LeMarchand L, Boice JD, Jr., Henderson BE. Thyroid cancer in the Pacific (letter). J Natl Cancer Inst 1997; 89:90-91.

78. Musolino SV, Greenhouse NA, Hull AP. An estimate by two methods of thyroid absorbed doses due to BRAVO fallout in several Northern Marshall Islands. Health Phys 1997; 73:651-662.

79. Simon SL, Graham JC. Findings of the first comprehensive radiological monitoring program of the Republic of the Marshall Islands. Health Phys 1997; 73:66-85.

80. Rallison ML, Lotz TM, Bishop M, Divine W, Haywood K, Lyon JL, Stevens W. Cohort study of thyroid disease near the Nevada test site - a preliminary report. Health Phys 1990; 59:739-746.

81. Kerber RA, Till JE, Simon SL, Lyon JL, Thomas DC, Prestonmartin S, Rallison ML, Lloyd RD, Stevens W. A cohort study of thyroid disease in relation to fallout from nuclear weapons testing. JAMA 1993; 270:2076-2082.

82. Rallison ML, Dobyns BM, Keating FR, Jr., Rall JE, Tyler FH. Thyroid nodularity in children. JAMA 1975; 233:1069-1072.

83. Rallison ML, Dobyns BM, Keating FR, Jr., Rall JE, Tyler FH. Thyroid disease in children: A survey of subjects potentially exposed to fallout radiation. JAMA 1974; 56:457-463.

84. Till JE, Simon SL, Kerber R, Lloyd RD, Stevens W, Thomas DC, Lyon JL, Prestonmartin S. The Utah thyroid cohort study: Analysis of the dosimetry results. Health Phys 1995; 68:472-483.

85. Boice JD, Jr., Land CE, Preston DL. "Ionizing Radiation," In: Schottenfeld D, Fraumeni Jr JF, eds. *Cancer Epidemiology and Prevention.* Second edition. New York: Oxford University Press, 1996; 319-354.

86. Shipler DB, Napier BA, Farris WT, Freshley MD. Hanford environmental dose reconstruction project: an overview. Health Phys 1996; 71:532-544.

87. Drozhko EG, Hohryakov VV. Exposure of population of Chelyabinsk-65 by 131-I release. Radiatsiia I risk 1995; 5:159-162.

88. Akleyev AV. "Experience with the Studies of Medical and Biological Effects of Radiation Incidents in the South Urals," In: Nagataki S, Yamashita S, eds. *Nagasaki Symposium Radiation and Human health: Proposal from Nagasaki.* Amsterdam: Elsevier Science B.V. 1996; 117-126.

89. Rozenson R, Gusev B, Hoshi M, Satow Y. "A Brief Summary of Results of Radiation Studies on residents in the Semipalatinsk Area, 1957-1993," In: Nagataki S, Yamashita S, eds. *Nagasaki Symposium Radiation and Human health: Proposal from Nagasaki.* Amsterdam: Elsevier Science B.V. 1996; 127-139.

90. Schofield GB. "Environmental health and the Windscale Incident," In: Hubner KF, Fry SA, eds. *The Medical Basis for Radiation Accident Preparedness.* Elsevier North Holland, Inc. 1980; 481-489.

91. Malone J, Unger J, Delange F, Lagasse R, Dumont JE. Thyroid consequences of Chernobyl accident in the countries of the European Community. J Endocrinol Invest 1991; 14:701-717.

92.   Mettler FA, Jr., Ricks RC. "Historical Aspects of Radiation Accidents," In: Mettler FA, Jr.,
      Kelsey CA, Ricks RC, eds. *Medical Management of Radiation Accidents*. Boca Raton, FL: CRC
      Press, 1990; 17-30.
93.   Dreicer M, Aarkog A, Alexakhin L, Anspaugh L, Arkhipov NP, Johansson K. "Consequences of
      the Chernobyl Accident for the Natural and Human Environment," In: *One Decade After
      Chernobyl. Summing Up the Consequences of the Accident*. Vienna, Austria: International Atomic
      Energy Agency, 1996; 319-361.
94.   Becker DV, Robbins J, Beebe GW, Bouville AC, Wachholz BW. Childhood thyroid cancer
      following the Chernobyl accident: A status report. Endocrinol Metab Clin North Am 1996;
      25:197-211.
95.   Kazakov VS, Demidchik EP, Astakhova LN. Thyroid cancer after Chernobyl. Nature 1992;
      359:21.
96.   Baverstock K, Egloff B, Pinchera A, Ruchti C, Williams D. Thyroid cancer after Chernobyl.
      Nature 1992; 359:21-22.
97.   Astakhova LN, Vorontsova TV, Drozd VM. "Thyroid nodule pathology in children of Belarus
      following the Chernobyl accident," In: Robbins J, ed. *Treatment of Thyroid Cancer in Childhood*.
      Springfield, VA: National Technical Information Service, 1994; 35-40.
98.   Oleynic VA, Cheban AK. "Thyroid cancer in children of Ukraine from 1981 to 1992," In:
      Robbins J, ed. *Treatment of Thyroid Cancer in Childhood*. Springfield, VA: National technical
      informatioin Service, 1994; 45-50.
99.   Karaoglou A, Desmet G, Kelly GN, Menzel HG, eds. *Proceedings of the First International
      Conference, The Radiological Consequences of the Chernobyl Accident. Pulication EUR 16544*.
      Brussels:. European Communities, 1996.
100. Williams ED, Cherstvoy ED, Egloff B, Hofler H, Vecchio G, Bogdanova T, Bragarnik M, Tronko
      ND. "Interaction of Pathology and Molecular Characterization of Thyroid Cancers," In:
      Karaoglou A, Desmet G, Kelly GN, Menzel HG, eds. *The Radiological Consequences of the
      Chernobyl Accident. Proceedings of the First International Conference, Minsk, Belarus, March
      18-22, 1996. Publication EUR 16544 EN*. Luxembourg: European Commission, 1996; 699-715.
101. Astakhova LN, Anspaugh LR, Beebe GW, Bouville A, Drozdovitch VV, Garber V, Gavrilin YI,
      Khrouch VT, Kuvshinnikov AV, Kuzmenekov YN, Minenko VP, Moschik SI, Nalivko AS,
      Robbins J, Shemiankina EV, Shinkarev S, Tochitskaya SI, Waclawiw MA. Chernobyl-related
      thyroid cancer in children of Belarus: A case-control study. Radiat Res , 1998; in press
102. Wachholz BW. "United States Cooperation with Belarus and Ukraine in the Development and
      Implementatioin of Scientific Protocols of Thyroid Cancer and Other Thyroid Disease Following
      the Chernobyl Accident," In: Nagataki S, ed. *Nagasaki Symposium on Chernobyl: Update and
      Future*. Amsterdam: Elsevier, 1994; 145-148.
103. Nauman J, Wolff J. Iodide prophylaxis in Poland after the Chernobyl reactor accident: Benefits
      and risks. Am J Med 1993; 94:524-532.
104. Williams ED, Becker DV, Dimidchik EP, Nagataki S, Pinchera A, Tronko ND. "Effects on the
      Thyroid in Populations Exposed to Radiation as a Result of the Chernobyl Accident," In: *One
      Decade After Chernobyl. Summing Up the Consequences of the Accident*. Vienna, Austria:
      International Atomic Energy Agency, 1996; 207-230.
105. Cardis E, Anspaugh L, Ivanov EK, Likhtarev IA, Mabuchi K, Okeanov AE, Prisyazhiuk AE.
      "Estimated Long Term Health Effects of the Chernobyl Accident," In: *One Decade After
      Chernobyl. Summing Up the Consequences of the Accident*. Vienna, Austria: International Atomic
      Energy Agency, 1996; 241-271.
106. Robbins J, ed. *Treatment of Thyroid Cancer in Childhood*. Springfield, VA:. National Technical
      Information Service, 1994.
107. Robbins J. "Characteristics of spontaneous and radiation induced thyroid cancers in children," In:
      Nagataki S, ed. *Nagasaki Symposium on Chernobyl: Update and Future*. Amsterdam: Elsevier,
      1994; 81-87.
108. Williams ED, Tronko ND, eds. *Molecular, Cellular, Biological Characterization of Childhood
      Thyroid Cancer. International Scientific Collaboration on Consequences of Chernobyl Accident*.
      Luxembourg:. European Commission, 1996.
109. Robbins J, Schneider AB. Radioiodine-induced thyroid cancer: Studies in the aftermath of the
      accident at Chernobyl. Trends Endocrinol Metab 1998; 8:in press.
110. Royal HD. "The Three Mile Island and Chernobyl Reactor Accidents," In: Mettler FA, Jr., Kelsey
      CA, Ricks RC, eds. *Medical Management of Radiation Accidents*. Boca Raton, FL: CRC Press,
      1990; 269-292.

111. Schneider AB, Fogelfeld L. "Radiation-induced endocrine tumors," In: Arnold A, ed. *Endocrine Neoplasms.* Norwell, MA: Kluwer Academic Publishers, 1997; 141-162.
112. Becker DV, Braverman LE, Dunn JT, Gaitan E, Gorman CA, Maxon HR, Schneider AB, van Middlesworth L, Wolff J. The use of iodine as a thyroid blocking agent in the event of a reactor accident. Report of the Environmental Hazards Committee of the American Thyroid Association. JAMA 1984; 659-661.
113. Becker DV, Zanzonico P. Potassium iodide for thyroid blockade in a reactor accident: Administrative policies that govern its use. Thyroid 1997; 7:193-197.
114. Wolff J. "Iodide Prophylaxis for Reactor Accidents," In: Nagataki S, Yamashita S, eds. *Nagasaki Symposium Radiation and Human health: Proposal from Nagasaki.* Amsterdam: Elsevier Science B.V. 1996; 227-237.
115. De Benedetti VMG, Travis LB, Welsh JA, van Leeuwen FE, Stovall M, Clarke E, Boice JD, Jr., Bennett WP. p53 mutations in lung cancer following radiation therapy for Hodgkin's disease. Cancer Epidem Biomarker Prev 1996; 5:93-98.
116. Schneider AB, Shore-Freedman E, Weinstein R. Radiation-Induced Thyroid and Other Head and Neck Tumors: Occurrence of Multiple Tumors And Analysis of Risk Factors. J Clin Endocrinol Metab 1986; 63:107-112.
117. Sznajder L, Abrahams C, Parry DM, Gierlowski TC, Shore-Freedman E, Schneider AB. Multiple schwannomas and meningiomas associated with irradiation in childhood. Arch Intern Med 1996; 156:1873-1878.
118. Swift M, Morrell D, Massey R, Chase C. Incidence of Cancer in 161 Families Affected by Ataxia-Telangiectasia. N Engl J Med 1991; 325:1831-1836.
119. Wong AKC, Pero R, Ormonde PA, Tavtigian SV, Bartel PL. RAD51 interacts with the evolutionarily conserved BRC motifs in the human breast cancer susceptibility gene brca2. J Biol Chem 1997; 272:31941-31944.
120. Scully R, Chen J, Plug A, Xiao Y, Weaver D, Feunteun J, Ashley T, Livingston DM. Association of BRCA1 with Rad51 in mitotic and meiotic cells. Cell 1997; 88:265-275.

3 MOLECULAR PATHOGENESIS OF TUMORS OF THYROID FOLLICULAR CELLS

James A. Fagin
University of Cincinnati
Cincinnati, Ohio

Introduction

This chapter will consider current information on the pathogenesis of tumors of follicular thyroid cells. The genetic events associated with medullary thyroid cancers will be described separately, as they are derived from a different cell type and have distinct characteristics (please see Chapter 4). In 1997, an estimated 16,100 patients were diagnosed with thyroid cancer in the U.S. Of the two major forms of differentiated cancer derived from thyroid follicular cells, papillary carcinomas are by far the most common. By contrast, follicular thyroid carcinomas are now quite rare (1). Iodide intake is a key environmental factor determining the relative incidence of follicular and papillary cancers. The association of follicular carcinomas with iodine deficiency suggests that this type of tumor often develops within glands subjected to a chronic proliferative drive. Many of them probably arise from pre-existing adenomas, and as such fit the paradigm of clonal evolution through a multistep process involving progressive transformation through somatic mutations of genes important in growth control. By contrast, papillary carcinomas do not have a readily identifiable benign precursor lesion. Although most cases of papillary carcinoma arise in patients with no known risk factor, a history of prior exposure to radiation as a child increases the relative risk for this disease, as discussed in Chapters 1 and 2.

GENETIC TARGETS OF THYROID TUMORIGENESIS:

Oncogenes:

Cell proliferation is stimulated through extracellular growth factors that activate specific signaling cascades that dictate the orderly sequence of events needed for DNA synthesis and cell division. Many of the intermediates in this signaling process are proto-oncogenes, in that they can inappropriately activate cell growth either when overexpressed, or through gain-of-function mutations. Thus, protein products acting at multiple steps along cellular signaling pathways can function as oncogenes when their abundance or structure is disrupted.

Growth Factors as Thyroid Oncogenes:

Increased synthesis of growth factors by tumor cells is observed in many forms of cancer. A well recognized example is the overexpression of v-*sis*, a product of the simian sarcoma virus that is structurally and functionally homologous to platelet-derived growth factor-B (PDGF-B). The constitutive and unregulated production of v-*sis* disrupts homeostatic growth control mechanisms by binding to and activating the specific PDGF receptor on the plasma membrane of the same cells, and inappropriately driving proliferation (2). Overexpression of growth factors has been observed in thyroid neoplasms, and may participate in the neoplastic process. Fibroblast growth factors (FGF) 1 and 2 are mitogens for thyroid follicular cells (3), and are overexpressed in multinodular goiters as well as benign and malignant thyroid neoplasms (4,5). Vascular endothelial cell growth factor (VEGF) is also expressed at higher levels in thyroid cancers than in normal or benign thyroid tumors (6,7). Although a role for these factors in the neoplastic process has not been rigorously established, their known angiogenic properties may be significant in determining thyroid tumor neovascularization. The emergence of new approaches to cancer therapy using anti-angiogenic compounds (8,9) should provide impetus to further clarify events involved in controlling new vessel formation in the different forms of thyroid malignancy.

Other growth factors, such as TGFα (or its close relative EGF), and IGF-I are also mitogens for thyroid follicular cells *in vitro*, and are locally expressed within the thyroid, but evidence for a primary role in neoplasia is lacking (10,11). What are the mechanisms by which tumor cells overexpress growth factors? This does not usually involve primary modifications of the growth factor genes themselves. Rather, growth factor overexpression is secondary to oncogenic activation of other signaling pathways. For instance, mutations of K-ras result in increased TGFα gene expression in rat thyroid FRTL-5 cells (12).

Abnormalities in Signal Reception:

Tyrosine Kinase Receptors: Growth factor receptors are common targets of oncogenesis. This can occur simply through gene amplification of a tyrosine kinase receptor of normal structure, resulting in an increase in the total number of receptors in the plasma membrane. For example, the epidermal growth factor (EGF) receptor is overexpressed in certain epithelial malignancies and in glioblastomas, and its close relative c-erb-B2/neu is amplified and overexpressed in breast and ovarian cancer (13). Even though these receptors are structurally intact, their increased abundance favors clustering, ligand-independent dimerization and tyrosine trans-phosphorylation of the receptor kinase domain, resulting in constitutive activation of downstream signaling pathways. So far, amplification of growth factor receptors has not proven to be a common finding in thyroid neoplasms. Overexpression of met, the receptor for hepatocyte growth factor (HGF) has been reported to be highly prevalent in papillary thyroid carcinomas (14,15). This is not due to amplification or other defects of the met gene, but may instead be secondary to induction of met gene expression, possibly as a result of illegitimate signaling from mutant ras or ret/PTC oncogenes (16). The resulting increase in responsiveness to HGF may participate in the tumorigenesis process (17).

Growth factor receptors can also lead to cell transformation when their structure is modified through activating mutations. One example relevant to the pathogenesis of thyroid papillary carcinomas is the *ret/PTC* oncogene (18), a mutant form of the tyrosine kinase receptor *ret*. Ret is the membrane receptor for glial-derived neurotrophic growth factor (19), and is not normally expressed in thyroid follicular cells. A chromosomal rearrangement linking the promoter/s of unrelated gene/s to the C-terminal fragment of ret (that is missing the extracellular and transmembrane domains) results in the aberrant production of a truncated form of the receptor in thyroid cells. This chimeric protein contains the region involved in the transmission of the growth signal, but lacks the sites allowing signal reception (ligand binding) and anchorage to the plasma membrane. The mutant *ret* is then able to signal in an unregulated fashion. There are several types of *ret* rearrangements found in human thyroid papillary carcinomas, formed by the fusion of the intracellular tyrosine kinase domain of the gene with different 5' gene fragments. *Ret/PTC1* is formed by a paracentric inversion of the long arm of chromosome 10 leading to fusion with a gene named *H4/D10S170* (18). *Ret/PTC2* is formed by a reciprocal translocation between chromosomes 10 and 17, resulting in the juxtaposition of the TK domain of c-ret with a portion of the regulatory subunit of *RIα* cAMP-dependent protein kinase A (20). *Ret/PTC3* is also a result of an intrachromosomal rearrangement and is formed by fusion with the *RFG/ELE1* gene (21,22). Recently several variants of *ret/PTC3* have been observed in papillary carcinomas arising in children exposed to radiation after Chernobyl (23,24). In addition a rearrangement in which the truncated *ret* has been coupled to a novel partner (RFG5) has been observed in two radiation-induced cases (25). In all cases, the truncated fragment of *ret* lacks the transmembrane domain, and the aberrant protein is located within the cytosol (21). The expression of this chimeric product is driven by the respective promoters of the genes upstream of the rearrangement. *Ret* rearrangements are found in less than half of papillary carcinomas in the adult population (reviewed in (26)). Ret rearrangements are particularly common in pediatric papillary thyroid carcinomas (27,28), and in cancers from children exposed to radiation after the Chernobyl nuclear accident (please see below). Rearrangements of another member of the tyrosine receptor family, the proto-oncogene trk, are also seen in papillary thyroid cancers, albeit with a far lower prevalence (29).

Curiously, the *ret* receptor is also the target of mutations in a different form of endocrine neoplasia, but through entirely different mechanisms (30). Whereas *ret* is not normally present in thyroid follicular cells, it is an important membrane receptor in cells of neuroendocrine lineage, such as the parafollicular C-cells (31). Heterozygous germ line mutations in *ret* have been identified in patients with multiple endocrine neoplasia type II, and familial medullary thyroid carcinoma (FMTC) (32), as described in detail in Chapter 4. In FMTC the mutant *ret* commonly has an alteration of one of the cysteine residues in the extracellular region of the receptor. Presumably this changes the conformation of the ligand-binding pocket, and results in constitutive activation. This signaling drive causes C-cell hyperplasia, and it is thought that secondary somatic genetic hits affecting other genes (not yet identified) determine the initiation of the neoplastic clone and its eventual malignant transformation. The *ret* gene is also subject to similar types of point mutations in sporadic MTC. The *ret* example illustrates ways in which the same membrane receptor can be illegitimately activated through distinct mechanisms in two different cell types (i.e. follicular thyroid cells, and parafollicular C cells).

G-protein Coupled Receptors: The growth of pituitary, thyroid and adrenal cells is controlled in part through ligands that activate G protein-coupled receptors of the seven-transmembrane domain family, and that signal in part through stimulation of adenylate cyclase activity. The TSH receptor can be activated in the absence of ligand by point mutations altering domains important in signal transmission (33). Germline mutations of this receptor are associated with syndromes of familial hyperthyroidism (34). More relevant to neoplasia, somatic mutations of the TSH receptor are observed in many hyperfunctioning thyroid adenomas. Progressive growth and the ability to synthesize hormones in the absence of TSH stimulation characterize these benign tumors. Activating mutations have been identified at multiple sites of the receptor protein, including the 3rd, 6th and 7th transmembrane domains, the 1st and 2nd extracellular loop, and the 3rd intracellular loop (35). The TSH receptor is quite extraordinary as an oncogene, in that gain-of-function mutations can be located at multiple sites in the molecule. Parma et al have proposed that this may be due to the fact that the unliganded wild-type TSH receptor has some degree of basal activity (as opposed to other members of this receptor family), and may be prone to further stimulation by a series of different mutational hits (35). The consensus from clinical studies is that autonomously functioning thyroid nodules have a low probability of malignant transformation (36). Accordingly, activating point mutations of the TSH receptor are quite rare in differentiated thyroid carcinomas (37-40).

Abnormalities in Signal Transmission:

Ras Oncogenes: After ligand binding, tyrosine kinase receptors dimerize, and become autophosphorylated on selected tyrosine residues within their cytoplasmic region. The phosphorylated tyrosines create a high affinity binding site for proteins containing Src homology 2 (SH2) domains, that are thus recruited to the receptor, and form the initial link in a chain of phosphorylation reactions culminating in the activation of one of a family of map kinases, which in turn activate a number of transcription factors. A critical signaling molecule in this cascade is *ras*, a membrane-associated protein that in its inactive state is bound to guanosine diphosphate (GDP). After activation, *ras* releases GDP and binds GTP, and becomes the bridge to a series of serine-threonine kinases that further transmit and distribute the signal (41). Point mutations in discrete domains within *ras* that increase its affinity for GTP, or inactivate the autocatalytic GTPase function of the protein, permanently switch the protein to the "on" position. Remarkably, thirty percent of all human tumors contain a mutation in a *ras* allele, making *ras* the most widely mutated human proto-oncogene (41). Mutations of *ras* oncogenes are found in both follicular adenomas and follicular carcinomas, which suggests that *ras* activation is an early step in thyroid tumor development (42-45).

What are the phenotypic implications of *ras* mutations in thyrocytes? Whereas normal thyroid cells have an absolute requirement for TSH for growth, well-differentiated rat thyroid cells (FRTL-5) transfected with mutant *ras* clones are able to grow in its absence (46). However, mutant *ras* is not by itself sufficient to induce thyroid cell transformation, as determined by the ability to form tumors in athymic mice or colonies in soft agar. In addition to its effects on growth, constitutive activation of *ras* is associated with a profound impairment in thyroid cell differentiation. Thyroid cell differentiated properties include the ability to respond to TSH, trap iodine, synthesize thyroglobulin (Tg) and thyroid peroxidase (TPO), and organize into follicular structures. Thyroid cells expressing mutant *ras* lose many of these properties (47).

Although the mechanism of *ras*-mediated dedifferentiation is not fully understood, it may occur in part by interference with cAMP-dependent signaling. Thus, *ras* activation is associated with exclusion of the catalytic domain of protein kinase A from the nucleus (48,49), and interference with phosphorylation and activation of TTF-1, a transcription factor necessary for expression of thyroid-specific genes such as the TSH receptor, Tg and TPO. The manner in which mutant *ras* may interfere with expression or function of the sodium-iodide symporter has not been studied. The potential impact of *ras* mutations on predisposition to malignant transformation will be discussed in the final section of this chapter.

The gsp Oncogene: The essential role of TSH in the control of thyroid cell proliferation has already been discussed. Furthermore, the TSH receptor is subject to somatic mutations in autonomously functioning thyroid adenomas, indicating that intermediates along the cAMP-dependent signal transduction cascade can function as oncogenes when their structure is modified in a manner that renders them constitutively active. After ligand activation, the TSH receptor associates with the heterotrimeric G-protein complex, which in turn transmits the signal by stimulating the catalytic activity of adenylate cyclase. The Gs α subunit of this complex is also a target of activating point mutations in autonomously functioning thyroid adenomas (50), as well as in growth hormone-secreting pituitary tumors (51). The resulting *gsp* oncogene has mutations that are confined to one of two possible hot spots, which either inactivate the intrinsic GTPase activity of the protein (Arg 201), or alter the affinity of Gs α for guanine nucleotides (Gln 227). Mutations of Gs α are quite uncommon in thyroid carcinomas (37-39,52), again attesting to the fact that constitutive activation of intermediates along the adenylate cyclase signaling cascade may not be a frequent harbinger of malignant transformation.

Other Candidate Oncogenes:

The oncogenes we have discussed so far have been clearly demonstrated to play a role in the pathogenesis of thyroid neoplasms. It is quite likely that others remain to be discovered. Protein kinase C (PKC) isozymes transduce extracellular signals for growth in many cell types, including thyrocytes. Prevostel et al have described a point mutation of PKC α in up to 50% of follicular adenomas (53). The mutant PKC α has been found to translocate to aberrant subcellular sites after activation, and confers cells with a degree of serum-independence for growth, and the ability to form small colonies in soft agar (54). However, in a recent comprehensive screen of thyroid neoplasms, we found no mutations of PKCα in any of the 82 tumors we examined, including 41 thyroid adenomas (Ward L et al. In preparation). Using the technique of comparative genomic hybridization, we recently defined several chromosomal regions that are amplified in human thyroid neoplasms. The chromosome 2p21 locus was amplified in a number of thyroid tumors, and in the follicular thyroid carcinoma cell line WRO (55). Indeed, by positional cloning we identified a fairly complex amplification and rearrangement of the gene for PKCϵ in WRO cells that resulted in the overexpression of a chimeric form of the PKC isozyme. This truncated form of PKCϵ functions as a dominant negative inhibitor of the wild-type form of the protein, and protects cells from apoptosis, thus contributing to tumorigenesis (56). At this point, however, it is preliminary to advocate a pathophysiological role for PKC isozymes in human thyroid tumorigenesis until there is more evidence demonstrating defects in their structure or function in primary tumors.

Of particular interest is the cytogenetic observation of translocations involving chromosome 19q13 in follicular adenomas, raising the possibility that a candidate oncogene for thyroid neoplasms may lie within that region (57). In support of this observation, we have found a high prevalence of amplification of the 19q13 in follicular neoplasms and to a lesser extent in papillary carcinomas as determined by comparative genomic hybridization (55).

Tumor Suppressor Genes:

Cells must breach a series of barriers that normally restrain growth in order to progress towards malignancy. Tumor suppressor genes code for proteins that normally inhibit or restrict cell division. Whereas oncogenes act in a dominant fashion, that is, a disruption in one allele is sufficient to evoke the neoplastic phenotype, tumor suppressor genes have a recessive mode of action. In familial syndromes, such as in congenital retinoblastoma or multiple endocrine neoplasia type I, one of the alleles of the tumor suppressor gene (i.e. *Rb, menin*) is already mutated in the germline, but cells remain normal unless the second allele is also damaged, which often takes place postnatally. Structural inactivation of both alleles of a tumor suppressor gene can also arise as an acquired event during the course of sporadic tumor evolution.

The normal counterparts of several tumor suppressor genes play important roles in control of cell cycle progression. The *Rb* gene, the first tumor suppressor to be identified (58), serves as a gatekeeper between the G1 and S phases of the cell cycle. During G_1, Rb is underphosphorylated, and prevents entry into S by binding and sequestering transcription factors needed to activate DNA synthesis. Rb is inactivated by phosphorylation only when the cell has completed the preparation to replicate its DNA (59). Inactivating mutations of both copies of Rb illegitimately release this cell cycle block. Rb mutations are seen not only in retinoblastomas, but in common cancers as well. Viral oncoproteins such as the SV40 large T antigen, adenoviral E1A, and the human papilloma virus E7 can also functionally inactivate Rb, in part by their ability to bind to the underphosphorylated domains of the protein (60-62). Final proof of the tumor suppressing properties of this gene is that cancer cell lines lacking functional Rb can be growth arrested by reintroduction of a normal copy of the gene (63). There have been no attempts to examine the role of Rb in thyroid tumors in a comprehensive fashion. Immunohistochemical studies failed to demonstrate significant changes in the pattern of Rb staining of thyroid cancers compared to normal thyroid tissues. However, it is unclear whether the Rb genes are the subject of more discrete defects in thyroid neoplasms. Another notable example of a tumor suppressor gene with an important cell cycle control function is p16/CDKN2, a cyclin dependent kinase inhibitor that prevents Rb phosphorylation by specifically antagonizing the effects of the holoenzyme complex of cyclin D with either cdk4 or cdk6. Mutations of p16 have been found in many thyroid cancer cell lines, but only rarely in primary tumors (64-67). Interestingly, the p16 gene is frequently hypermethylated in thyroid tumors, suggesting that loss of expression of this critical cell cycle checkpoint gene may occur more commonly as an epigenetic event during tumor evolution (67).

p53 is the most commonly mutated gene in human cancer (68). The fact that many cancers have lost p53 function points to the cardinal role it plays in the maintenance of cell homeostasis. Why is the function of p53 so vital? The p53 protein is a transcriptional activator, and this property is needed for preservation of its tumor suppressing properties. Most inactivating mutations of the gene nullify one of the sequence-specific DNA binding domains of the protein. In some cell types, a single mutant p53 allele can generate a product that complexes with the wild-type form of the protein to functionally inactivate it.   In this circumstance, p53 has a dominant negative effect, and violates the paradigm that tumor suppressor genes are invariably recessive (i.e. both copies must be mutated for the phenotype to manifest). The p53 protein is involved with the cell cycle machinery, largely by its ability to transactivate expression of genes coding for proteins such as p21/WAF1, that induce G_1 arrest by inhibiting cyclin-dependent kinase complexes (69,70). In addition, p53 can help trigger a program of apoptosis. The ability to arrest the cell cycle, and under certain conditions, to activate a program of cell death place p53 at a major crossroads in the determination of cell survival. A fuller picture emerges by understanding the conditions that lead to p53 expression. Levels of p53 increase after exposure to agents that induce DNA damage, such as ionizing radiation and certain drugs used in cancer chemotherapy. Presumably, p53 acts to allow DNA repair to proceed under more favorable conditions (71). However, if the damage is overwhelming, p53 can initiate apoptosis so as to prevent perpetuation of the flawed cell. Interestingly, mice with homozygous disruption of both p53 alleles develop normally, but get cancers at many sites after birth (72). Affected members of families with Li-Fraumeni syndrome inherit a single mutant p53 allele, and have a high predisposition to cancers of several organs (these tumors exhibit somatic mutations in the other p53 allele). Thus, it appears that the presence of p53 is needed in cellular emergencies. In its absence, cells that would normally be removed are able to survive, and occasionally give rise to cancers.

Inactivating point mutations of the p53 tumor suppressor gene are highly prevalent in anaplastic and poorly differentiated thyroid tumors, but not in well-differentiated papillary or follicular carcinomas (73-76). These data implicate p53 inactivation as an important step in late-stage progression of thyroid cancer. Besides impairing apoptosis and removing an important cell cycle checkpoint, loss-of-function of p53 predisposes cells to additional genetic damage, and is therefore commonly associated with cancers displaying aggressive behavior (77).   In addition, mutations of p53 may interfere directly with thyroid cell differentiated gene expression. Introduction of mutant p53 expression vectors into the well-differentiated thyroid cell line PCCL3 results in loss of expression of Tg, TPO and the TSH receptor, and preferential impairment of expression of the thyroid-specific transcription factor Pax-8 (78).   Conversely, re-expression of wild-type p53 in undifferentiated thyroid carcinoma cell lines is associated with restoration of Pax-8 production, and of expression of thyroid peroxidase (79,80).

As mentioned above, loss of function of tumor suppressor genes usually requires structural inactivation of both alleles. One of these is usually lost as part of a large deletion of chromosomal material. Based on this paradigm, the hunt for tumor suppressor genes has been conducted using approaches to identify regions of genetic or chromosomal loss that are common in particular forms of tumors. Papillary carcinomas have a low prevalence of chromosomal or allelic losses (81). By contrast, follicular adenomas, and in particular follicular carcinomas exhibit more frequent allelic deletions. Using polymorphic molecular probes to scan the genome, some of the regions preferentially affected lie within chromosomes 2p, 2q, 3p, 7q, 10q, 11q, 17p (82-87). There has been considerable effort to identify potential tumor suppressor genes lying within those regions. No mutations of either the von Hippel-Lindau (VHL) or the FHIT genes were found in follicular neoplasms with 3p deletions, possibly excluding these candidate tumor suppressors as significant in the pathogenesis of thyroid cancer (85). Recently, the gene conferring predisposition to Cowden's disease was identified (PTEN) and localized to chromosome 10q23.3. Cowden's disease is characterized by widespread development of hamartomas in multiple organs, and increased risk of breast, thyroid and other cancers (88,89). The PTEN gene codes for a dual specificity phosphatase, and is mutated in the germline in patients with Cowden's disease. Hamartomas and cancers developing in these patients develop somatic mutations or deletions affecting the remaining normal PTEN allele (90,91). Somatic mutations of PTEN have been reported in atypical follicular adenomas, but not follicular carcinomas, suggesting that loss of function of this gene may not be significant in the adenoma-carcinoma transition (92).

Disruption of Programmed Cell Death:

Tissue homeostasis is maintained in part by factors that control the appropriate balance between cell proliferation and cell death. Apoptosis is a physiological process that requires sequential expression of gene products that induce chromatin condensation, DNA cleavage and cytosolic shrinkage. Within endocrine tissues, for instance, apoptosis is required for breast and prostatic involution after lactation, and androgen withdrawal, respectively. As mentioned previously, apoptosis is triggered to prevent proliferation of damaged cells, such as occurs after exposure to ionizing radiation. If tumors are to arise they must successfully bypass the cell-killing program that is activated in response to particular cues. In certain cancers, mutations of genes involved in the regulation of cell death appear to be primary mediators of tumorigenesis. Perhaps the most significant example is the overexpression of *bcl-2* in follicular lymphomas, that occurs as a result of a translocation between the immunoglobulin heavy chain gene promoter and the *bcl-2* gene (93,94). The normal function of *bcl-2* in B-lymphocytes is to promote cell survival, presumably as a mechanism to perpetuate immune memory. Illegitimate overexpression of *bcl-2* is not in itself sufficient to induce tumorigenesis, but favors the perpetuation of a neoplastic clone by impairing apoptosis, and allowing the survival of cells that accumulate mutations affecting genes involved in growth control.

Apoptotic mechanisms appear to be significant in the pathogenesis of thyroid cell destruction in autoimmune thyroiditis. This may occur in part through local activation of Fas, a membrane protein that belongs to the tumor necrosis factor receptor family of proteins (95). There is presently only sketchy information on the possible role of apoptosis in thyroid tumor evolution. However, initiation of programmed cell death is a key protective mechanism evoked after oncogene activation (96). For tumor clones to develop and expand it is likely that the apoptotic program must be disabled through secondary genetic or epigenetic events that are yet to be identified.

Factors that Maintain the Integrity of the Genome:

Hereditary nonpolyposis colorectal cancer (HNPCC) is an autosomal dominant disease associated with early onset of colorectal cancer. The genes responsible for conferring this predisposition, hMSH2, hMLH1, hPMS1 and hPMS2, code for enzymes that correct nucleotide mismatches that occur during DNA synthesis (97,98). A homozygous disruption of one of these genes (one allele mutated in the germline, the other as an acquired somatic event) results in microsatellite instability (RER), a tendency to acquire alterations at mononucleotide, dinucleotide or trinucleotide repeat sequences (microsatellites), that are widespread throughout the genome. These regions are more prone to error during DNA replication, and the defects cannot be appropriately corrected in the absence of the appropriate enzymatic machinery. It is thought that the RER genome will eventually result in mutations affecting genes important in growth control, as has been demonstrated for the TGFβII receptor (99). Recent studies failed to show evidence of microsatellite instability in either sporadic or radiation-induced papillary thyroid carcinomas (100). A subset of the latter did exhibit somatic *mini*satellite instability (i.e.manifesting as mutations of tandem repeats with unit sizes of 6-100 bp), that probably originate through mechanisms not involving the same family of mismatch repair enzymes whose dysfunction cause *micro*satellite instability.

Genetic instability more commonly manifests as alterations in chromosome number (aneuploidy) (101). Here, the fundamental abnormality is not known, but is likely to affect mechanisms controlling chromosome segregation during mitosis (102). Normally a checkpoint control monitors the proper assembly of the mitotic spindle, a step essential to ensure that chromosomes are attached stably to the microtubules prior to the onset of anaphase. Mutations in *Bub1*, a gene coding for a protein involved in this mitotic checkpoint, have recently been reported in colorectal cell lines with chromosomal instability (103). Loss of heterozygosity and alterations of chromosome number are prevalent in follicular thyroid carcinomas, whereas these defects are not seen in the more common papillary thyroid cancers (81,84,85,87). It is tempting to speculate that the former have acquired a genetic defect that predisposes them to large-scale chromosomal instability, but this remains to be established.

Events Predisposing to Thyroid Neoplasia:

Genetic Predisposition to Non-medullary Thyroid Cancer:

There are several familial syndromes of neoplasia that exhibit increased incidence of tumors of thyroid follicular cells (Table 1). An increased predisposition to papillary carcinoma is well established in certain families with adenomatous polyposis, an autosomal condition characterized by the presence of multiple adenomatous polyps of the intestine (104-106). The association with thyroid cancer extends to Gardner's syndrome, a variant of FAP characterized by numerous intestinal adenomas, osteomas, soft tissue lesions, and other extracolonic neoplasms (107,108). Thyroid cancers in FAP exhibit a marked female preponderance (female: male ratio 8:1), and are more common under the age of 30. Women below 35 years of age with FAP have been estimated to have a 160-fold higher risk of thyroid carcinoma than normal individuals (104). Papillary carcinomas from patients with FAP are commonly multifocal, well-encapsulated, and often display unusual histopathological features, such as areas of cribriform, solid and spindle cells within the tumors (109). Predisposition to FAP is conferred by germline inactivating mutations of the APC gene, that maps to chromosome 5q21 (110,111). Colorectal neoplasms from patients with FAP frequently exhibit loss-of-heterozygosity at this locus, consistent with a role for APC as a tumor suppressor gene, requiring loss of function of both alleles in order for the recessive phenotype to emerge. It is not known whether thyroid carcinomas from patients with FAP also have somatic mutations of the wild-type allele of the APC gene. The presence of extracolonic neoplasms in patients with FAP is also genetically determined, and is not due to the nature of the structural defect of the APC gene itself. This predicts that one or more "modifier" genes may act in concert with APC to alter the predisposition to tumor formation at extracolonic sites, such as the thyroid gland. Indeed, there is good evidence for the existence of such "modifier" genes, capable of modulating the expression of the FAP phenotype. Examination of FAP kindreds demonstrates that family members inheriting the same APC mutation differ dramatically in tumor burden (i.e. number of polyps). To determine the possible genetic basis for this variability, MacPhee et al have used a mouse strain with multiple intestinal neoplasia (*Min*) (112), harboring a nonsense mutation in exon 15 of APC, a defect also found frequently in human FAP kindreds. When *Min* mice were crossed with different mouse strains, there was a dramatic difference in the number of intestinal polyps in the F1 progeny of animals harboring the *Min* mutation according to the genetic background. The genetic locus conferring the difference in tumor burden was then mapped by interspecific backcross analysis to mouse chromosome 4, and a candidate "modifier" gene, that for secretory phospholipase A2, identified (112). Localization of gene modifiers in humans or in mice with adenomatous polyposis may prove to be an expedient way to identify candidate genes conferring predisposition to familial thyroid cancer. It is noteworthy that mutations of APC are not prevalent in sporadic thyroid neoplasms, indicating that inactivation of this gene is not likely by itself to predispose to sporadic thyroid tumor formation (113,114).

Table 1: Familial syndromes associated with tumors of thyroid follicular cells

Disease entity	Manifestations	Chromosomal location	Gene	Function
Familial polyposis coli	Polyps in large intestine papillary thyroid cancer	5q21	APC	Cell adhesion
Gardner's syndrome	Polyps in small and large intestine, osteomas, fibromas, lipomas, ampullary cancers papillary thyroid cancer	5q21, others?	APC	Cell adhesion
Turcot's syndrome	Polyps in large intestine, brain tumors papillary thyroid cancer	5q21, others?	APC	Cell adhesion
Multiple endocrine neoplasia type I	Parathyroid adenomas, pituitary adenomas, pancreatic endocrine tumors follicular adenomas?	11q13	menin	Unknown
Cowden's disease	Multiple hamartomas Follicular adenomas, goiter follicular carcinomas	10q22-23	PTEN	Dual specificity phosphatase
Carney complex	Spotty skin pigmentation, myxomas, schwannomas, pigmented adrenocortical nodules hypercortisolism, follicular adenomas, follicular carcinomas	2p16, 17q23	Unknown	
Familial non-medullary thyroid cancer	Papillary thyroid carcinoma	Unknown		

Thyroid tumors have also been reported in other familial syndromes. They are the most frequent extracutaneous manifestation of Cowden's disease (multiple hamartoma syndrome), being observed in two thirds of patients; they include benign thyroid lesions (adenomas, goiter, thyroglossal duct cyst), and follicular thyroid carcinoma (115). As mentioned above, the gene for Cowden's disease has recently been identified (PTEN), and found to function as a dual specificity phosphatase. Mutations of PTEN have been found in sporadic atypical follicular adenomas (88-91). There are case reports describing the association of thyroid carcinoma in patients with Peutz-Jeghers syndrome (116), and ataxia-telangiectasia (117). In patients with multiple endocrine neoplasia type1 (MEN1), thyroid disease is observed mostly as benign lesions (nodular hyperplasia, goiter, adenoma), and far more rarely as a malignancy (118). The gene conferring predisposition to MEN1 (*menin*) is located on chromosome 11q13, is believed to function as a tumor suppressor, through mechanisms that have not been worked out (119,120). Pancreatic, pituitary and parathyroid tumors from patients with MEN1 frequently exhibit loss of heterozygosity at this locus, presumably resulting in loss-of-function of the normal allele. Loss of heterozygosity at chromosome 11q13 is also found in sporadic follicular thyroid neoplasms, but to our knowledge there are no studies in which the structure of menin has been examined in these tumors (82,83).

Over the years, there have been multiple reports of clustering of cases of papillary carcinomas in families (121-125). Most of the literature consists of descriptions of individual family pedigrees. This has resulted in uncertainty as to whether the familial association represents evidence of genetic predisposition to the disease, exposure to a common environmental triggering event, increased susceptibility to environmental effects, or a chance occurrence. A comprehensive analysis of families of all cases of papillary carcinoma diagnosed in Iceland between 1955 and 1984 revealed that 3.8% of the propositi had a first degree relative with thyroid carcinoma, a higher than expected frequency that was not, though, statistically significant (although there was a significantly increased risk in male relatives) (126). Stoffer et al studied families from 226 consecutive papillary thyroid carcinoma patients from a private practice, and concluded that between 3.5 and 6.2% had at least one affected relative (127). Four individuals with familial papillary carcinoma had a history of radiation in childhood that may have contributed to the expression of the phenotype. Some of the pedigrees reported by Stoffer et al had multiple affected individuals (127). Ron et al reported a population-based case-control study of the Connecticut Tumor Registry, in which a 5-fold excess risk of non-medullary thyroid cancer was found in close relatives (128,129). These three studies are the most informative concerning the existence of familial predisposition to non-medullary thyroid carcinoma, and yielded results consistent with this notion. There are several groups actively pursuing studies to explore a possible genetic basis for familial non-medullary thyroid cancer.

Radiation Induced Thyroid Cancer:

The major known risk factor for papillary thyroid carcinoma is prior exposure to radiation (please see Chapters 1 and 2). The effects of radiation on cancer risk are dose-dependent. Relative risk (RR) of thyroid cancer was 4.0 among children exposed to a mean dose to the thyroid of 9 rads (130). In a separate study, the RR was 12.9 for children exposed to 1-49 rads, and 196 for greater than 600 rads (131). A lower age at the time of exposure has been consistently associated with a higher RR for thyroid cancer, a phenomenon that was strikingly apparent in the pediatric thyroid carcinomas arising after the Chernobyl nuclear disaster (132). Exposure to a common environmental insult, such as external radiation, may represent an alternative mechanism for the familial clustering of patients with papillary thyroid carcinoma. The most significant sources of exposure have been after therapeutic irradiation, and through environmental disasters (133). As a result of the accident at the Chernobyl nuclear power plant in 1986 millions of Curies of short-lived radioiodine isotopes were released in the fallout. The absorption of radioiodines from ingestion of contaminated food and water and through inhalation led to internal exposure to the thyroid gland, which was 3-10 times higher in children than in adults. An increased incidence of thyroid cancer in children from the most contaminated areas of Belarus (i.e. Gomel region) was noted as early as 3 years after the accident (134). Between 1991 and 1992, the incidence of childhood thyroid cancer in Belarus was 60-fold greater than prior to the disaster (135), and this increase now extends to contaminated regions of Ukraine and Southwest Russia. In Belarus, the risk of thyroid carcinoma was inversely associated with the distance of residence location from the source of radioactive contamination, and with age at the time of exposure: the greatest number of children subsequently developing thyroid cancer were less than 4 years of age at the time of the accident (132). Radiation is known to induce DNA strand breaks, but the precise genetic targets are likely to vary according to the cell type. Recent studies suggest that activating mutations of the *ret* proto-oncogene resulting in the aberrant expression of the tyrosine kinase domain of the *ret* receptor (i.e. *ret*/PTC rearrangements) are common in post-Chernobyl papillary thyroid carcinomas (28,136,137). However, *ret*/PTC is also found with high prevalence in children without a history of radiation exposure (28), although the precise types of *ret* rearrangement differ. It is possible that rearrangements of *ret* may occur as a direct result of radiation damage to thyroid cells, either through exposure of individuals to high doses (e.g. as in the case of Chernobyl patients), or increased susceptibility to radiation effects (e.g. in pediatric thyroid carcinomas found in the general population). Alternatively, other DNA damaging agents may account for the high prevalence of ret/PTC in sporadic childhood papillary thyroid cancer.

Epigenetic Changes: Changes in DNA Methylation:

The majority of human gene promoters lie within chromosome areas rich in CG dinucleotides, referred to as CG islands. Most of these CG sites are demethylated, with the exception of genes located on the X chromosome, and certain imprinted loci (138). CG island methylation results in heritable inhibition of gene transcription, and has been proposed as an alternative mechanism of gene inactivation in neoplasia (139,140). Increased DNA methylation has been reported to inhibit expression of tumor suppressor genes (141), and to predispose to transitional point mutations at methylated cytosines (142). Abnormal CpG methylation is a common event in neoplasia, usually occurring as an early event (140,143). The mechanism for these methylation changes is unknown. Thyroid tumors are no exception to this paradigm, as they exhibit a very high prevalence of methylation abnormalities, occurring early in tumor progression (144).

Hypothesis: An Integrated Perspective of Thyroid Tumor Pathogenesis:

It may be enlightening to attempt to recreate the natural history of thyroid cancers based on available epidemiological and genetic information. However, it is important to emphasize that there is much we do not know. Progression of thyroid tumors is mostly interrupted when they are removed at surgery, making data on prognostic implications of particular genotypes difficult to evaluate. Some of the histotypes can be difficult to interpret, complicating the comparison between different patient series. Although in part speculative, this remains a worthwhile exercise, as it may point to some unresolved questions, and areas of opportunity for the future.

Papillary thyroid carcinomas:

A general assumption in tumor genetics is that a single oncogenic mutation is not sufficient to induce malignant transformation. It follows that sequential abnormalities must take place (Figure 1). There is no recognizable histological precursor for papillary carcinomas, and it is therefore difficult to reconstruct the genetic steps that may be involved in tumor evolution. Ret/PTC rearrangements may occur as initiating events (145). It appears that ret/PTC is not in itself sufficient to evoke malignant transformation, as demonstrated by inability of human fetal thyroid explants with radiation-induced ret/PTC1 rearrangements to form tumors in athymic nude mice (146). Overexpression of ret/PTC1 in thyroid glands of transgenic mice results in tumors with a papillary histotype (147). Although this experiment indicates that ret/PTC1 overexpression can initiate the path towards papillary carcinoma formation, it does not prove that ret/PTC is sufficient for induction of malignancy, as secondary genetic events may take place during cancer development. Based on the Chernobyl experience (136,137,148), and *in vitro* data (146,149), it is reasonable to postulate that radiation may directly lead to DNA strand breaks, and to ret activation through gene rearrangements. The precise nature of possible secondary genetic changes resulting in further progression is unclear. Mutations of *ras* have been observed in papillary carcinomas, in some cases associated with gene amplification of the mutant ras gene (43,150). It is possible that *ras* mutations are secondary changes in a subset of papillary carcinomas, as opposed to their role in the follicular adenoma-carcinoma progression, in which *ras* activation occurs in precursor lesions. Other contributing factors to papillary carcinoma development include changes in gene expression of proteins important in growth control. As found in almost all thyroid tumors, the DNA of papillary carcinomas shows abnormal patterns of methylation (144). Hypermethylation of CpG islands in critical promoter regions has the potential to silence expression of tumor suppressor genes such as CDKN2/p16 (67). Overexpression of the tyrosine kinase receptor met has been reported in papillary thyroid carcinomas, but its role in tumor progression is unclear (16,151).

This much is known: papillary carcinomas have a low rate of aneuploidy (152,153), loss of heterozygosity (81,87) and microsatellite instability (100). This predicts that the tumor clone will remain fairly homogeneous, and explains in part the excellent prognosis and response to therapy of this type of thyroid cancer.

Follicular thyroid carcinomas:

Follicular carcinomas are believed to arise from benign adenomas. Absolute proof of the adenoma-carcinoma transition is lacking, however the existence of intermediate phenotypes (i.e. minimally invasive follicular carcinomas) is consistent with this microevolution. Follicular carcinomas are more common in iodine deficiency regions, suggesting that the proliferative drive may be a factor in their

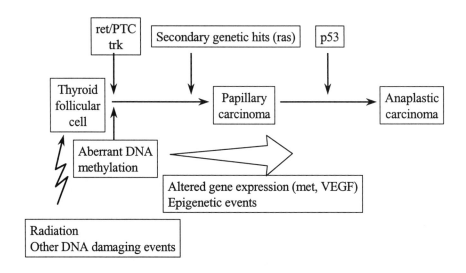

Figure 1: Genetic events in progression to thyroid papillary carcinomas. Please see text for details.

development. Mutations of all three mammalian ras genes (H-ras, N-ras, and to a lesser extent K-ras) are seen in follicular adenomas and carcinomas. Ras mutations may be involved in initiating clonal expansion, or they may occur as a fairly early event after its development (Figure 2). Transition to malignancy is a low probability event, and it is unclear if ras activation may favor transformation. It is possible that effects of mutant *ras* on cell transformation may be indirect, and result from promotion or facilitation of additional genetic defects (154-157). Mouse fibroblasts engineered to express activated human H-*ras* under the control of a bacterial lactose regulatory system, in such a manner that the expression of the mutant *ras* only takes place in the presence of the lactose analog isopropyl-1-thio-β-galactopyranoside (IPTG), have been used to test the mechanisms of cell transformation by ras. Cells expressing activated H-*ras* show a markedly increased frequency of development of methotrexate resistance, primarily due to amplification of the dihydrofolate reductase gene. Expression of mutant H-*ras* was also associated with resistance to PALA, conferred by amplification of the CAD gene, indicating that the increased propensity for amplification was not locus-specific. The tendency towards development of genomic instability conferred by expression of activated H-*ras* was already apparent within the first cell cycle after expression of the mutant oncogene (155,156). The precise mechanisms that might explain how constitutive *ras* activation impairs chromosomal stability are not known, but may relate to accelerated traverse through cell cycle check points and premature entry into S phase, prior to appropriate repair of DNA damage arising from endogenous sources. Using an analogous system, we have also observed that thyroid cells conditionally expressing mutant ras develop large-scale chromosomal abnormalities manifesting within 48h (Elisei R, Saavedra H, Knauf J, Stambrook P, Fagin J, unpublished). It is unclear whether the high rate of aneuploidy seen in follicular carcinomas can be attributed to mutations of *ras*. It will be of interest to establish whether follicular carcinomas develop abnormalities in mitotic checkpoint controls, and in particular whether these may be due to mutations of genes coding for proteins involved in this process.

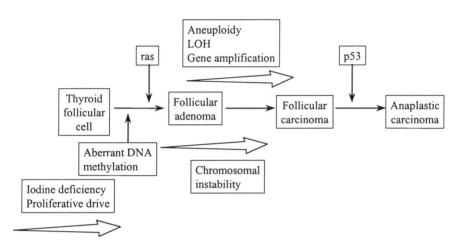

Figure 2: Genetic events in progression to follicular carcinomas. Please see text for details.

Undifferentiated or anaplastic thyroid carcinomas:

The end stage forms of thyroid cancer are characterized by loss of differentiated properties, greater tumor invasiveness and metastatic spread. Tumor clones are genetically heterogeneous, a manifestation of genomic instability. This cellular heterogeneity confers tumors with a poor prognosis, and resistance to all treatment modalities. Mutations of the p53 tumor suppressor gene are a common feature of undifferentiated thyroid cancers (73-76), and could be responsible for their aggressive phenotype. Many of the experimental gene therapy protocols to treat advanced forms of cancer are directed to tumors with inactivating mutations of p53, and anaplastic carcinomas may prove to be good candidates for clinical trials if these strategies prove to be successful.

References:

1.   LiVolsi VA, Asa SL. The demise of follicular carcinoma of the thyroid gland. [Review] [36 refs]. THYROID 1994; 4(2):233-6.

2.   Leal F, Williams LT, Robbins KC, Aaronson SA. Evidence that the v-sis gene product transforms by interaction with the receptor for platelet-derived growth factor. Science 1985; 230(4723):327-30.

3.   Black EG, Logan A, Davis JR, Sheppard MC. Basic fibroblast growth factor affects DNA synthesis and cell function and activates multiple signalling pathways in rat thyroid FRTL-5 and pituitary GH3 cells. Journal of Endocrinology 1990; 127(1):39-46.

4.   Shingu K, Sugenoya A, Itoh N, Kato R. Expression of basic fibroblast growth factor in thyroid disorders. World Journal of Surgery 1994; 18(4):500-5.

5.   Eggo MC, Hopkins JM, Franklyn JA, Johnson GD, Sanders DS, Sheppard MC. Expression of fibroblast growth factors in thyroid cancer. Journal of Clinical Endocrinology & Metabolism 1995; 80(3):1006-11.

6.   Viglietto G, Maglione D, Rambaldi M, Cerutti J, Romano A, Trapasso F, Fedele M, Ippolito P, Chiappetta G, Botti G. Upregulation of vascular endothelial growth factor (VEGF) and downregulation of placenta growth factor (PlGF) associated with malignancy in human thyroid tumors and cell lines. Oncogene 1995; 11(8):1569-79.

7.   Soh EY, Duh QY, Sobhi SA, Young DM, Epstein HD, Wong MG, Garcia YK, Min YD, Grossman RF, Siperstein AE, et al. Vascular endothelial growth factor expression is higher in differentiated thyroid cancer than in normal or benign thyroid. Journal of Clinical Endocrinology & Metabolism 1997; 82(11):3741-7.

8.   O'Reilly MS, Boehm T, Shing Y, Fukai N, Vasios G, Lane WS, Flynn E, Birkhead JR, Olsen BR, Folkman J. Endostatin: an endogenous inhibitor of angiogenesis and tumor growth. Cell 1997; 88(2):277-85.

9.   Folkman J. Angiogenesis and angiogenesis inhibition: an overview. [Review] [39 refs]. EXS 1997; 79:1-8:1-8.

10. Driman DK, Kobrin MS, Kudlow JE, Asa SL. Transforming growth factor-alpha in normal and neoplastic human endocrine tissues. Hum Pathol 1992; 23(12):1360-5.

11. van der Laan BF, Freeman JL, Asa SL. Expression of growth factors and growth factor receptors in normal and tumorous human thyroid tissues. THYROID 1995; 5(1):67-73.

12. Colletta G, Cirafici AM, Di Carlo A, Ciardiello F, Salomon DS, Vecchio G. Constitutive expression of transforming growth factor alpha does not transform rat thyroid epithelial cells. Oncogene 1991; 6(4):583-7.

13. Slamon DJ, Godolphin W, Jones LA, Holt JA, Wong SG, Keith DE, Levin WJ, Stuart SG, Udove J, Ullrich A. Studies of the HER-2/neu proto-oncogene in human breast and ovarian cancer. Science 1989; 244(4905):707-12.

14. Di Renzo MF, Olivero M, Ferro S, Prat M, Bongarzone I, Pilotti S, Belfiore A, Costantino A, Vigneri R, Pierotti MA, et al. Overexpression of the c-MET/HGF receptor gene in human thyroid carcinomas. Oncogene 1992; 7(12):2549-53.

15. Belfiore A, Gangemi P, Costantino A, Russo G, Santonocito GM, Ippolito O, Di Renzo MF, Comoglio P, Fiumara A, Vigneri R. Negative/low expression of the Met/hepatocyte growth factor receptor identifies papillary thyroid carcinomas with high risk of distant metastases. Journal of Clinical Endocrinology & Metabolism 1997; 82(7):2322-8.

16. Ivan M, Bond JA, Prat M, Comoglio PM, Wynford-Thomas D. Activated ras and ret oncogenes induce over-expression of c-met (hepatocyte growth factor receptor) in human thyroid epithelial cells. Oncogene 1997; 14(20):2417-23.

17. Dremier S, Taton M, Coulonval K, Nakamura T, Matsumoto K, Dumont JE. Mitogenic, dedifferentiating, and scattering effects of hepatocyte growth factor on dog thyroid cells. Endocrinology 1994; 135(1):135-40.

18. Grieco M, Santoro M, Berlingieri MT, Melillo RM, Donghi R, Bongarzone I, Pierotti MA, Porta GD, Fusco A, Vecchio G. PTC is a Novel Rearranged Form of the ret Proto-Oncogene and Is Frequently Detected In Vivo in Human Thyroid Papillary Carcinomas. Cell 1990; 60:557-63.

19. Sanicola M, Hession C, Worley D, Carmillo P, Ehrenfels C, Walus L, Robinson S, Jaworski G, Wei H, Tizard R, et al. Glial cell line-derived neurotrophic factor-dependent RET activation can be mediated by two different cell-surface accessory proteins. Proceedings of the National Academy of Sciences of the United States of America 1997; 94(12):6238-43.

20. Bongarzone I, Monzini N, Borrello MG, Carcano C, Ferraresi G, Arighi E, Mondellini P, Della Porta G, Pierotti MA. Molecular characterization of a thyroid tumor-specific transforming sequence formed by the fusion of ret tyrosine kinase and the regulatory subunit RI alpha of cyclic AMP-dependent protein kinase A. Mol Cell Biol 1993; 13(1):358-66.

21. Minoletti F, Butti MG, Coronelli S, Miozzo M, Sozzi G, Pilotti S, Tunnacliffe A, Pierotti MA, Bongarzone I. The two genes generating RET/PTC3 are localized in chromosomal band 10q11.2. Genes, Chromosomes & Cancer 1994; 11(1):51-7.

22. Santoro M, Dathan NA, Berlingieri MT, Bongarzone I, Paulin C, Grieco M, Pierotti MA, Vecchio G, Fusco A. Molecular characterization of RET/PTC3: a novel rearranged version of the RETproto-oncogene in a human thyroid papillary carcinoma. Oncogene 1994; 9(2):509-16.

23. Klugbauer S, Demidchik EP, Lengfelder E, Rabes HM. Molecular analysis of new subtypes of ELE/RET rearrangements, their reciprocal transcripts and breakpoints in papillary thyroid carcinomas of children after Chernobyl. Oncogene 1998; 16(5):671-5.

24. Klugbauer S, Lengfelder E, Demidchik EP, Rabes HM. A new form of RET rearrangement in thyroid carcinomas of children after the Chernobyl reactor accident. Oncogene 1996; 13(5):1099-102.

25. Klugbauer S, Demidchik EP, Lengfelder E, Rabes HM. Detection of a novel type of RET rearrangement (PTC5) in thyroid carcinomas after Chernobyl and analysis of the involved RET-fused gene RFG5. Cancer Research 1998; 58(2):198-203.

26. Sugg SL, Zheng L, Rosen IB, Freeman JL, Ezzat S, Asa SL. ret/PTC-1, -2, and -3 oncogene rearrangements in human thyroid carcinomas: implications for metastatic potential? [see comments]. Journal of Clinical Endocrinology & Metabolism 1996; 81(9):3360-5.

27. Bongarzone I, Fugazzola L, Vigneri P, Mariani L, Mondellini P, Pacini F, Basolo F, Pinchera A, Pilotti S, Pierotti MA. Age-related activation of the tyrosine kinase receptor protooncogenes RET and NTRK1 in papillary thyroid carcinoma. Journal of Clinical Endocrinology & Metabolism 1996; 81(5):2006-9.

28. Nikiforov YE, Rowland JM, Bove KE, Monforte-Munoz H, Fagin JA. Distinct pattern of ret oncogene rearrangements in morphological variants of radiation-induced and sporadic thyroid papillary carcinomas in children. Cancer Research 1997; 57(9):1690-4.

29. Greco A, Pierotti MA, Bongarzone I, Pagliardini S, Lanzi C, Della Porta G. TRK-T1 is a novel oncogene formed by the fusion of TPR and TRK genes in human papillary thyroid carcinomas. Oncogene 1992; 7(2):237-42.

30. Ponder BA, Smith D. The MEN II syndromes and the role of the ret proto-oncogene. [Review] [194 refs]. Advances in Cancer Research 1996; 70:179-222:179-222.

31. Santoro M, Rosati R, Grieco M, Berlingieri MT, D'Amato GL, de Franciscis V, Fusco A. The ret proto-oncogene is consistently expressed in human pheochromocytomas and thyroid medullary carcinomas. Oncogene 1990; 5(10):1595-8.

32. Santoro M, Carlomagno F, Romano A, Bottaro DP, Dathan NA, Grieco M, Fusco A, Vecchio G, Matoskova B, Kraus MH, et al. Activation of RET as a dominant transforming gene by germline mutations of MEN2A and MEN2B. Science 1995; 267(5196):381-3.

33. Parma J, Duprez L, Van Sande J, Cochaux P, Gervy C, Mockel J, Dumont J, Vassart G. Somatic mutations in the thyrotropin receptor gene cause hyperfunctioning thyroid adenomas. Nature 1993; 365:649-51.

34. Duprez L, Parma J, Van Sande J, Allgeier A, Leclere J, Schvartz C, Delisle M, Decoulx M, Orgiazzi J, Dumont J, et al. Germline mutations in the thyrotropin receptor gene cause non-autoimmune autosomal dominant hyperthyroidism. Nature Genetics 1994; 7:396-401.

35. Parma J, Duprez L, Van Sande J, Hermans J, Rocmans P, Van Vliet G, Costagliola S, Rodien P, Dumont JE, Vassart G. Diversity and prevalence of somatic mutations in the thyrotropin receptor and Gs alpha genes as a cause of toxic thyroid adenomas. Journal of Clinical Endocrinology & Metabolism 1997; 82(8):2695-701.

36. Mazzaferri EL. Management of a solitary thyroid nodule [see comments]. [Review]. New England Journal of Medicine 1993; 328(8):553-9.

37. Matsuo K, Friedman E, Gejman PV, Fagin JA. The thyrotropin receptor (TSH-R) is not an oncogene for thyroid tumors: structural studies of the TSH-R and the alpha-subunit of Gs in human thyroid neoplasms. Journal of Clinical Endocrinology & Metabolism 1993; 76(6):1446-51.

38. Spambalg D, Sharifi N, Elisei R, Gross JL, Medeiros-Neto G, Fagin JA. Structural studies of the thyrotropin receptor and Gs alpha in human thyroid cancers: low prevalence of mutations predicts infrequent involvement in malignant transformation. Journal of Clinical Endocrinology & Metabolism 1996; 81(11):3898-901.

39. Esapa C, Foster S, Johnson S, Jameson JL, Kendall-Taylor P, Harris PE. G protein and thyrotropin receptor mutations in thyroid neoplasia. Journal of Clinical Endocrinology & Metabolism 1997; 82(2):493-6.

40. Russo D, Arturi F, Schlumberger M, Caillou B, Monier R, Filetti S, Suarez HG. Activating mutations of the TSH receptor in differentiated thyroid carcinomas. Oncogene 1996; 11:1907-11.

41. Medema RH, Bos JL. The role of p21ras in receptor tyrosine kinase signaling. [Review] [470 refs]. Critical Reviews in Oncogenesis 1993; 4(6):615-61.

42. Lemoine NR, Mayall ES, Wyllie FS, Williams ED, Goyns M, Stringer B, Wynford-Thomas D. High frequency of ras oncogene activation in all stages of human thyroid tumorigenesis. Oncogene 1989; 4(2):159-64.

43. Namba H, Rubin SA, Fagin JA. Point mutations of ras oncogenes are an early event in thyroid tumorigenesis. Molecular Endocrinology 1990; 4(10):1474-9.

44. Suarez HG, du Villard JA, Severino M, Caillou B, Schlumberger M, Tubiana M, Parmentier C, Monier R. Presence of Mutations in all Three Ras Genes in Human Thyroid Tumors. Oncogene 1990; 5:565-70.

45. Karga H, Lee J-K, Vickery AL, Thor A, Gaz RD, Jameson JL, Suarez HG. Ras Oncogene Mutations in Benign and Malignant Thyroid Neoplasms. J Clin Endocrinol Metab 1991; 73:832-6.

46. Fusco A, Berlingieri MT, Di Fiore PP, Portella G, Grieco M, Vecchio G. One- and Two-Step Transformations of Rat Thyroid Epithelial Cells by Retroviral Oncogenes. Molecular and Cellular Biology 1987; 3365-70.

47. Francis-Lang H, Zannini M, De Felice M, Berlingieri MT, Fusco A, Di Lauro R. Multiple mechanisms of interference between transformation and differentiation in thyroid cells. Mol Cell Biol 1992; 12(12):5793-800.

48. Avvedimento VE, Musti AM, Ueffing M, Obici S, Gallo A, Sanchez M, DeBrasi D, Gottesman ME. Reversible inhibition of a thyroid-specific trans-acting factor by Ras. Genes & Development 1991 5(1):22-8.

49. Gallo A, Benusiglio E, Bonapace IM, Feliciello A, Cassano S, Garbi C, Musti AM, Gottesman ME, Avvedimento EV. v-Ras and protein kinase C dedifferentiate thyroid cells by down-regulating nuclear cAMP-dependent protein kinase A. Genes and Development 1992; 6:1621-30.

50. Lyons J, Landis CA, Harsh G, Vallar L, Grunewald K, Feichtinger H, Duh Q, Clark OH, Kawasaki E, Bourne HR, et al. Two G protein oncogenes in human endocrine tumors. Science 1990; 249:655-9.

51. Landis CA, Masters SB, Spada A, Pace AM, Bourne HR, Vallar L. GTPase inhibiting mutations activate the ? chain of G$_s$ and stimulate adenylyl cyclase in human pituitary tumours. Nature 1989; 340:692-6.

52. O'Sullivan C, Barton CM, Staddon SL, Brown CL, Lemoine NR. Activating point mutations of the gsp oncogene in human thyroid adenomas. Molecular Carcinogenesis 1991; 4(5):345-9.

53. Prevostel C, Alvaro V, Boisvilliers F, Martin A, Jaffol C, Joubert D. The natural protein kinase Cα mutant is present in human thyroid neoplasms. Oncogene 1995; 11:669-74.

54. Alvaro V, Prevostel C, Joubert D, Slosberg E, Weinstein BI. Ectopic expression of a mutant form of PKCalpha originally found in human tumors: aberrant subcellular translocation and effects on growth control. Oncogene 1997; 14(6):677-85.

55. Chen XN, Knauf JA, Gonsky R, Wang M, Lai EH, Chissoe S, Fagin JA, Korenberg JR. From amplification to gene in thyroid cancer: a high resolution mapped BAC resource for cancer chromosome aberrations guides gene discovery after comparative genome hybridization (CGH). Am J Hum Genet 1998; In press.

56. Knauf JA, Elisei R, Mochly-Rosen D, Liron T, Chen XN, Gonsky R, Korenberg JR, Fagin JA. Involvement of a rearrangement of protein kinase C epsilon in thyroid cell tumorigenesis. 1998; manuscript submitted.

57. Belge G, Garcia E, Rippe V, Fusco A, Bartnitzke S, Bullerdiek J. Breakpoints of 19q13 translocations of benign thyroid tumors map within a 400 kilobase region. Genes, Chromosomes & Cancer 1997; 20(2):201-3.

58. Friend SH, Bernards R, Rogelj S, Weinberg RA, Rapaport JM, Albert DM, Dryja TP. A human DNA segment with properties of the gene that predisposes to retinoblastoma and osteosarcoma. Nature 1986; 323(6089):643-6.

59. Chen PL, Scully P, Shew JY, Wang JY, Lee WH. Phosphorylation of the retinoblastoma gene product is modulated during the cell cycle and cellular differentiation. Cell 1989; 58(6):1193-8.

60. Dyson N, Bernards R, Friend SH, Gooding LR, Hassell JA, Major EO, Pipas JM, Vandyke T, Harlow E. Large T antigens of many polyomaviruses are able to form complexes with the retinoblastoma protein. Journal of Virology 1990; 64(3):1353-6.

61. Whyte P, Buchkovich KJ, Horowitz JM, Friend SH, Raybuck M, Weinberg RA, Harlow E. Association between an oncogene and an anti-oncogene: the adenovirus E1A proteins bind to the retinoblastoma gene product. Nature 1988; 334(6178):124-9.
62. Chellappan S, Kraus VB, Kroger B, Munger K, Howley PM, Phelps WC, Nevins JR. Adenovirus E1A, simian virus 40 tumor antigen, and human papillomavirus E7 protein share the capacity to disrupt the interaction between transcription factor E2F and the retinoblastoma gene product. Proceedings of the National Academy of Sciences of the United States of America 1992; 89(10):4549-53.
63. Huang HJ, Yee JK, Shew JY, Chen PL, Bookstein R, Friedmann T, Lee EY, Lee WH. Suppression of the neoplastic phenotype by replacement of the RB gene in human cancer cells. Science 1988; 242(4885):1563-6.
64. Tung WS, Shevlin DW, Bartsch D, Norton JA, Wells SA, Jr., Goodfellow PJ. Infrequent CDKN2 mutation in human differentiated thyroid cancers. Molecular Carcinogenesis 1996; 15(1):5-10.
65. Jones CJ, Shaw JJ, Wyllie FS, Gaillard N, Schlumberger M, Wynford-Thomas D. High frequency deletion of the tumour suppressor gene P16INK4a (MTS1) in human thyroid cancer cell lines. Molecular & Cellular Endocrinology 1996; 116(1):115-9.
66. Calabro V, Strazzullo M, La Mantia G, Fedele M, Paulin C, Fusco A, Lania L. Status and expression of the p16INK4 gene in human thyroid tumors and thyroid-tumor cell lines. International Journal of Cancer 1996; 67(1):29-34.
67. Elisei R, Shiohara M, Koeffler HP, Fagin JA. Genetic and epigenetic alterations of the cyclin-dependent kinase inhibitors p15INK^{4b} and p16^{INK4a} in human thyroid carcinoma cell lines, and in primary thyroid cancers. Cancer 1998; in press.
68. Greenblatt MS, Bennett WP, Hollstein M, Harris CC. Mutations in the p53 tumor suppressor gene: clues to cancer etiology and molecular pathogenesis. [Review] [288 refs]. Cancer Research 1994; 54(18):4855-78.
69. el-Deiry WS, Harper JW, O'Connor PM, Velculescu VE, Canman CE, Jackman J, Pietenpol JA, Burrell M, Hill DE, Wang Y. WAF1/CIP1 is induced in p53-mediated G1 arrest and apoptosis. Cancer Research 1994; 54(5):1169-74.
70. el-Deiry WS, Tokino T, Velculescu VE, Levy DB, Parsons R, Trent JM, Lin D, Mercer WE, Kinzler KW, Vogelstein B. WAF1, a potential mediator of p53 tumor suppression. Cell 1993; 75(4):817-25.
71. Lane DP. Cancer. p53, guardian of the genome [news; comment] [see comments]. Nature 1992; 358(6381):15-6.
72. Donehower L, Donehower LA, Harvey M, Slagle BL, McArthur MJ, Montgomery CA, Butel JS, Bradley A. Mice deficient for p53 are developmentally normal but susceptible to spontaneous tumours. Nature 1992; 356:215-20.
73. Ito T, Seyama T, Mizuno T, Tsuyama N, Hayashi Y, Dohi K, Nakamura N, Akiyama M. Genetic alterations in thyroid tumor progression: association with p53 gene mutations. Japanese Journal of Cancer Research 1993; 84(5):526-31.
74. Ito T, Seyama T, Mizuno T, Tsuyama N, Hayashi T, Hayashi Y, Dohi K, Nakamura N, Akiyama M. Unique Association of p53 Mutations with Undifferentiated but not with Differentiated Carcinomas of the Thyroid Gland. Cancer Res 1992; 52:1369-71.
75. Fagin JA, Matsuo K, Karmakar A, Chen DL, Tang SH, Koeffler HP. High prevalence of mutations of the p53 gene in poorly differentiated human thyroid carcinomas. Journal of Clinical Investigation 1993; 91(1):179-84.
76. Donghi R, Longoni A, Pilotti S, Michieli P, Porta GD, Pierotti MA. Gene p53 Mutations are Restricted to Poorly Differentiated and Undifferentiated Carcinomas of the Thyroid Gland. J Clin Invest 1993; 91:1753-60.
77. Livingstone LR, White A, Sprouse J, Livanos E, Jacks T, Tlsty TD. Altered Cell Cycle Arrest and Gene Amplification Potential Accompany Loss of Wild-Type p53. Cell 1992; 70:923-35.
78. Battista S, Martelli ML, Fedele M, Chiappetta G, Trapasso F, De Vita G, Battaglia C, Santoro M, Viglietto G, Fagin JA, et al. A mutated p53 gene alters thyroid cell differentiation. Oncogene 1995; 11:2029-37.
79. Fagin JA, Tang SH, Zeki K, Di Lauro R, Fusco A, Gonsky R. Reexpression of thyroid peroxidase in a derivative of an undifferentiated thyroid carcinoma cell line by introduction of wild-type p53. Cancer Research 1996; 56(4):765-71.

80. Moretti F, Farsetti A, Soddu S, Misiti S, Crescenzi M, Filetti S, Andreoli M, Sacchi A, Pontecorvi A. p53 re-expression inhibits proliferation and restores differentiation of human thyroid anaplastic carcinoma cells. Oncogene 1997; 14(6):729-40.

81. Califano JA, Johns MM, 3rd, Westra WH, Lango MN, Eisele D, Saji M, Zeiger MA, Udelsman R, Koch WM, Sidransky D. An allelotype of papillary thyroid cancer. International Journal of Cancer 1996; 69(6):442-4.

82. Matsuo K, Tang SH, Fagin JA. Allelotype of human thyroid tumors: loss of chromosome 11q13 sequences in follicular neoplasms. Molecular Endocrinology 1991; 5(12):1873-9.

83. Zedenius J, Wallin G, Svensson A, Grimelius L, Hoog A, Lundell G, Backdahl M, Larsson C. Allelotyping of follicular thyroid tumors. Hum Genet 1995; 96:27-32.

84. Tung WS, Shevlin DW, Kaleem Z, Tribune DJ, Wells SA, Jr., Goodfellow PJ. Allelotype of follicular thyroid carcinomas reveals genetic instability consistent with frequent nondisjunctional chromosomal loss. Genes, Chromosomes & Cancer 1997; 19(1):43-51.

85. Grebe SK, McIver B, Hay ID, Wu PS, Maciel LM, Drabkin HA, Goellner JR, Grant CS, Jenkins RB, Eberhardt NL. Frequent loss of heterozygosity on chromosomes 3p and 17p without VHL or p53 mutations suggests involvement of unidentified tumor suppressor genes in follicular thyroid carcinoma. Journal of Clinical Endocrinology & Metabolism 1997; 82(11):3684-91.

86. Herrmann MA, Hay ID, Bartelt DH, Jr., Ritland SR, Dahl RJ, Grant CS, Jenkins RB. Cytogenetic and molecular genetic studies of follicular and papillary thyroid cancers. Journal of Clinical Investigation 1991; 88(5):1596-604.

87. Ward LS, Brenta G, Medvedovic M, Fagin JA. Studies of allelic loss in thyroid tumors reveal major differences in chromosomal instability between papillary and follicular carcinomas. Journal of Clinical Endocrinology & Metabolism 1998; 83(2):525-30.

88. Eng C. Genetics of Cowden syndrome: through the looking glass of oncology. [Review] [52 refs]. International Journal of Oncology 1998; 12(3):701-10.

89. Liaw D, Marsh DJ, Li J, Dahia PL, Wang SI, Zheng Z, Bose S, Call KM, Tsou HC, Peacocke M, et al. Germline mutations of the PTEN gene in Cowden disease, an inherited breast and thyroid cancer syndrome. Nature Genetics 1997; 16(1):64-7.

90. Marsh DJ, Dahia PL, Coulon V, Zheng Z, Dorion-Bonnet F, Call KM, Little R, Lin AY, Eeles RA, Goldstein AM, et al. Allelic imbalance, including deletion of PTEN/MMACI, at the Cowden disease locus on 10q22-23, in hamartomas from patients with Cowden syndrome and germline PTEN mutation. Genes, Chromosomes & Cancer 1998; 21(1):61-9.

91. Lynch ED, Ostermeyer EA, Lee MK, Arena JF, Ji H, Dann J, Swisshelm K, Suchard D, MacLeod PM, Kvinnsland S, et al. Inherited mutations in PTEN that are associated with breast cancer, cowden disease, and juvenile polyposis. American Journal of Human Genetics 1997; 61(6):1254-60.

92. Marsh DJ, Zheng Z, Zedenius J, Kremer H, Padberg GW, Larsson C, Longy M, Eng C. Differential loss of heterozygosity in the region of the Cowden locus within 10q22-23 in follicular thyroid adenomas and carcinomas. Cancer Research 1997; 7(3):500-3.

93. McDonnell TJ, Korsmeyer SJ. Progression from lymphoid hyperplasia to high-grade malignant lymphoma in mice transgenic for the t(14; 18). Nature 1991; 349(6306):254-6.

94. Hockenbery D, Nunez G, Milliman C, Schreiber RD, Korsmeyer SJ. Bcl-2 is an inner mitochondrial membrane protein that blocks programmed cell death. Nature 1990; 348(6299):334-6.

95. Giordano C, Stassi G, De Maria R, Todaro M, Richiusa P, Papoff G, Ruberti G, Bagnasco M, Testi R, Galluzzo A. Potential involvement of Fas and its ligand in the pathogenesis of Hashimoto's thyroiditis [see comments]. Science 1997; 275(5302):960-3.

96. Bissonnette RP, Echeverri F, Mahboubi A, Green DR. Apoptotic cell death induced by c-myc is inhibited by bcl-2. Nature 1992; 359(6395):552-4.

97. Nicolaides NC, Papadppoulos N, Liu B, Wel YF, Carter KC, Ruben SM, Rosen CA, Haseltine WA, Fleischmann RD, Fraser CM, et al. Mutations of two PMS homologues in hereditary nonpolyposis colon cancer. Nature 1994; 371:75-80.

98. Parsons R, Li GM, Longley M, Modrich P, Liu B, Berk T, Hamilton SR, Kinzler KW, Vogelstein B. Mismatch Repair Deficiency in Phenotypically Normal Human Cells. Science 1995; 268:738-40.

99. Markowitz S, Wang J, Myeroff L, Parsons R, Sun L, Lutterbaugh J, Fan RS, Zborowska E, Kinzler KW, Vogelstein B. Inactivation of the type II TGF-beta receptor in colon cancer cells with microsatellite instability [see comments]. Science 1995; 268(5215):1336-8.

100. Nikiforov YE, Brenta G, Nikiforova MN, Fagin JA. Prevalence of microsatellite and minisatellite instability in thyroid carcinomas from children exposed to radiation after the Chernobyl nuclear accident. Oncogene 1998; In press.
101. Lengauer C, Kinzler KW, Vogelstein B. Genetic instability in colorectal cancers. Nature 1997; 386(6625):623-7.
102. Orr-Weaver TL, Weinberg RA. A checkpoint on the road to cancer [news; comment]. Nature 1998; 392(6673):223-4.
103. Cahill DP, Lengauer C, Yu J, Riggins GJ, Willson JK, Markowitz SD, Kinzler KW, Vogelstein B. Mutations of mitotic checkpoint genes in human cancers [see comments]. Nature 1998; 392(6673):300-3.
104. Plail RO, Bussey HJR, Glazer G, Thomson JPS. Adenomatous Polyposis: An Association with Carcinoma of the Thyroid. Br J Surg 1987; 74:377-80.
105. Iwama T, Mishima Y, Utsunomiya J. The Impact of Familial Adenomatous Polyposis on the Tumorigenesis and Mortality at the Several Organs. Its Rational Treatment. Annals of Surg 1993; 217(2):101-8.
106. Bell B, Mazzaferri EL. Familial Adenomatous Polyposis (Gardner's Syndrome) and Thyroid Carcinoma. Digestive Diseases and Sciences 1993; 38:185-90.
107. Camiel MR, Mule JE, Alexander LL, Benninghoff DL. Association of Thyroid Carcinoma with Gardner's Syndrome in Siblings. N Engl J Med 1968; 278:1056-9.
108. Bell B, Mazzaferri EL. Familiar Adenomatous Polyposis (Gardner's Syndrome) and Thyroid Carcinoma. A Case Report and Review of the Literature. Dig Dis Sci 1993; 38(1):185-90.
109. Harach HR, Williams GT, Williams ED. Familial adenomatous polyposis associated thyroid carcinoma: a distinct type of follicular cell neoplasm. [Review]. Histopathology 1994; 25(6):549-61.
110. Groden J, Thliveris A, Samowitz W, Carlson M, Gelbert L, Albertsen H, Joslyn G, Stevens J, Spirio L, Robertson M, et al. Identification and Characterization of the Familial Adenomatous Polyposis Coli Gene. Cell 1991; 66:589-600.
111. Kinzler KW, Nilbert MC, Su NKL. Identification of FAP locus genes from chromosome 5q21. Science 1991; 253:661-4.
112. MacPhee M, Chepenik KP, Liddell RA, Nelson KK, Siracusa LD, Buchberg AM. The Secretory Phospholipase A2 Gene is a Candidate for the Mom1 Locus, a Major Modifier of APC^{min}-Induced Intestinal Neoplasia. Cell 1995; 81:957-66.
113. Zeki K, Spambalg D, Sharifi N, Gonsky R, Fagin JA. Mutations of the adenomatous polyposis coli gene in sporadic thyroid neoplasms. Journal of Clinical Endocrinology & Metabolism 1994; 79(5):1317-21.
114. Colletta G, Sciacchitano S, Palmirotta R, Ranieri A, Zanella E, Cama A, Costantini RM, Battista P, Pontecorvi A. Analysis of adenomatous polyposis coli gene in thyroid tumours. British Journal of Cancer 1994; 70(6):1085-8.
115. Mallory SB. Cowden Syndrome (Multiple Hamartoma Syndrome). Dermatologic Clinics 1995; 13:27-31.
116. Reed MWR, Harris SC, Quayle AR, Talbot CH. The association between thyroid neoplasia and intestinal polyps. Annals of the Royal College of Surgeons of England 1990; 72:357-9.
117. Ohta S, Katsura T, Shimada M, Shima A, Chishiro H, Matsubara H. Ataxia-Telangiectasia with Papillary Carcinoma of the Thyroid. Am J Ped Hem/Onc 1986; 8:255-68.
118. DeLellis RA. Biology of Disease. Multiple Endocrine Neoplasia Syndromes Revisited. Lab Invest 1995; 72:494-505.
119. Larsson C, Skogseid B, Oberg K, Nakamura Y. Multiple Endocrine Neoplasia Type 1 Gene Maps to Chromosome 11 and is Lost in Insulinoma. Nature 1988; 332:85-7.
120. Chandrasekharappa SC, Guru SC, Manickam P, Olufemi SE, Collins FS, Emmert-Buck MR, Debelenko LV, Zhuang Z, Lubensky IA, Liotta LA, et al. Positional cloning of the gene for multiple endocrine neoplasia-type 1. Science 1997; 276(5311):404-7.
121. Ozaki O, Ito K, Kobayashi K, Suzuki A, Manabe Y, Hosoda Y. Familial Occurrence of Differentiated, Nonmedullary Thyroid Carcinoma. World J Surg 1988; 12:565-71.
122. Nemec J, Soumar J, Zamrazil V, Pohunkova D, Motlik K, Mirejovsky P. Familial Occurrence of Differentiated (Non-Medullary) Thyroid Cancer. Oncology 1975; 32:151-7.
123. Samaan NA. Papillary Carcinoma of the Thyroid: Hereditary or Radiation-Induced? Cancer Invest 1996; 7(4):399-400.
124. Lote K, Andersen K, Nordal E, Brennhovd IO. Familial Occurrence of Papillary Thyroid Carcinoma. Cancer 1980; 46:1291-7.

125. Kwok CG, McDougall IR. Familial Differentiated Carcinoma of the Thyroid: Report of Five Pairs of Siblings. Thyroid 1995; 5:395-7.
126. Hrafnkelsson J, Tulinius H, Jonasson JG, Olafsdottir G, Sigvaldason H. Papillary Thyroid Carcinoma in Iceland. Acta Oncologica 1989; 28:785-8.
127. Stoffer SS, Van Dyke DL, Vaden Bach J, Szpunar W, Weiss L. Familial Papillary Carcinoma of the Thyroid. Am J Med Genet 1986; 25:775-82.
128. Ron E, Kleinerman RA, Boice JD, Jr., LiVolsi VA, Flannery JT, Fraumeni JF, Jr. A Population-Based Case-Control Study of Thyroid Cancer. JNCI 1987; 79:1-12.
129. Ron E, Kleinerman RA, LiVolsi VA, Fraumeni, Jr. Familial Nonmedullary Thyroid Cancer. Oncology 1991; 48:309-11.
130. Ron E, Modan B, Preston D, Alfandary E, Stovall M, Boice JD, Jr. Thyroid Neoplasia Following Low-Dose Radiation in Childhood. Radiation Res 1989; 120:516-31.
131. Shore RE, Woodard E, Hildreth N, Dvoretsky P, Hempelmann L, Pasternack B. Thyroid Tumors Following Thymus Irradiation. JNCI 1985; 74:1177-84.
132. Nikiforov Y, Gnepp DR, Fagin JA. Thyroid lesions in children and adolescents after the Chernboyl disaster:Implications for the study of radiation carcinogenesis. J Clin Endocrinol Metab 1996; 81:9
133. Nikiforov YE, Fagin JA. Mechanisms of radiation-induced carcinogenesis: The thyroid model. In: Advances in Molevular and Cellular Endocrinology. D. LeRoith (Ed). JAI Press. 1998; Vol 2:169-196.
134. Kazakov VS, Demidchik EP, Astakhova LN. Thyroid Cancer after Chernobyl. Nature 1992; 359:21
135. Nikiforov Y, Gnepp DR. Pediatric thyroid cancer after the Chernobyl disaster. Pathomorphologic study of 84 cases (1991-1992) from the Republic of Belarus. Cancer 1994; 74(2):748-66.
136. Klugbauer S, Lengfelder E, Demidchik EP, Rabes HM. High Prevalence of RET Rearrangement in Thyroid Tumors of Chlidren from Belarus After the Chernobyl Reactor Accident. Oncogene 1995; 11:2459-61.
137. Fugazzola L, Pilotti S, Pinchera A. Oncogenic rearrangements of the RET proto-oncogene in papillary thyroid carcinomas from children exposed to the Chernobyl nuclear accident. Cancer Res 1995; 55:5617-20.
138. Eden S, Cedar H. Genomic imprinting. Action at a distance [news; comment]. Nature 1995; 375(6526):16-7.
139. Issa JP, Vertino PM, Wu J, Sazawal S, Celano P, Nelkin BD, Hamilton SR, Baylin SB. Increased cytosine DNA-methyltransferase activity during colon cancer progression. J Natl Cancer Inst 1993; 85(15):1235-40.
140. Baylin SB, Herman JG, Graff JR, Vertino PM, Issa JP. Alterations in DNA methylation: a fundamental aspect of neoplasia. [Review] [248 refs]. Advances in Cancer Research 1998; 72:141-196.
141. Herman JG, Merlo A, Mao L, Lapidus RG, Issa JP, Davidson NE, Sidransky D, Baylin SB. Inactivation of the CDKN2/p16/MTS1 gene is frequently associated with aberrant DNA methylation in all common human cancers. Cancer Research 1995; 55(20):4525-30.
142. Rideout WM, 3d, Coetzee GA, Olumi AF, Jones PA. 5-Methylcytosine as an endogenous mutagen in the human LDL receptor and p53 genes. Science 1990; 249(4974):1288-90.
143. Counts JL, Goodman JI. Alterations in DNA methylation may play a variety of roles in carcinogenesis. [Review] [18 refs]. Cell 1995; 83(1):13-5.
144. Matsuo K, Tang SH, Zeki K, Gutman RA, Fagin JA. Aberrant deoxyribonucleic acid methylation in human thyroid tumors. Journal of Clinical Endocrinology & Metabolism 1993; 77(4):991-5.
145. Viglietto G, Chiappetta G, Martinez-Tello FJ, Fukunaga FH, Tallini G, Rigopoulou D, Visconti R, Mastro A, Santoro M, Fusco A. RET/PTC oncogene activation is an early event in thyroid carcinogenesis. Oncogene 1995; 11(6):1207-10.
146. Mizuno T, Kyoizumi S, Suzuki T, Iwamoto KS, Seyama T. Continued expression of a tissue specific activated oncogene in the early steps of radiation-induced human thyroid carcinogenesis. Oncogene 1997; 15(12):1455-60.
147. Jhiang SM, Sagartz JE, Tong Q, Parker-Thornburg J, Capen CC, Cho J, Xing S, Ledent C. Targeted Expression of the ret/PTC1 Onogene Induces Papillary Thyroid Carcinomas. Endocrinology in Press 1995;

148.   Johnson MR, DeClue JE, Felzmann S, Vass WC, Xu G, White R, Lowy DR. Neurofibromin can inhibit Ras-dependent growth by a mechanism independent of its GTPase-accelerating function. Molecular & Cellular Biology 1994; 14(1):641-5.

149.   Ito T, Seyama T, Iwamoto KS, Hayashi T, Mizuno T, Tsuyama N, Dohi K, Nakamura N, Akiyama M. *In vitro* irradiation is able to cause RET oncogene rearrangement. Cancer Research 1993; 53:2940-3.

150.   Namba H, Gutman RA, Matsuo K, Alvarez A, Fagin JA. H-ras protooncogene mutations in human thyroid neoplasms. Journal of Clinical Endocrinology & Metabolism 1990; 71(1):223-9.

151.   Ruco LP, Ranalli T, Marzullo A, Bianco P, Prat M, Comoglio PM, Baroni CD. Expression of Met protein in thyroid tumours. Journal of Pathology 1996; 180(3):266-70.

152.   Joensuu H, Klemi P, Eerola E. DNA aneuploidy in follicular adenomas of the thyroid gland. American Journal of Pathology 1986; 124(3):373-6.

153.   Joensuu H, Klemi P, Eerola E, Tuominen J. Influence of cellular DNA content on survival in differentiated thyroid cancer. Cancer 1986; 58(11):2462-7.

154.   Wani MA, Xu X, Stambrook PJ. Increased methotrexate resistance and dhfr gene amplification as a consequence of induced Ha-ras expression in NIH 3T3 cells. Cancer Research 1994; 54(9):2504-8.

155.   Denko NC, Giacca AJ, Stringer JR, Stambrook PJ. The human Ha-*ras* oncogene induces genomic instability in murine fibroblasts within one cell cycle. Proc Natl Acad Sci USA 1994; 91:5124-8.

156.   Denko N, Stringer J, Wani M, Stambrook P. Mitotic and Post Mitotic Consequences of Genomic Instability Induced by Oncogenic Ha-*Ras* . Somatic Cell and Molecular Genetics 1995; 21(4):241-53.

157.   Finney RE, Bishop JM. Predisposition to neoplastic transformation caused by gene replacement of H-ras1. Science 1993; 260(5113):1524-7.

4 PATHOGENESIS OF MEDULLARY THYROID CARCINOMA

Robert F. Gagel
Gilbert J. Cote
*University of Texas
M.D. Anderson Cancer Center
Houston, Texas*

Introduction

Medullary thyroid carcinoma (MTC) is a neoplasm derived from the calcitonin producing or C cells of the thyroid gland. The C cell is a neuroendocrine cell that is distributed throughout the thyroid gland in mammalian species with the greatest concentration of cells located centrally at the junction of the upper one-third and lower two-thirds of each lobe. In birds and bony fish the C cells are located in a single discrete gland called the ultimobranchial body. These cells migrate during embryologic life from the neural crest (1,2). The recent discovery of a molecular basis for approximately one-half of all medullary thyroid carcinomas has not only provided insight into the process of transformation, but has also elucidated a potential mechanism for directing migration of neural crest cells to several different anatomic locations.

Mapping of the Causative Gene for Multiple Endocrine Neoplasia Type 2

Multiple endocrine neoplasia type 2 (MEN 2) is a rare hereditary neoplastic syndrome (fewer than 1000 reported kindreds worldwide) characterized by autosomal dominant transmission of MTC, parathyroid neoplasia, and pheochromcytoma. There are several variants. MEN 2A or Sipple syndrome is the association of MTC, parathyroid neoplasia, and pheochromcytoma (3). MEN 2B is the association of MTC and pheochromocytoma with neuromas in the oral mucosa and throughout the gastrointestinal tract. In addition, affected individuals have thickened nerves, and certain features of Marfan's syndrome such as long, thin arms, an altered upper body-lower body ratio, and pectus abnormalities (4-6). Familial medullary thyroid carcinoma (FMTC) is MTC transmitted as an autosomal dominant trait without other manifestations of MEN 2 (7). MEN 2A with Hirschsprung disease (8) or cutaneous lichen amyloidosis over the upper back are rare variants (9,10).

The presence of large and well-defined families with this disorder made it an early target for genetic linkage analysis. In 1987 two groups mapped the causative gene to centromeric chromosome 10 (11, 12). Successive studies refined the locus and in 1993 mutations of the *c-ret* proto-oncogene were identified in MEN 2A (13), FMTC (14), and MEN 2B (15, 16). Studies performed by multiple groups during the 6 years since have confirmed the original observations (17), provided a broader understanding of how these mutations cause neoplastic transformation, and have defined a potential role for the Ret receptor complex in normal embryonic development.

The c-ret *Proto-oncogene*

The *c-ret* proto-oncogene is a 21 exon gene that encodes a tyrosine kinase receptor (18-20). This receptor is characterized by a cadherin-like region in the extracellular domain, a cysteine-rich region immediately external to the membrane, and an intracellular tyrosine kinase domain (Figure 1). Two broad classes of mutations are associated with hereditary medullary thyroid carcinoma .

Mutations of the c-ret Proto-oncogene in Hereditary Medullary Thyroid Carcinoma

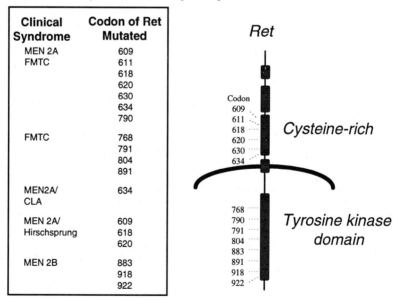

Clinical Syndrome	Codon of Ret Mutated
MEN 2A	609
FMTC	611
	618
	620
	630
	634
	790
FMTC	768
	791
	804
	891
MEN2A/ CLA	634
MEN 2A/ Hirschsprung	609
	618
	620
MEN 2B	883
	918
	922

Figure 1. Mutations of the *c-ret* proto-oncogene associated with hereditary medullary thyroid carcinoma. Abbreviations: MEN 2A, multiple endocrine neoplasia type 2A; FMTC, familial medullary thyroid carcinoma; MEN 2A/CLA, MEN 2A and cutaneous lichen amyloidosis; MEN 2A/Hirschsprung, MEN 2A in association with Hirschsprung disease; and MEN 2B, multiple endocrine neoplasia type 2B.

Extracellular Domain Mutations

The most common are missense mutations affecting the cysteine-rich extracellular domain which convert highly-conserved cysteines to another amino acid. Codon 634, in exon 11, is most commonly mutated, accounting for approximately 75-80% of all mutations in hereditary medullary thyroid carcinoma (17). Three codon changes (arg > tyr > trp) account for more than 90% of mutations at this codon. Mutation of the cysteine at codon 630, also in exon 11, has been reported although it is rare. Mutations at codons 609, 611, 618, 620, all located within exon 10, account for approximately 10-15% of all mutations (21).

A mutation of codon 634 is most commonly associated with classic MEN 2A or Sipple's syndrome. Mutations of codons 609, 611, 618, 620, or 630 have been associated either with FMTC or MEN 2A, although FMTC is more commonly associated with this group of mutations (14). The MEN 2A/Hirschsprung disease variant has been found in kindreds with codon 609, 618, and 620 mutations only (17, 22) (23). The MEN 2A/CLA variant has been found only in individuals with a codon 634 mutation (24, 25) (Table 1).

The extracellular domain mutations cause constitutive activation and dimerization of the Ret receptor. In vitro studies in which mutant (codon 634) or normal c-ret cDNA was expressed in NIH 3T3 cells showed a transforming effect of these mutations (26, 27) and, more importantly, demonstrated dimerization of mutant receptor in the absence of ligand (Figure 2). What these studies did not predict was the identification of the second component of the receptor complex (GFRα-1, Figure 2), discovered approximately 3 years later.

Intracellular Domain Mutations

Intracellular missense mutations comprise the second major class of mutations found in hereditary MTC (Figure 1). The most common is a met918thr mutation, affecting the catalytic region of the tyrosine kinase domain and found as a germline mutation in 95% of patients with MEN 2B (16, 17). This mutation is also found as a somatic mutation in approximately 25% of sporadic MTCs (22). There is evolving evidence that tumors with this mutation are more aggressive and associated with a shorter survival time (28). Expression of a mutant receptor with the met918thr substitution also causes transformation of NIH 3T3 cells, but without dimerization of the receptor (26, 27), leading to the proposal that the point mutation activates the catalytic unit directly. Other rare (fewer than 5 reported cases) intracellular mutations associated with MEN 2B involve codons 883 (29) and 922 (30) (Table 1).

Table 1. Mutations of the RET Proto-oncogene Associated with MEN 2 and
Hereditary Medullary Thyroid Carcinoma

Affected Codon/ Exon	Amino Acid Change Normal›Mutant	Nucleotide Change Normal›Mutant	Clinical Syndrome	% of Total
609/10	cys›arg	TGC›CGC	MEN 2A/	0-1
	cys›gly	TGC›GGC	FMTC	
	cys›tyr	TGC›TAC	MEN 2A &	
			Hirschsprung	
611/10	cys›ser	TGC›AGC	MEN 2A/	2-3
	cys›arg	TGC›CGC	FMTC	
	cys›tyr	TGC›TAC		
	cys›phe	TGC›TTC		
	cys›trp	TGC›TGG		
618/10	cys›ser	TGC›AGC	MEN 2A/	
	cys›arg	TGC›CGC	FMTC	
	cys›gly	TGC›GGC		3-5
	cys›tyr	TGC›TAC	MEN 2A/	
	cys›ser	TGC›TCC	Hirschsprung	
	cys›phe	TGC›TTC		
620/10	cys›ser	TGC›AGC	MEN 2A/	
	cys›arg	TGC›CGC	FMTC	6-8
	cys›gly	TGC›GGC		
	cys›tyr	TGC›TAC	MEN 2A/	
	cys›ser	TGC›TCC	Hirschsprung	
	cys›phc	TGC›TTC		
	cys›trp	TGC›TGG		
630/11	cys›tyr	TGC›TAC	MEN 2A/	0-1
	cys›ser	TGC›TCC	FMTC	
	cys›phe	TGC›TTC		
634/11	cys›ser	TGC›AGC	MEN 2A	
	cys›arg	TGC›CGC		
	cys›gly	TGC›GGC	MEN 2A/	
	cys›tyr	TGC›TAC	CLA	75-85
	cys›ser	TGC›TCC		
	cys›phe	TGC›TTC		
	cys›trp	TGC›TGG		
635/11	thr ser cys ala	ACGAGCTGTGCC	MEN 2A	rare
637/11	cys arg thr	TGCCGCACG	MEN 2A	rare
768/13	glu›asp	GAG›GAC	FMTC	0-1
790/13	leu›phe	TTG›TTC	MEN 2A/	0-1
	leu›phe	TTG›TTT	FMTC	
791/13	tyr›phe	TAT›TTT	FMTC	0-1
804/13	val›met	GTG›ATG	MEN 2A/	0-1
	val›leu	GTG›TTG	FMTC	
883/15	ala›phe	GCT›TTT	MEN 2B	rare
891/15	ser›ala	TCG›GCG	FMTC	rare
918/16	met›thr	ATG›ACG	MEN 2B	3-5
922/16	ser›tyr	TCC›TAC	MEN 2B	rare

Mutations of the intracellular domain associated solely with FMTC include codon 768 (31), 791 (32), 804 (33), and 891 (34). A few kindreds with each of these mutations have been described. Both FMTC and MEN 2A have been identified in kindreds with a codon 790 mutation (32). There has been no independent demonstration of transforming capability for any of the intracellular domain mutations other than codon 918 (26, 27), although genotype-phenotype correlation provides compelling evidence for a causal effect.

The Ret/GFRα Receptor System and Proposed Effects of Mutations on Signaling

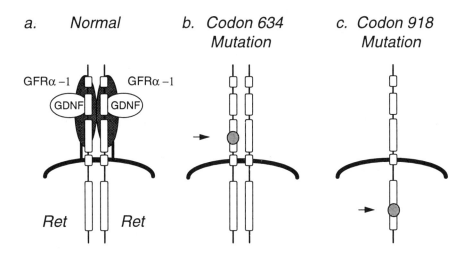

Figure 2. The Ret/GFR signaling system and the effect of Ret mutations on activation and dimerization. Panel (a) shows the interaction of glial cell-derived neurotrophic factor (GDNF) with the receptor complex formed by GFRα-1 and Ret. Interaction of GDNF with this complex causes dimerization, autophosphorylation of the Ret receptor, and activation of several kinase pathways (see Figure 5). Panel (b) depicts the impact of a *c-ret* codon 634 mutation on receptor activation. *In vitro* studies described in the text have shown this mutation to cause dimerization and activation of the receptor, in the absence of either GFRα-1 or GDNF. Panel (c) shows the impact of a codon 918 mutation on receptor activation. There is no evidence of receptor dimerization and no evidence that either GFRα-1 or GDNF is needed for activation. There is compelling evidence that the extracellular domain mutations activate a different set of downstream substrate proteins than is activated in the presence of a codon 918 mutation.

Recognition that Glial Cell-derived Neurotrophic Factor (GDNF) is a Ligand for the RET Receptor

Glial cell-derived neurotrophic factor (GDNF) is a small peptide isolated from brain that functions to promote neuronal survival (35). The interesting biological properties of this peptide led several groups to create mouse knockout models in which a functional copy of the GDNF gene was deleted (36-38). The phenotype observed in these animals was, surprisingly, similar to that observed in mice in which the *c-ret* proto-oncogene had been deleted. The lethal phenotype was characterized by profound defects in the neuronal development of the gastrointestinal tract, analogous to Hirschsprung disease, and defective kidney development (39). There were also abnormalities of the sympathetic nervous system, including underdevelopment of the superior cervical ganglion in both knockout models.

These findings led to experiments that demonstrated GDNF functioned as a ligand for the Ret tyrosine kinase receptor (40-42). In a completely independent line of investigation, a search for a receptor for GDNF led to the identification of a completely different receptor protein (43), a glycophosphatydlinositol-anchored extracellular protein which was initially given the name GDNF receptor-alpha (GDNFR-α) and recently renamed GFRα-1 (44). Additional variants named GFRα-2 and GFRα-3 have been identified (45-48). Ret and GFRα-1 form a receptor complex for GDNF and the peptides neurturin and persephin (48), peptides with similar biologic functions as GDNF (Table 2). GFRα-1 and GFRα-2 can mediate GDNF or neurturin-induced activation of Ret, but GDNF binds more efficiently to GFRα-1, whereas neurturin binds more efficiently to GFRα-2 (49). Studies have further demonstrated that there is a rank order of binding of GDNF to Ret/GFR complexes in which GFRα-1> GFRα-2> GFRα-3. Further specific biologic functions for these 3 GFR variants is suggested by overlapping but distinct patterns of expression for these 3 receptor variants. Table 2 provides an overview of a rapidly growing but incomplete literature on the RET/GFR receptor complex (44).

The GDNF (36-38) and *c-ret* (39, 50) knockout mice provide insight into the role of this receptor signaling system during embyronic development. During early embryologic life, Ret (and by inference GFRα-1) is normally expressed in the developing ureteric bud, whereas GDNF is expressed in the metanephric blastema (Figure 3) (36-38). The interaction between GDNF and the Ret/ GFRα-1 receptor system results in migration and branching of the ureteric bud into the metanephric blastema, thereby creating the highly branched collecting system for the glomeruli, which are derived from the metanephric blastema. In either the *c-ret* or GDNF knockout animals, there is a failure of the ureteric bud to branch into the metanephric blastema leading to a nonfunctional kidney and lethality. In one experimental paradigm in the GDNF knockout animal, a pellet containing GDNF was inserted into the metanephric blastema of a developing embryo, resulting in normal branching of the ureteric bud, providing compelling evidence for the importance of the interaction between GNDF and the Ret/GFRα-1 receptor (37).

Table 2. Expression of GDNF, NT, PSP and the GFR/Ret receptor complexes

Gene	Chromosome Location	Expression	Receptor	Ligand
Glial cell-derived neurotrophic factor (GDNF)	5p13.1-p13.3	brain, thyroid, lung, kidney, GI tract,	GFRα-1 GFRα-2, Ret	
Neurturin (NTN)	19p13.3	brain, PNS, thyroid,heart, lung, GI tract, kidney, liver, Sertoli cells, oviduct	GFRα-1 GFRα-2	
Persephin (PSP)		brain, heart, kidney, liver	Unknown	
GFRα-1	10q26	brain, PNS, thyroid,heart, lung, GI tract, kidney, liver		GDNF >> Neurturin
GFRα-2	8p21-22	brain, PNS, thyroid,heart, lung, GI tract, kidney, liver, gonadal germ cells		Neurturin > GDNF
GFRα-3	5q31.1-q31.3	PNS, thyroid, heart, lung, GI tract, kidney, liver		Unknown
c-ret proto-oncogene	10q11.2	brain, PNS, thyroid, heart, lung, GI tract, kidney, liver		GDNF Neurturin

Abbreviations: GDNF, glial cell-derived neurotrophic factor; NTN, neurturin; GFRα-1 = GDNFR-α; and GFRα2 = TmR-2 = NTNR-α = RETL2 = GDNFR-β.

Ret/GDNF Interactions in the Developing Kidney

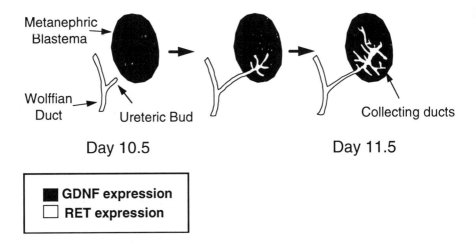

Figure 3. Interaction between Ret and GDNF (glial cell-derived neurotrophic factor) causes normal branching of the ureteric bud. Expression of GDNF in the developing metanephric blastema leads to invasion by the Ret expressing ureteric bud. In the absence of either GDNF or Ret there is a failure of normal branching of the ureteric bud, leading to a nonfunctional kidney and death in the early neonatal period.

A Functional Role for the RET/GFR Receptor in Normal Embyronic Nervous System Development

A similar pattern of expression is likely to explain the normal development of the enteric nervous system. During early embryonic life there is migration of Ret containing cells from the neural crest derived from somites 1-5 into the developing gastrointestinal tract (Figure 4). Although not demonstrated as clearly, there is the belief that GDNF is expressed in the developing GI tract and functions as a trophic factor to promote migration of neural crest cells into the gastrointestinal tract.

The situation in the brain is far more complicated. Although there are overlapping areas of RET and the GFR family receptors, distinct differences in expression occur. For example, there are areas where RET and GDNF or NTRN is found without expression of the GFR family of receptors and other areas where the GFR family of proteins is solely expressed without Ret. There are also differences in the expression of the 3 GFR family members in developing or adult brain, although details are sketchy at this point (46,48,51-53). It is clear that this is a receptor system of incredible complexity and is important in the normal development of the nervous system.

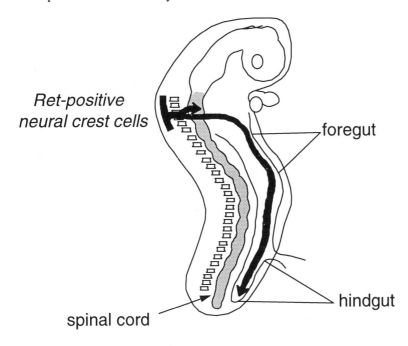

Ret-positive neural crest cells

foregut

hindgut

spinal cord

Figure 4. Migration of Ret positive neural crest cells into the developing gastrointestinal tract. During normal embryonic development there is migration of cells expressing Ret from the neural crest (somites 1-5) into the developing gastrointestinal tract. Mutations of the *c-ret* proto-oncogene cause several abnormalities of neural innervation. Codon 883, 918, and 922 activating mutations (Table 1) cause neuromas in the distribution of Ret expression. Inactivating mutations and a few activating mutations (codons 609, 618, 620, Table 1) cause Hirschsprung disease, a condition characterized by a lack of normal gastrointestinal innervation.

Intracellular Signaling Pathways for the RET/GFR Receptor

Current evidence indicates that at least two different intracellular signaling pathways are coupled to Ret activation. Dimerization of the RET/GFR receptor complex occurs in the presence of either GNDF or an extracellular activating mutation (such as a codon 634 mutation), a process which results in autophosphorylation of the RET receptor and activation of several signaling cascades (Figure 5). The available evidence indicates that MAP (mitogen-activated protein) kinase (ERK 1/2) is activated through a Shc, Grb2, SOS and RAS-mediated pathway. It is thought that Ret tyrosine 1062, which forms the Shc recognition domain, is necessary to activate this pathway (Figure 5) (54).

Activation of the Ret receptor complex by GDNF or by the presence of a codon 634 mutation also activates the JNK (*c-jun* kinase) pathway (Figure 5). Activation of this pathway is abrogated by the presence of an inactivating mutation of RET

(R972G), a mutation which also reverses the transforming effects of either a codon 634 or 918 mutation, whereas mutation of the RET tyrosine 1062, necessary for MAP kinase activation, has no effect on JNK activation. Further studies have demonstrated that Rac1 and Cdc42, Rho-like GTPases, are involved in activation of JNK (55-57). Furthermore, activation of the Ret receptor by a codon 918 mutation, which does not cause receptor dimerization, also activates the JNK pathway (56).

The specific cellular processes activated by these tyrosine kinase pathways have not been fully elucidated, although there is substantial general evidence for linkage to cellular pathways involved in cell growth and death. In addition, evidence has accumulated that activating mutations of *c-ret* may result in altered cellular adhesion leading to enhanced metastatic potential of cells expressing these mutations (56,58). One gap-junction protein, connexin 43, has been shown to be upregulated by mutant Ret (58).

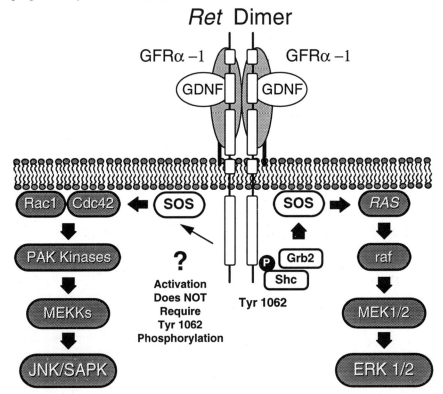

Figure 5. Intracellular signaling pathways activated by the GDNF-GFRα-1/Ret signaling system. Two different intracellular signaling pathways (JNK/SAPK and ERK 1/2) are activated by the GDNF-GFRα-1/Ret receptor complex. Abbreviations for the receptor complex are as outlined in Figure 2. Abbreviations for the JNK/SAPK and ERK 1/2 pathways are described in the text.

Clinical Use of Genetic Information in the Management of Medullary Thyroid Carcinoma

Strategies for Mutation Detection

Two features of this clinical syndrome make it feasible to utilize genetic information for management of patients at risk for hereditary medullary thyroid carcinoma. The first is the finite number of mutations associated with this clinical syndrome. Mutation of a single codon, 634, is responsible for more than 80% of all hereditary medullary thyroid carcinoma and when mutation of 5 other codons (609, 611, 618, 620, and 918) is included a molecular defect for more than 95% of all hereditary MTC can be identified. The second feature is that these codons are found in 3 relatively small exons (exon 10, 11, and 16) (Figure 6). These features make polymerase chain reaction amplification and direct DNA sequencing straightforward and practical.

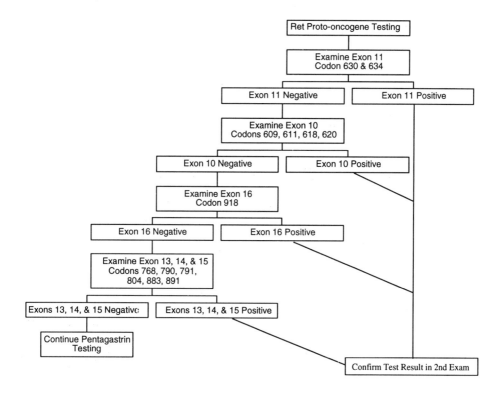

Figure 6. Strategy for mutational analysis in kindreds with proven hereditary medullary thyroid carcinoma. Initial genetic testing should focus on exon 11 where more than 75% of all mutations causing hereditary MTC are found.

These features suggest a strategy for prioritization of mutation detection (59). Mutation detection should focus initially on exon 11 (codon 634) followed in order by exon 10 (609, 611, 618, 620) and then by exon 16 (codon 918). In most cases examination of exon 16 could be eliminated by clinical correlation, but systematic screening of all patients for this mutation may be advisable because of the occasional patient with MEN 2B (Table 1) without the distinctive clinical features associated with MEN 2B. In kindreds with proven transmission of hereditary MTC, analysis of these 6 codons will identify a mutation in most. If no mutation is identified it is important to sequence *c-ret* exons 13, 14, and 15 to identify other rare mutations. In patients with MEN 2B with no identifiable mutation at codon 918, examination of codon 883, 922, and 634 (one case) should be pursued.

Although there are several laboratories in the United States and abroad offering mutational analysis, only a handful analyze for the less common mutations (for a listing of commercial sources of MEN 2 mutational analysis see the web site at: http://endocrine.mdacc.tmc.edu). The clinician utilizing genetic testing information should also be aware of the inaccuracies associated with genetic testing. A variety of causes (technical and sample-mix-up) lead to an error rate of approximately 5% (60). If genetic testing is to be considered the sole basis for a clinical decision, it should be repeated on two independently obtained blood samples and preferably in two different laboratories. Although the cost of two independent analyses may seem prohibitive ($500-750/analysis), an error leading to failure of correct diagnosis is of great concern.

Impact of Genetic Testing Errors

Two different types of errors can be anticipated. The first is assignation of mutant gene carrier status to a normal child leading to unnecessary removal of the thyroid gland. Although this error is of concern because of the necessity for lifelong thyroid hormone replacement and risks for recurrent laryngeal nerve damage and hypoparathyroidism, the actual rate of this type of error is certainly less than has been associated with calcitonin stimulation by pentagastrin, estimated to be at least 10% (60). The second type of error, of greatest concern, is the failure to identify children who carry a mutant gene. If genetic testing is used as the sole screening procedure, failure to identify a gene carrier in childhood will result in presentation as an adult with a palpable MTC and likely metastasis.

Use of Negative Genetic Test Results

A negative *c-ret* analysis in a kindred with a known mutation should be repeated twice on a separately obtained DNA sample and the individual excluded from further analysis. It is important, where possible, to include a family member with a known mutation in the analysis as a positive control.

Use of Positive Genetic Test Results

During the first 2 years after the discovery of *c-ret* mutations in MEN 2 there was hesitance regarding the use of genetic test results as the sole determinant for making a treatment decision, largely related to the uncertain significance of mutations. By the time of the 6th International Workshop on Multiple Endocrine Neoplasia in 1997, there was remarkable consensus regarding the use of this testing. More than 90% of participants agreed that *c-ret* testing should be performed in children by the age of 5 years and that total thyroidectomy should be performed in children with a mutant gene, preferably before the age of 6 years. There are several reasons for choosing this age. The identification of a child with MEN 2A who had metastasis at age 6 and several others with microscopic MTC provides the most compelling reason (61, 62). A second reason is the failure of total thyroidectomy, performed at a mean age of 13 years, to cure 100% of children with this disorder (62). There is evidence of metastasis or persistent calcitonin elevations in approximately 10-15% of individuals from this study an average of 20-25 years following thyroidectomy (60).

Although there is a belief that surgical intervention at an earlier age will improve the cure rate, there is currently no proof and it is likely that another 20-25 years will pass before such evidence becomes available. The evidence favoring a positive effect of earlier thyroidectomy is the improvement in cure rate seen previously when the age of diagnosis and surgical intervention was lowered from a mean of 35 to 13 years. Greater than fifty percent of patients had evidence of metastatic disease at the time of surgery prior to prospective screening (63), whereas detectable metastatic disease is uncommon in patients identified during childhood by pentagastrin testing (62).

A second mechanism for recurrence could be an incomplete thyroidectomy combined with subsequent transformation of residual normal C cells. This argument has been advanced to justify a complete thyroidectomy, including the posterior capsule, in hereditary MTC (64).

There are a few investigators who advocate the continued use of pentagastrin testing in individuals with a positive genetic test and base the timing of surgery on a positive pentagastrin test result (65). The major reason for advocating this approach is the ability to defer surgery until the child is older, facilitating management of hypothyroidism and potential hypoparathyroidism. This management approach may make sense for the handful of families with codon 768, 804, and 891 mutations where the virulence of the MTC appears to be less than that associated with the exon 10 (codon 609, 611, 618, 620) or exon 11 (codon 634) mutations. It seems imprudent to consider this approach in children with exon 10 or 11 *c-ret* mutations for the aforementioned reasons.

It will be important to continue ongoing surveillance of children treated by thyroidectomy at an early age to determine with certainty whether earlier intervention further improves the cure rate.

Acceptance of Genetic Testing by Kindreds with Hereditary Medullary Thyroid Carcinoma

The application of genetic testing in MEN 2 kindreds has provided insight into the use of genetic testing in hereditary malignancy (66-68). In contrast to the controversy associated with the use of genetic testing in breast, ovarian, and colon carcinoma, the implementation of testing in MEN 2 kindreds has proceeded very smoothly. This is likely the result of a 20 year experience with prospective screening and treatment for this disease. Family members have long accepted early thyroidectomy as the treatment of choice for this disease and the current recommendation for earlier thyroidectomy is a direct extension of an accepted logic. In fact, the general experience has been that young children do remarkably well following thyroidectomy, except in those rare cases where hypoparathyroidism has developed. The sense of relief among parents is nearly universal. Unlike the experience with genetic testing for disease in which the test result does not lead to a specific treatment, parents of children at risk for hereditary MTC learn that some of their children are not gene carriers and that they have facilitated definitive treatment for the thyroid carcinoma in those who are.

Future Trends

The rapid development of *in vitro* fertilization and preimplantation screening techniques makes it possible to consider this approach in hereditary MTC. Application of this technique utilizes *in vitro* fertilization of eggs harvested from the mother following hyperovulation (69). A single cell is microdissected from the early embryo at a pluripotential stage (16-32 cell stage) and analyzed for the presence of a *c-ret* mutation by polymerase chain reaction-based techniques. Only embryos with two normal *c-ret* alleles are implanted into the mother's uterus. Although this technique has been applied to a single couple with MEN 2 (author's experience), there is currently no widespread experience. Issues related to its low rate of use include the current low success rate of *in vitro* fertilization, the debate over the ethical and moral issues surrounding use of this technology, and the cost of the *in vitro* fertilization procedure. A compelling societal argument for use of this technology can be made based on cost. Cumulative lifetime costs of caring for a single patient with MEN 2A currently exceed $100,000 in the United States, whereas application of this technology currently costs less than $50,000/ fertilization attempt. The cost of the procedure will be recouped in the first generation with continued economic and family benefits accruing in each succeeding generation. An argument advanced against the use of this technology is that unlike other genetic diseases where there is currently no accepted form of therapy, adequate treatment currently exists for each component of the MEN 2 syndrome, making it unlikely that premature death will occur in patients receiving adequate conventional treatment.

Mutation analysis in sporadic medullary thyroid carcinoma

Mutations of the *c-ret* proto-oncogene contribute to the development of approximately 30-40% of sporadic MTCs. Reports from multiple investigators have identified somatic mutations, most commonly of codon 918 (103/265 = 38%) (21,22) and less commonly of codon 634 (4/131), 618 (1/150), 768 (4/72), or 883 (4/111) (21). In addition, germline mutations of the *c-ret* proto-oncogene are found in approximately 6% of patients with apparent sporadic MTC, most commonly in exon 10; reviewed in (22). In most of these examples, however, there was a greater benefit because other asymptomatic gene carriers were identified and treated. Four *de novo* germline mutations have been identified in individuals with MEN 2-like syndromes but no family history; reviewed in (22). The collective studies have led most investigators in this field to advocate testing for germline mutations of the *c-ret* proto-oncogene in patients with apparent sporadic MTC.

Mutations of the c-ret proto-oncogene in sporadic pheochromocytoma

Mutations of the *c-ret* proto-oncogene have been identified in a handful of sporadic pheochromocytomas (codons 620, 630, 634, and 918) (21). Although no large scale studies have been performed, there is general consensus that this oncogene will play less of a role in pheochromocytoma than in MTC.

Acknowledgements.

The authors would like to acknowledge Donna L. Williams for manuscript preparation.

References

1.   Le Douarin NM, Dupin E. Cell lineage analysis in neural crest ontogeny. J Neurobiol 1993; 24:146-161.
2.   Le Douarin N, Le Lievre C. Demonstration de l'origine neurales des cellules a calcitonine du corps ultimobranchial chez l'embryon de poulet. Compt Rend 1970; 270:2857-2860.
3.   Sipple JH The association of pheochromocytoma with carcinoma of the thyroid gland. Am J Med 1961; 31:163-166.
4.   Carney JA, Go VL, Sizemore GW, Hayles AB. Alimentary-tract ganglioneuromatosis. A major component of the syndrome of multiple endocrine neoplasia, type 2b. N Engl J Med 1976; 295:1287-1291.
5.   Rashid M, Khairi MR, Dexter RN, Burzynski NJ, Johnston CC, Jr. Mucosal neuroma, pheochromocytoma and medullary thyroid carcinoma: multiple endocrine neoplasia type 3. Medicine (Baltimore) 1975; 54:89-112.
6.   Carney JA, Sizemore GW, Hayles AB. Multiple endocrine neoplasia, type 2b. Pathobiol Annu 1978; 8:105-153.
7.   Farndon JR, Leight GS, Dilley WG, Baylin SB, Smallridge RC, Harrison TS, Wells SA, Jr. Familial medullary thyroid carcinoma without associated endocrinopathies: a distinct clinical entity. Br J Surg 1986; 73:278-281.
8.   Verdy M, Lacroix A, Sturtridge W, Kuchel O, Cadotte M, Schurch W, Cantin J, Cholette JP, Bolte E. Type II multiple endocrine neoplasia (Sipple syndrome): study of a family. Union Med Can 1985; 114:49-59.
9.   Gagel RF, Levy ML, Donovan DT, Alford BR, Wheeler T, Tschen JA. Multiple endocrine

neoplasia type 2a associated with cutaneous lichen amyloidosis. Ann Intern Med 1989; 111:802-806.

10. Nunziata V, Giannattasio R, di Giovanni G, D'Armiento MR, Mancini M. Hereditary localized pruritus in affected members of a kindred with multiple endocrine neoplasia type 2A (Sipple's syndrome). Clin Endocrinol 1989; 30:57-63.

11. Simpson NE, Kidd KK, Goodfellow PJ, McDermid H, Myers S, Kidd JR, Jackson CE, Duncan AM, Farrer LA, Brasch K. Assignment of multiple endocrine neoplasia type 2A to chromosome 10 by linkage. Nature 1987; 328:528-530.

12. Mathew CG, Chin KS, Easton DF, Thorpe K, Carter C, Liou GI, Fong SL, Bridges CD, Haak H, Kruseman AC, Schifter S, Hansen HH, Telenius H, Telenius-Berg M, Ponder BAJ. A linked genetic marker for multiple endocrine neoplasia type 2A on chromosome 10. Nature 1987; 328:527-528.

13. Mulligan LM, Kwok JB, Healey CS, Elsdon MJ, Eng C, Gardner E, Love DR, Mole SE, Moore JK, Papi L, et al. Germ-line mutations of the RET proto-oncogene in multiple endocrine neoplasia type 2A. Nature 1993; 363:458-460.

14. Donis-Keller H, Dou S, Chi D, Carlson KM, Toshima K, Lairmore TC, Howe JR, Moley JF, Goodfellow P, Wells SA, Jr. Mutations in the RET proto-oncogene are associated with MEN 2A and FMTC. Hum Mol Genet 1993; 2:851-856.

15. Carlson KM, Dou S, Chi D, Scavarda N, Toshima K, Jackson CE, Wells SA, Jr., Goodfellow PJ, Donis-Keller H. Single missense mutation in the tyrosine kinase catalytic domain of the RET protooncogene is associated with multiple endocrine neoplasia type 2B. Proc Natl Acad Sci USA 1994; 91:1579-1583.

16. Hofstra RM, Landsvater RM, Ceccherini I, Stulp RP, Stelwagen T, Luo Y, Pasini B, Hoppener JW, van Amstel HK, Romeo G, Ponder BAJ. A mutation in the RET proto-oncogene associated with multiple endocrine neoplasia type 2B and sporadic medullary thyroid carcinoma. Nature 1994; 367:375-376.

17. Eng C, et al. The relationship between specific RET proto-oncogene mutations and disease phenotype in multiple endocrine neoplasia type 2. International RET mutation consortium analysis. JAMA 1996; 276:1575-1579.

18. Takahashi M, Ritz J, Cooper GM. Activation of a novel human transforming gene, ret, by DNA rearrangement. Cell 1985; 42:581-588.

19. Takahashi M, Buma Y, Iwamoto T, Inaguma Y, Ikeda H, Hiai H. Cloning and expression of the ret proto-oncogene encoding a tyrosine kinase with two potential transmembrane domains. Oncogene 1988; 3:571-578.

20. Takahashi M. Structure and expression of the ret transforming gene. Iarc Sci Publ 1988; 92:189-197.

21. Eng C, Mulligan LM. Mutations of the RET proto-oncogene in the multiple endocrine neoplasia type 2 syndromes, related sporadic tumours, and hirschsprung disease. Human Mutation 1997; 9:97-109.

22. Wohllk N, Cote GJ, Bugalho MMJ, Ordonez N, Evans DB, Goepfert H, Khorana S, Schultz PS, Richards CS, Gagel RF. Relevance of RET Proto-Oncogene Mutations in Sporadic Medullary Thyroid Carcinoma. J Clin Endocrinol Metab 1996; 81:3740-3745.

23. Decker RA, Peacock ML. Occurrence of MEN 2a in familial Hirschsprung's disease: a new indication for genetic testing of the RET proto-oncogene. Journal of Pediatric Surgery 1998; 33:207-214.

24. Ceccherini I, Romei C, Barone V, Pacini F, Martino E, Loviselli A, Pinchera A, Romeo G. Identification of the cys 634-to-tyr mutation of the RET proto-oncogene in a pedigree with mutliple endocrine neoplasia type 2A and localized cutaneous lichen amyloidosis. J Endocr Invest 1994; 17:201-204.

25. Hofstra RM, Sijmons RH, Stelwagen T, Stulp RP, Kousseff BG, Lips CJ, Steijlen PM, Van Voorst Vader PC, Buys CH. RET mutation screening in familial cutaneous lichen amyloidosis and in skin amyloidosis associated with multiple endocrine neoplasia. Journal of Investigative Dermatology 1996; 107:215-218.

26. Asai N, Iwashita T, Matsuyama M, Takahashi M. Mechansims of activation of the ret proto-oncogene by multiple endocrine neoplasia 2A mutations. Molec Cell Biol 1995; 15:1613-1619.

27. Santoro M, Carlomagno F, Romano A, Bottaro DP, Dathan NA, Grieco M, Fusco A, Vecchio G,

Matoskova B, Kraus MH, Di Fiiore PP. Activation of RET as a dominant transforming gene by germline mutations of MEN 2A and MEN 2B. Science 1995; 267:381-383.

28. Zedenius J, Larsson C, Bergholm U, Bovee J, Svensson A, Hallengren B, Grimelius L, Backdahl M, Weber G, Wallin G. Mutations of codon 918 in the RET proto-oncogene correlate to poor prognosis in sporadic medullary thyroid carcinomas. J Clin Endocrinol Metab 1995; 80:3088-3090.

29. Gimm O, Marsh DJ, Andrew SD, Frilling A, Dahia PL, Mulligan LM, Zajac JD, Robinson BG, Eng C. Germline dinucleotide mutation in codon 883 of the RET proto-oncogene in multiple endocrine neoplasia type 2B without codon 918 mutation. Journal of Clinical Endocrinology & Metabolism 1997; 82:3902-3904.

30. Kitamura Y, Goodfellow PJ, Shimizu K, Nagahama M, Ito K, Kitagawa W, Akasu H, Takami H, Tanaka S, Wells SA, Jr. Novel germline RET proto-oncogene mutations associated with medullary thyroid carcinoma (MTC): mutation analysis in Japanese patients with MTC. Oncogene 1997; 14:3103-3106.

31. Eng C, Smith DP, Mulligan LM, Healey CS, Zvelebil MJ, Stonehouse TJ, Ponder MA, Jackson CE, Waterfield MD, Ponder BA. A novel point mutation in the tyrosine kinase domain of the RET proto-oncogene in sporadic medullary thyroid carcinoma and in a family with FMTC. Oncogene 1995; 10:509-513.

32. Berndt I, Reuter M, Saller B, Frankraue K, Groth P, Grussendorf M, Raue F, Ritter M, Hoppner W. A new hot spot for mutations in the ret protooncogene causing familial medullary thyroid carcinoma and multiple endocrine neoplasia type 2A. J Clin Endocrinol Metab 1998; 83:770-774.

33. Bolino A, Schuffenecker I, Luo Y, Seri M, Silengo M, Tocco T, Chabrier G, Houdent C, Murat A, Schlumberger M, Tourniaire J, Lenoir GM, Romeo G. RET mutations in exons 13 and 14 of FMTC patients. Oncogene 1995; 10:2415-2419.

34. Hofstra RM, Fattoruso O, Quadro L, Wu Y, Libroia A, Verga U, Colantuoni V, Buys CH. A novel point mutation in the intracellular domain of the ret protooncogene in a family with medullary thyroid carcinoma. Journal of Clinical Endocrinology & Metabolism 1997; 82:4176-4178.

35. Lin LF, Doherty DH, Lile JD, Bektesh S, Colline F. GDNF: a glial cell line-derived neurotrophic factor for midbrain dopaminergic neurons. Science 1993; 260:1130-1132.

36. Sanchez M, Silos-Santiago I, Frisen J, He B, Lira S, Barbacid M. Newborn mice lacking GDNF display renal agenesis and absence of enteric neurons, but no deficits in midbrain dopaminergic neurons. Nature 1996; 382:70-73.

37. Pichel JG, Shen L, Sheng HZ, Granholm A-C, Drago J, Grinberg A, Lee EJ, Huang SP, Saarma M, Hoffer BJ, Sariola H, Westphal H. Defects in enteric innervation and kidney development in mice lacking GDNF. Nature 1996; 382:73-76.

38. Moore MW, Klein RD, Farinas I, Sauer H, Armanini M, Phillips H, Reichardt LF, Ryan AM, Carver-Moore K, Rosenthal A. Renal and neuronal abnormalities in mice lacking GDNF. Nature 1996; 382:76-79.

39. Schuchardt A, D'Agati V, Larsson-Blomberg L, Costantini F, Pachnis V. Defects in the kidney and enteric nervous system of mice lacking the tyrosine kinase receptor Ret. Nature 1994; 367:380-383.

40. Trupp M, Arenas E, Falnzilber M, Nilsson AS, Sieber BA, Grigoriou M, Kilkenny C, Salazar-Grueso E, Pachnis V, Arumae U, Sarlola H, Saarma M, Ibanez CF. Functional receptor for GDNF encoded by the c-ret proto-oncogene. Nature 1996; 381:785-788.

41. Durbec P, Marcos-Gutierrez CV, Kilkenny C, Suvanto P, Smith D, Ponder B, Costantini F, Saarma M, Sarlola H, Pachnis V. GDNF signalling through the ret receptor tyrosine kinase. Nature 1996; 381:789-793.

42. Treanor JJS, et al. Characterization of a multicomponent receptor for GDNF. Nature 1996; 382:80-83.

43. Jing S, Wen D, Yu Y, Holst PL, Luo Y, Fang M, Tamir R, Antonio L, Hu Z, Cupples R, Louis JC, Hu S, Altrock BW, Fox GM. GDNF-induced activation of the Ret protein tyrosine kinase is mediated by GDNFR-a, a novel receptor for GDNF. Cell 1996; 85:1113-1124.

44. GFRα Nomenclature Committee. Nomenclature of GPI-linked receptors for the GDNF ligand family. Neuron 1997; 19:485.

45. Trupp M, Raynoschek C, Belluardo N, Ibanez C. Multiple GPI-anchored receptors control GDNF-dependent and independent activation of the c-ret receptor tyrosine kinase. Mol Cell Neurosci 1998;11:47-63.

46. Baloh R, Gorodinsky A, Golden J, Tansey M, Keck C, Popescu N, Johnson E, Milbrandt J.

GFR-alpha-3 is an orphan member of the GDNF/neurturin/persephin rececptor family. Proc Natl Acad Sci USA 1998; 95:5801-5806.

47.   Baloh RH, Tansey MG, Golden JP, Creedon DJ, Heuckeroth RO, Keck CL, Zimonjic DB, Popescu NC, Johnson EM, Jr., Milbrandt J. TrnR2, a novel receptor that mediates neurturin and GDNF signaling through Ret. Neuron 1997; 18:793-802.

48.   Milbrandt J, et al. Persephin, a novel neurotrophic factor related to GDNF and neurturin. Neuron 1998; 20:245-253.

49.   Jing S, Yu Y, Fang M, Hu Z, Holst PL, Boone T, Delaney J, Schultz H, Zhou R, Fox GM. GFRalpha-2 and GFRalpha-3 are two new receptors for ligands of the GDNF family. Journal of Biological Chemistry 1997; 272:33111-33117.

50.   Schuchardt A, D'Agati V, Larsson-Blombert L, Costantini F, Pachnis V. RET-deficient mice: an animal model for Hirschsprung's disease and renal agenesis. J Int Med 1995; 238:327-332.

51.   Naveilhan P, Baudet C, Mikaels A, Shen L, Westphal H, Ernfors P. Expression and regulation of GFRalpha3, a glial cell line-derived neurotrophic factor family receptor. Proceedings of the National Academy of Sciences of the United States of America 1998; 95:1295-1300.

52.   Nomoto S, Ito S, Yang LX, Kiuchi K. Molecular cloning and expression analysis of GFR alpha-3, a novel cDNA related to GDNFR alpha and NTNR alpha. Biochem Biophys Res Commun 1998; 244:849-853.

53.   Yu T, Scully S, Yu Y, Fox G, Jing S, Zhou R. Expression of GDNF family receptor components during development: implications in the mechanisms of interactions. J Neurosci 1998; 18:4684-4696.

54.   Ohiwa M, Murakami H, Iwashita T, Asai N, Iwata Y, Imai T, Funahashi H, Takagi H, Takahashi M. Characterization of Ret-Shc-Grb2 complex induced by GDNF, MEN 2A, and MEN 2B mutations. Biochem Biophys Res Commun 1997; 237:747-751.

55.   Xing S, Furminger TL, Tong Q, Jhiang SM. Signal transduction pathways activated by RET oncoproteins in PC12 pheochromocytoma cells. Journal of Biological Chemistry 1998; 273:4909-4914.

56.   Marshall GM, Peaston AE, Hocker JE, Smith SA, Hansford LM, Tobias V, Norris MD, Haber M, Smith DP, Lorenzo MJ, Ponder BA, Hancock JF. Expression of multiple endocrine neoplasia 2B RET in neuroblastoma cells alters cell adhesion in vitro, enhances metastatic behavior in vivo, and activates Jun kinase. Cancer Research 1997; 57:5399-5405.

57.   Chiariello M, Visconti R, Carlomagno F, Melillo R, Bucci C, Defranciscis V, Fox G, Jing S, Coso O, Gutkind J, Fusco A, Santoro M. Signalling of RET receptor tyrosine kinase through the C-Jun NH2-terminal protein kinases (JNKS) - evidence for a divergence of the erks and jnks pathways induced by RET. Oncogene 1998 ; 16:2435-2445.

58.   Xing S, Smanik PA, Oglesbee MJ, Trosko JE, Mazzaferri EL, Jhiang SM. Characterization of ret oncogenic activation in MEN2 inherited cancer syndromes. Endocrinology 1996; 137:1512-1519.

59.   Decker RA, Peacock ML, Borst MJ, Sweet JD, Thompson NW. Progress in genetic screening of multiple endocrine neoplasia type 2A: Is calcitonin testing obsolete? Surgery 1995; 118:257-264.

60.   Gagel RF, Cote GJ, Martins Bugalho MJG, Boyd AE, Cummings T, Goepfert H, Evans DB, Cangir A, Khorana S, Schultz PN. Clinical use of molecular information in the management of multiple endocrine neoplasia type 2A. J Int Med 1995; 238:333-341.

61.   Graham SM, Genel M, Touloukian RJ, Barwick KW, Gertner JM, Torony C. Provocative testing for occult medullary carcinoma of the thyroid: findings in seven children with multiple endocrine neoplasia type IIa. J Pediatr Surg 1987; 22:501-503.

62.   Gagel RF, Tashjian AH, Jr., Cummings T, Papathanasopoulos N, Kaplan MM, DeLellis RA, Wolfe HJ, Reichlin S. The clinical outcome of prospective screening for multiple endocrine neoplasia type 2a: An 18-year experience. N Engl J Med 1988 ; 318:478-484.

63.   Melvin KEW, Tashjian AH, Jr., Miller HH. Studies in familial (medullary) thyroid carcinoma. Recent Prog Horm Res 1972; 28:399-470.

64.   Wells SA, Chi DD, Toshima K, Dehner LP, Coffin CM, Dowton B, Ivanovich JL, DeBenedetti MK, Dilley WG, Moley JF, Norton JA, Donis-Keller H. Predictive DNA testing and prophylactic thyroidectomy in patients at risk for multiple endocrine neoplasia type 2A. Ann Surg 1994 ; 220:237-250.

65.   Utiger RD. Medullary thyroid carcinoma, genes, and the prevention of cancer [editorial;

comment]. N Engl J Med 1994; 331:870-871.

66. Lips CJ, Landsvater RM, Hoppener JW, Geerdink RA, Blijham G, van Veen JM, van Gils AP, de Wit MJ, Zewald RA, Berends MJ, et al. Clinical screening as compared with DNA analysis in families with multiple endocrine neoplasia type 2A. N Engl J Med 1994; 331:828-835.

67. Frank-Raue K, Hoppner W, Buhr H, Herfarth C, Ziegler R, Raue F. Application of genetic screening in families with hereditary medullary thyroid carcinoma. Experimental & Clinical Endocrinology & Diabetes 1996; 104:108-110.

68. Chi DD, Toshima K, Donis-Keller H, Wells SA, Jr. Predictive testing for multiple endocrine neoplasia type 2A (MEN 2A) based on the detection of mutations in the RET protooncogene. Surgery 1994 ; 116:124-132; discussion 132-133.

69. Handyside AH, Lesko JG, J.J. T, Winston RM, Hughes MR. Birth of a normal girl after in vitro fertilization and preimplantation diagnostic testing for cystic fibrosis. 1992; N Engl J Med 32:905-909.

5 PATHOLOGIC FEATURES OF THYROID TUMORS

Paul Biddinger, MD
Yuri E. Nikiforov, MD, PhD
University of Cincinnati
Cincinnati, Ohio

Introduction

Thyroid tumors include those arising from follicular epithelium, C cells, mesenchymal elements and lymphoid cells. The majority of thyroid neoplasms derive from follicular cells. The classification and understanding of thyroid neoplasms has evolved during the last century from a relatively simple model (1) to one more complex and clinically helpful. The most widely used and accepted classifications are those issued by the World Health Organization (WHO) and the Armed Forces Institute of Pathology (AFIP). The Armed Forces Institute of Pathology issued the series one fascicle of thyroid tumors in 1953 (2) and the WHO published its first histologic classification of thyroid tumors in 1974 (3). Since then, the second edition of the WHO publication appeared in 1988 (4) and the third series of the AFIP fascicle series in 1992 (5).

The two classifications are similar but some discrepancies exist. The prime example is the separate category of poorly differentiated carcinoma used in the AFIP classification. In our opinion, the separation of poorly differentiated carcinoma from well differentiated and anaplastic (undifferentiated) carcinomas represents a significant evolutionary event in the classification of thyroid tumors. The AFIP classification also separates oncocytic (Hürthle cell) neoplasms from conventional follicular neoplasms. Whether oncocytic neoplasms should be classified separately or simply as variants of follicular neoplasms is controversial. We have elected to follow the AFIP format and consider oncocytic neoplasms distinct clinicopathologic entities.

Much of this chapter will address variants of conventional forms of thyroid neoplasms. The attention given to some of these variants is arguably excessive given their rarity. However, some of these variants behave significantly different than their conventional counterparts, and their definition has constituted some of the more recent developments in thyroid pathology.

Table 1. Classification of Thyroid Tumors

Primary Tumors

Epithelial Tumors

Tumors of Follicular Cells

- Papillary Carcinoma
- Follicular Neoplasms
    - Follicular Adenoma
    - Follicular Carcinoma
- Oncocytic Neoplasms
    - Oncocytic Adenoma
    - Oncocytic Carcinoma
- Poorly Differentiated Carcinoma
- Anaplastic (Undifferentiated) Carcinoma

Tumors of C (parafollicular) cells

- Medullary Carcinoma

Malignant Lymphoma

Rare Primary Tumors

Secondary Tumors

Tumor-like Lesions

Papillary Carcinoma

Papillary carcinoma is defined as a malignant epithelial tumor showing evidence of follicular cell differentiation, typically with papillary and follicular structures as well as characteristic nuclear features (4). It is the most common form of thyroid malignancy, comprising approximately 80% of the cases (6). Current relative percentages tend to be higher than in the past. This may in part reflect more frequent recognition of certain tumors with follicular architecture as variants of papillary carcinoma. The vast majority of tumors classified as papillary carcinoma are well differentiated and have an excellent prognosis.

Papillary carcinomas are usually solid, whitish with shades of gray or tan, and have ill defined, infiltrative margins. They range in size from microscopic to large with extrathyroidal extension. The cut surface may show granularity that reflects papillary formation. Less common gross features include encapsulation, diffuse involvement of the gland, calcification or cyst formation.

Microscopically, the tumors exhibit papillary and/or follicular architecture (Figure 1). Papillary growth is characterized by fibrovascular cores covered by a single layer of neoplastic cells. The cells are cuboidal to columnar and papillae can be straight or branched. Most have a mixture of papillary and follicular growth patterns. It is inappropriate to use the term mixed papillary-follicular carcinoma if the follicular component has typical nuclear features of papillary carcinoma.

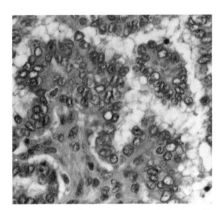 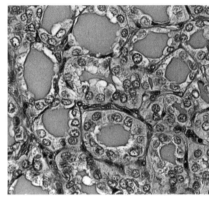

Figure 1. Papillary carcinomas. Typical papillary architecture illustrated in left photomicrograph ; follicular variant in right.

Papillary carcinomas have nuclear features which help distinguish this neoplasm from other neoplasms and tumor-like conditions. The nuclei are enlarged. They outmeasure normal follicular cells and those found in nodular hyperplasia and follicular neoplasms. They also tend to appear crowded and overlapping. The nuclei are hypochromatic, unlike most malignant neoplasms in which the nuclei appear hyperchromatic. These hypochromatic nuclei have finely dispersed chromatin ("ground glass appearance") or appear optically clear ("Orphan Annie eye nuclei). The nuclei may contain rounded, relatively clear areas known as pseudoinclusions. These are due to cytoplasmic invagination into a cup-shaped nucleus. The nuclei also tend to have irregular nuclear outlines. Due to these irregularities and infolding of the membrane, nuclei sometimes exhibit linear streaks, or grooves, along the long axis. These grooves give the nuclei an appearance comparable to coffee beans. Nucleoli may or may not be identifiable. If present, they are often peripherally located, abutting the nuclear membrane.

Psammoma bodies are found in about 50% of cases (5,6). They represent a form of dystrophic calcification arising from damaged papillae. Thrombosis or damage of the blood vessels of the fibrovascular cores is considered to be the initiating event (6,7). These calcified foci have a distinctive laminated appearance and are extrafollicular. True psammoma bodies are almost pathognomonic for papillary carcinoma. Their sole presence in a gland or lymph node usually means that papillary carcinoma is elsewhere. Psammoma bodies have been described rarely in other conditions including Graves' disease (8), Hashimoto's thyroiditis (9), and medullary carcinoma (5). Psammoma-like bodies can be seen in other thyroid lesions. While laminated, basophilic and sometimes calcified, they are distinguished from true psammoma bodies by their intrafollicular location. Oncocytic tumors are particularly prone to contain psammoma-like bodies.

Fibrosis is common and usually seen at the periphery of the neoplasm. Lymphocytic infiltration is present in about one third of cases and tends to be most pronounced at the periphery. Explanations for this finding include immune response to tumor or preexisting autoimmune thyroiditis. Mitoses are rarely found. If readily identifiable, they raise suspicion that a more aggressive, less differentiated neoplasm is evolving (10). Multicentricity is observed in about 20% of cases (11), Higher percentages are reported with more thorough examination. Multicentricity may reflect intrathyroidal lymphatic spread or multiple primary sites.

Approximately 25% of cases exhibit focal areas with solid growth pattern (12). These foci seem to have little clinical significance and should not be interpreted as emergence of a poorly differentiated carcinoma as long as the nuclei have typical features of papillary carcinoma (5). Focal squamous differentiation is relatively common, observed in 15-45% of cases (5,6). Overt keratinization may or may not be seen.

Immunostaining for thyroglobulin reveals cytoplasmic positivity, but the staining is usually weak and less intense than that exhibited by follicular neoplasms. Papillary carcinomas exhibit positivity for cytokeratin. They usually express low molecular weight cytokeratins. Some investigators have found that papillary carcinomas also stain for high molecular weight cytokeratins whereas follicular neoplasms and normal follicular epithelium are typically positive only for low molecular weight cytokeratins (13,14). The use of high and low molecular cytokeratins as diagnostic discriminators, however, has not proven to be reliable (6). Immunoreactivity with antibodies for CD44 cell adhesion protein, and especially its v6 variant, has been reported in most papillary carcinomas as opposed to nearly all follicular carcinomas and non-neoplastic thyroid cells which were negative (15,16).

The differential diagnosis includes a wide variety of thyroid lesions with papillary-like structures. Papillary-like infolding of follicular epithelium is seen in nodular hyperplasia, diffuse toxic hyperplasia (Graves' disease) and follicular neoplasms. The absence of typical nuclear features is the most important feature distinguishing them from papillary carcinoma.

Papillary carcinoma spreads via lymphatics, hematogenously and by direct extension. Intraglandular spread via lymphatic channels is one explanation for multicentricity. Cervical lymph node metastasis is relatively common, and affected nodes frequently undergo cystic transformation. Hematogenous spread occurs in 4-14% of cases with lung being the most frequent site (5). Other relatively common sites of metastasis include bone, liver and brain. Extension into the soft tissues of the neck is seen in 10-34% of cases (5), with a smaller number of cases involving the larynx, trachea, esophagus or skin.

Papillary carcinoma is seen more commonly in glands with chronic lymphocytic thyroiditis or Hashimoto's thyroiditis (17). Whether there is a causal relationship is unresolved. It may be that thyroiditis simply increases the odds that this generally indolent neoplasm is found.

The prognosis is generally excellent with 10 year mortality of 5% or less (11,18, 20). Adverse prognostic indicators are older age (>40 years for men, >50 years for women), male sex, size greater than 5 cm and extrathyroidal extension (11,18,19,21,22). Most investigators have not found multicentricity to be a significant prognostic factor (18,21,22). However, one study of 241 cases found multicentricity was associated with an increased incidence of metastasis and decreased disease free survival time, but had minimal impact on death rate (11). Certain histological variants including tall cell, columnar cell and diffuse sclerosing have been associated with a worse prognosis as will be discussed below.

Variants

Follicular variant of papillary carcinoma. Appreciation for this variant arose from clinicopathologic studies which found that follicular tumors with nuclear features of papillary carcinoma behaved like papillary carcinomas, particularly in their predilection for having cervical lymph node metastasis (23,25). This variant of papillary carcinoma exhibits follicular architecture exclusively, or almost exclusively. The allowable percentage of papillary architecture has not been set specifically, but typical papillae should be rare and hard to find.

A capsule is usually absent or incomplete. Those that are encapsulated or well circumscribed can be especially difficult to distinguish from a true follicular neoplasm (see below under encapsulated variant). Recognition of diagnostic nuclear features is the key to diagnosis. This is sometimes easier said than done, as the nuclear features can be focal. The threshold for accepting nuclear changes as diagnostic seems to vary among pathologists, and the opinion of an expert may be necessary to resolve differences of opinion. The prognosis of this variant is similar to conventional papillary carcinoma.

Papillary microcarcinoma. Papillary microcarcinoma is defined as papillary carcinoma measuring one centimeter or less in diameter (4). Microcarcinomas have an irregular, scar-like appearance and usually exhibit a follicular or solid growth pattern. They are often an incidental finding and most cases previously termed occult sclerosing papillary carcinoma fall under this subcategory. The prognosis is excellent and distant metastasis are extremely rare.

Encapsulated variant of papillary carcinoma. The histologic criteria for this variant are a well defined capsule surrounding the entire tumor and typical nuclear features of papillary carcinoma (4,5). Capsular invasion may or may not be present. The growth pattern can be papillary or follicular. Some subdivide the encapsulated variants according to the growth pattern. This variant accounts for about 10% of cases of papillary carcinoma (11,26,27), particularly if encapsulated follicular variants of papillary carcinoma are included. Encapsulated variants with papillary architecture alone are rare. In the past, these tumors were sometimes called papillary adenoma. However, no reliable criteria were identifiable that differentiated cases with metastasis from those without, and this term is not recommended.

The prognosis for these neoplasm is excellent with survival almost 100%, even though regional lymph node metastasis is present in 25% or more of the cases (27,28). Capsular invasion does not alter prognosis either. The differential includes follicular adenoma and follicular carcinoma. Some encapsulated lesions with follicular growth pattern, invasion, and nuclear features suggestive of papillary carcinoma can be difficult to distinguish between minimally invasive follicular carcinoma and encapsulated variant of papillary carcinoma. In light of this difficulty and interobserver variation among pathologists, Rosai and colleagues have suggested the use of the term "well differentiated carcinoma, not otherwise specified" (5). In the absence of capsular or vascular invasion, distinguishing encapsulated variant of papillary carcinoma from follicular adenoma can pose a similar problem. In this case, the pathologist must decide between malignant and benign diagnoses. Some cases may indeed represent a follicular variant of papillary carcinoma arising in a follicular adenoma. Fortunately, the excellent prognosis of this variant offsets virtually all of the adverse impact of underdiagnosis.

Diffuse sclerosing variant. The diffuse sclerosing variant of papillary carcinoma is characterized by diffuse involvement of one or both lobes, dense sclerosis with scattered foci of papillary carcinoma, and numerous foci of lymphatic invasion. No distinct mass lesion is identifiable (Figure 2). Psammoma bodies are generally abundant and foci of squamous metaplasia are common, sometimes extensive. Lymphocytic infiltrates may be seen.

This variant is associated with a higher incidence of cervical lymph node metastasis, pulmonary metastasis, and lower rate of disease free survival (29-31). The prognosis is less favorable although the death rate is still very low. This variant tends to occur in younger patients which may in part explain the low mortality rate despite other adverse factors.

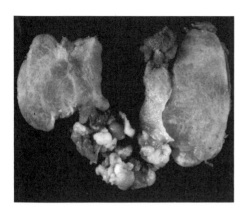 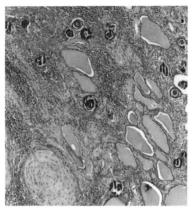

Figure 2. Gross and microscopic photographs of diffuse sclerosing variant of papillary carcinoma.

Solid/trabecular variant. This variant is characterized by tumor growth in solid sheets or trabecular nests divided by usually thin fibrous bands (Figure 3). Foci of solid or trabecular growth may be seen in the diffuse-sclerosing variant, in papillary carcinomas from patients with familial adenomatous polyposis (32), and in conventional papillary carcinomas. However, in order to be classified as solid/trabecular variant, the tumor must exhibit exclusive or predominantly solid/trabecular growth. Importantly, typical nuclear features of papillary carcinoma must be seen. This variant should be distinguished from poorly differentiated thyroid carcinoma based on the presence of typical papillary nuclear features, and lack of high mitotic activity, tumor necrosis, or extensive local invasion and distant metastases.

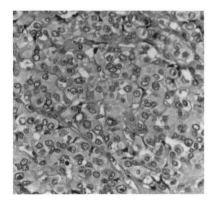 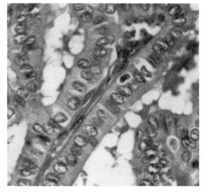

Figure 3. Photomicrograph of solid
cell variant of papillary carcinoma.

Figure 4. Photomicrograph of tall
variant of papillary carcinoma.

This variant is rare in the general population. It has been reported occasionally in children (33,34), and in some geographic areas (35). Recently, a high prevalence of solid variant was found in papillary carcinomas from children exposed to radiation after the Chernobyl nuclear accident (36,37). In these populations, more than one-third of all papillary carcinomas exhibited predominantly solid growth pattern. It has been shown recently that the solid variants of papillary carcinoma are associated with *ret*/PTC3 rearrangements, whereas typical papillary carcinoma more often harbors *ret*/PTC1 type of rearrangement of the *ret* tyrosine kinase receptor gene (38).

Biological behavior of tumors with these features is not clear. In a series from Japan, patients with the trabecular type of papillary carcinoma demonstrated lower five and ten year survival rates compared to conventional papillary carcinomas (35). In a pediatric population exposed to Chernobyl fallout, tumors with solid growth pattern and *ret*/PTC3 rearrangement had larger tumor size at presentation and higher prevalence of extrathyroidal extension (39), but overall outcome was similar to typical papillary carcinoma after a limited follow-up.

Tall cell variant. Tall cell variant of papillary carcinoma is composed of cells whose height is at least twice their width (Figure 4). They have eosinophilic cytoplasm that can be relatively abundant and resemble oncocytes. Nuclei tend to be located in the central or basal regions and frequently contain pseudoinclusions. These tumors have predominately papillary architecture although other patterns such as microfollicular, solid, glandular or cribriform can be seen. Thresholds vary regarding the relative percentage of tall cells necessary to make this diagnosis. Some require greater than 70% (40) or 50% (41) while Johnson et al. defined tall cell variants as having at least 30% (42). The effect of these differing criteria on the various studies is difficult to assess.

This variant was first described by Hawk and Hazard in 1976 (26). They noted that this variant accounted for 12% of their papillary carcinomas and that 4 of 18 patients died of disease within a few years of diagnosis. The mortality rate was higher than that associated with other types of papillary carcinoma. Other studies since then have found that this variant has a poorer prognosis (40,42). These neoplasms tend to occur in older individuals, tend to be larger (>5 cm) in size, and are more likely to exhibit mitotic activity, vascular invasion and extrathyroidal extension. Affected individuals have a higher incidence of recurrent and metastatic disease, and higher mortality rates.

Is the tall cell morphology a poor prognostic indicator by itself? This question arises because cases of this variant tend to have features that are poor prognostic indicators for conventional papillary carcinoma. Extrathyroidal extension at the time of diagnosis is a particularly ominous finding for virtually all cases of papillary carcinoma. Ostrowski and Merino (40) reported significantly higher expression of Leu M1 (CD 15) and CEA (ZC-23) in tall cell variants compared to conventional papillary carcinomas. CEA (ZC-23) is a monoclonal anti-carcinoembryonic antigen with cross-reactivity to nonspecific cross-reacting antigen and biliary glycoprotein antigen. They felt that these differences in immunoreactivity support the concept of tall cell variant as a distinct form of papillary carcinoma. However, the explanation for the expression of these antigens and what, if any, relationship they have to aggressive biologic behavior is unclear at this time. If one simply views the relative incidence of extrathyroidal extension as an indicator of aggressiveness, tall cell carcinoma clearly meets this standard even though the molecular connection between tall cell morphology and aggressive behavior remains to be elucidated.

Columnar cell variant. Columnar cell carcinoma was initially described by Evans in 1986 (43) when he reported two cases of an aggressive variant of thyroid carcinoma. This is a rare entity with a limited number of subsequent reports (6,44-48). These neoplasms tend to be large (> 5 cm) and range from encapsulated to minimally invasive to widely invasive with extrathyroidal extension. They usually have a papillary growth pattern although microfollicular, solid and cribriform growth patterns can be seen. The most distinctive feature of this variant is prominent nuclear stratification, giving them an appearance similar to adenomatous tumors of the colon. Most cells are at least twice as tall as wide, but their nuclear stratification distinguishes them from the tall cell variant. Some cases exhibit subnuclear cytoplasmic vacuolization similar to that seen in secretory endometrium.

The mitotic rate reported by the various studies ranges from rare to frequent. Most reports indicate that they are readily found, more so in solid foci than the more typical papillary regions. The cells are positive for thyroglobulin. Colloid is rare or absent. Some report finding typical nuclear features of papillary carcinoma in this variant (47) while others do not. Whether or not it should be considered a variant of papillary carcinoma is debatable. The absence or paucity of typical nuclear features and the aggressive biologic behavior of this neoplasm has sparked a debate whether or not it should be considered a variant of papillary carcinoma, a subtype of poorly differentiated carcinoma (44,46), or a separate category of thyroid neoplasia (43). This issue is yet to be resolved.

Most cases are sufficiently distinctive to allow ready diagnosis. Problems are most likely to occur with cases having clear cell (secretory-like) changes. Differential diagnosis in these cases includes follicular carcinomas with clear cell features, medullary carcinoma with clear cell features and metastatic renal cell carcinoma. Another potential problem could be recognizing this tumor in a metastatic location without knowledge of the thyroid primary. Confusion with metastatic colonic adenocarcinoma is quite possible in this situation.

In contrast to conventional papillary carcinoma, most cases have involved males. The age range is from the early 20's to mid 60's with the median age around 45. Patients have a high incidence of extrathyroidal extension and metastasis at the time of diagnosis. Metastases are found in regional lymph nodes as well as bone, lung, brain and adrenal glands. Most cases have proven to be fatal. Exceptions to the generally poor prognosis are encapsulated columnar neoplasms which have a good prognosis similar to conventional papillary carcinoma (49,50).

Oncocytic cell type. The histopathologic criteria for this unusual variant are not settled. The WHO defines this neoplasm as having typical papillary architecture, a cell population composed entirely of oncocytic cells, and typical nuclear features usually absent (4). Others advocate restricting this variant to oncocytic tumors that exhibit typical nuclear features of papillary carcinoma. In their study of 15 oncocytic tumors having either a papillary or follicular growth pattern and typical nuclear features in more than 75% of the cells, Berho and Suster report biologic behavior and prognosis similar to conventional papillary carcinoma (51). Lack of uniform histopathologic criteria probably explains the variable behavior of this tumor in other reports (52,53). The key question is whether or not one requires this variant to have typical nuclear features of papillary carcinoma. We prefer to consider tumors having abundant granular eosinophilic cytoplasm, but lacking typical nuclear of papillary carcinoma, under the separate category of oncocytic tumors.

Follicular Neoplasms

Follicular neoplasms encompass a group of benign and malignant tumors most of which bear cytological and architectural resemblance to normal thyroid follicles. The vast majority of these neoplasms are encapsulated, and evaluation for invasion through the capsule or into blood vessels is the critical step in distinguishing adenomas from most carcinomas.

Follicular Adenoma

Follicular adenomas are benign, relatively common neoplasms of the thyroid. They are encapsulated, usually solitary, and can vary greatly in size. Most are solid although cyst formation is sometimes evident. Adenomas range from light tan to orange to reddish brown in color. The color may be homogeneous or variegated, the latter appearance usually reflecting degenerative changes. The fibrous capsule is usually thin, and a thickened capsule increases the suspicion of follicular carcinoma.

Microscopic examination reveals a relatively uniform growth pattern in most cases. The growth patterns observed in conventional follicular adenomas include microfollicular (fetal), normofollicular, macrofollicular, trabecular or solid. These terms relate to the size, or absence, of follicular structures formed by the neoplastic cells. These histologic differences have no prognostic significance.

The cells bear close resemblance to normal follicular cells. The nuclei are round with regular outlines, and nucleoli are usually small or undetectable. The nuclei are surrounded by a modest amount of lightly eosinophilic to amphophilic cytoplasm. Mitoses are rare or absent. Degenerative changes are sometimes seen, especially following fine needle aspiration. These changes include hemorrhage, fibrosis, cyst formation, calcification and even focal ossification.

Immunohistochemical studies reveal positivity for thyroglobulin and cytokeratin. Thyroglobulin positivity is seen in the cytoplasm and colloid, and is usually less intense than that evident in the surrounding non-neoplastic thyroid tissue. The cells are typically positive for low molecular weight cytokeratins but negative for high molecular weight cytokeratins (5). Vimentin is coexpressed frequently. Ultrastructurally, the neoplastic cells exhibit features similar to non-neoplastic follicular cells (5).

Approximately 25% of follicular adenomas studied by flow cytometric analysis contain aneuploid cell populations (54-56). As with other endocrine neoplasms, aneuploidy has not proven to be a useful discriminator between follicular adenomas and carcinomas. Additionally, no significant difference in S phase percentage has been found between the benign and malignant versions of follicular neoplasms.

The differential diagnosis is primarily with two lesions, nodular hyperplasia (adenomatous hyperplasia or nodular goiter) and the minimally invasive form of follicular carcinoma. Distinguishing follicular adenomas from these other lesions can be quite challenging. Thyroid glands with nodular hyperplasia grossly may have a dominant nodule which appears well circumscribed and even encapsulated. Non-uniformity of the microscopic growth pattern, lack of complete encapsulation, and smaller hyperplastic nodules in the surrounding thyroid tissue favor nodular hyperplasia.

The differentiation of adenoma from minimally invasive follicular carcinoma entails careful examination of the interface between the tumor and adjacent non-neoplastic tissue. The diagnosis of carcinoma requires invasion of neoplastic cells through the capsule or into blood vessels of the tumor capsule or beyond (4-6). Cytologic differentiation between conventional follicular adenomas and carcinomas is impossible. Other considerations in the differential diagnosis include the follicular variant of papillary carcinoma and medullary carcinoma. The distinguishing features of these two neoplasms are discussed elsewhere in the chapter.

Variants

Oncocytic adenoma. Oncocytic adenoma, also known as Hürthle cell or oxyphilic adenoma, is characterized by the majority of the cells (≥ 75%) exhibiting oncocytic features (5,6). Oncocytic features are manifest by relatively abundant granular eosinophilic cytoplasm. Whether oncocytic adenomas and carcinomas should be classified as variants of follicular neoplasms or as separate tumor entities is controversial. We have chosen to consider them separately under the category of oncocytic neoplasms.

Hyalinizing trabecular adenoma. Carney et al. coined this term in 1987 (57) for a group of distinctive lesions characterized by encapsulation or circumscription, trabecular or alveolar (nested) growth pattern, and hyalinization of fibrovascular stroma (figure 5). Some of the neoplastic cells also exhibit cytoplasmic hyalinization, and studies have shown that the intra- and extracellular hyalinization is due to abundant basement membrane material (58,59). Follicles and colloid are minimal or absent. Nuclei range from round to spindled and may have grooves or pseudoinclusions. Psammoma-like bodies are sometimes seen. The surrounding non-neoplastic thyroid tissue commonly has features of chronic lymphocytic thyroiditis.

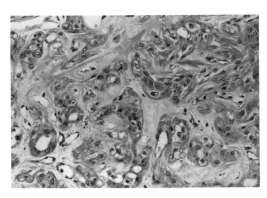

Figure 5. Photomicrograph of hyalinizing trabecular adenoma.

Differential diagnosis includes paraganglioma, medullary carcinoma, and papillary carcinoma. An alternative name once used for hyalinizing trabecular adenoma was paraganglioma-like adenoma (60) Immunohistochemistry is very helpful in distinguishing between hyalinizing trabecular adenoma and paraganglioma as the former is positive for thyroglobulin and the latter negative. Hyalinization mimics the amyloid stroma of medullary carcinoma, but stains for amyloid are negative in cases of hyalinizing trabecular adenoma. The trabecular architecture, absence of follicles and presence of spindle cells also bear resemblance to medullary carcinoma. Medullary carcinomas stain positively for calcitonin and are negative for thyroglobulin, while hyalinizing trabecular adenomas have the reverse staining pattern.

Nuclear grooves and pseudoinclusions are features hyalinizing trabecular adenoma shares with papillary carcinoma, but only a small minority of papillary carcinomas are encapsulated and trabecular architecture is uncharacteristic. Papillary carcinomas usually contain relatively large overlapping "ground glass" nuclei which help to distinguish them. Nevertheless, similar distribution of intracellular and extracellular basement membrane material and reports of tumors with mixed features have led some to hypothesize that hyalinizing trabecular adenoma may be a variant of papillary carcinoma (58).

Hyalinizing trabecular adenomas are benign and treatment is the same as with a conventional follicular adenoma. Minimally invasive malignant counterparts have been reported (61) so careful examination for capsular penetration or vascular invasion is mandatory.

Follicular Adenoma with Clear Cells. This rare variant of follicular adenoma is characterized by cells with clear cytoplasm due to accumulation of glycogen, lipid, thyroglobulin or dilated mitochondria (4,5). The growth pattern is usually follicular. The cells exhibit thyroglobulin positivity, but it is commonly focal and weak. Most cells are PAS positive, diastase sensitive which reflects their glycogen content. Many of these tumors seem to represent a progression from oncocytic adenomas.

The differential diagnosis includes follicular, papillary and medullary carcinomas with clear cells, parathyroid tissue or neoplasms, and metastatic renal cell carcinoma. Differentiation from follicular carcinoma follows the usual invasive criteria. Thyroglobulin positivity is helpful in distinguishing this tumor from parathyroid tissue or renal cell carcinoma. Papillary carcinoma is ruled out primarily on the absence of characteristic nuclear features. Treatment is as for conventional adenomas.

Follicular Adenoma with Signet Ring Cells. This extremely rare variant contains cells with eosinophilic intracytoplasmic vacuoles that displace and compress the nucleus to the side (4,5). The vacuoles are due to thyroglobulin accumulation, and thus the cells usually stain strongly positive for this substance. The vacuoles also stain positively with mucin stains, particularly PAS (diastase resistant) and alcian blue at pH 2.5. The signet ring cells have the potential to be mistaken for metastatic carcinoma, but immunostaining for thyroglobulin can resolve this issue.

Atypical Follicular Adenoma. Atypical follicular adenoma is so named due to nuclear atypia, prominent nucleoli and increased mitotic activity (62). They often have thick capsules and increased cellularity in the capsular region, thus heightening suspicion for malignancy. However, evaluation for malignancy is based on the same invasive criteria as for conventional adenomas (4-6). Tumors not meeting these criteria for malignancy can be treated as benign lesions despite their disturbing atypical features.

Follicular Carcinoma

Follicular carcinomas are defined as malignant epithelial tumors showing evidence of follicular cell differentiation but lacking diagnostic features of other malignant thyroid tumors (4,5). Follicular carcinoma is the second most common type of thyroid malignancy, comprising 5 to 15% of malignant neoplasms (5,6,63). The relative incidence is higher in iodine deficient regions (64,65). The WHO classification (4) acknowledges and accepts marked morphologic variation of follicular carcinomas, and mentions the existence of a group of poorly differentiated carcinomas with worse prognoses. In accordance with the AFIP classification (5), we prefer to reserve the term follicular carcinoma for well differentiated neoplasms, and place poorly differentiated carcinomas derived from follicular epithelia into a separate category.

Separation of follicular carcinomas into minimally invasive and widely invasive subtypes is important. The majority of follicular carcinomas are encapsulated, minimally invasive tumors that are indistinguishable grossly from follicular adenomas . They exhibit the same cytologic features and range of histologic patterns as their benign counterparts. Immunohistochemical and ultrastructural studies reveal features similar to adenomas (5). Mitoses are scant or absent. A thickened and irregular capsule as well as increased cellularity and nuclear atypia are suspicious for carcinoma, but not diagnostic per se.

The distinction of carcinoma from adenoma is based only on the presence of invasion completely through the capsule and/or invasion of blood vessels in the capsule or beyond (Figure 6). The presence of tumor cells within the blood vessels of the tumor nodule itself is of no diagnostic significance. Thus far no cytologic or molecular marker has proven to be a practical and reliable discriminator. Evaluation requires adequate sampling and careful examination of the tumor interface as invasion is often focal and subtle. Blood vessel invasion is considered a more reliable sign of carcinoma, but pathologists have to avoid interpreting artifactual tumor emboli caused by sectioning as true invasion. Neoplastic cells should be adherent to the vessel wall and, preferably, covered by endothelial cells (66).

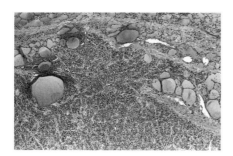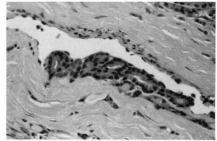

Figure 6. Photomicrographs of minimally invasive follicular carcinoma showing capsular penetration (left) and blood vessel invasion (right).

The widely invasive subtype exhibits gross extension of tumor into the surrounding thyroid gland. A capsule is not always identifiable. In contrast to the minimally invasive subtype, most widely invasive carcinomas exhibit nuclear atypia, significant mitotic activity and foci of necrosis. Areas of solid or trabecular growth pattern may be present. These features overlap with those of poorly differentiated carcinoma and distinguishing between the two may be quite difficult.

On a practical basis, this distinction is not critical given their similar prognosis and method of treatment (67). Differential diagnosis also includes follicular variant of papillary carcinoma and oncocytic carcinoma. Distinguishing features of these lesions are described under papillary carcinoma and oncocytic tumors, respectively.

Follicular carcinomas disseminate hematogenously with lung and bone being the most common sites of metastasis (68-70). Lymph node metastases are rare. Most lymph node metastases exhibiting follicular architecture represent metastatic follicular variant of papillary carcinoma (5,6).

The prognosis for minimally invasive follicular carcinoma is excellent with ten year survival rates similar to papillary carcinoma (71,72). Adverse factors include metastasis, multiple sites of metastasis and absence of radioactive iodine uptake by metastasis. Widely invasive carcinoma, in contrast, has a much poorer prognosis with ten year survival rates in the 50-80% range (66,71,73).

Oncocytic Neoplasms

Oncocytic neoplasms are composed of cells of follicular derivation that are also known as Hürthle, Askanazy, oxyphilic or eosinophilic cells. Their characteristic feature is relatively abundant, finely granular eosinophilic cytoplasm due to the presence of numerous mitochondria (Figure 7). To qualify as an oncocytic tumor, all or a high percentage of cells must exhibit oncocytic features. Greater than 75% is a common criterion (5,6). The WHO classification uses the adjective oxyphilic, indicative of their cytoplasmic affinity for acidic dyes (4). Use of the term Hürthle cell tumor is problematic because the cells Hürthle described appear to be C cells (74).

Oncocytic neoplasms are usually solitary and encapsulated. The cut surface typically has a solid appearance and a light brown or reddish brown color that is rather characteristic and allows one to suspect an oncocytic tumor. They sometimes exhibit hemorrhage, infarction, cystic change or calcification. Infarction is commonly associated with prior fine needle aspiration.

Microscopically, oncocytic tumors demonstrate follicular, trabecular or solid patterns of growth. The nuclei of oncocytes often show significant variation in size with occasional large hyperchromatic forms. Nucleoli are present and may be quite prominent. Oncocytic neoplasms commonly contain cells with relatively clear cytoplasm (5). The clear cell change may be focal or widespread.

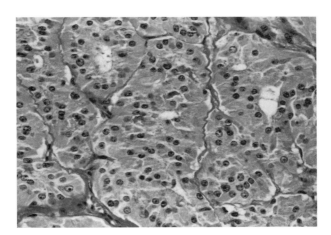

Figure 7. Photomicrograph of oncocytic adenoma.

The distinction between oncocytic adenomas and carcinomas is the same as for typical follicular neoplasms (4-6). The presence of invasion through the capsule or into blood vessels of the capsule or beyond is diagnostic for carcinoma. Oncocytic carcinomas commonly have a solid or trabecular growth pattern while most adenomas have a predominately follicular pattern, but growth pattern is not diagnostic per se. Likewise, adenomas and carcinomas cannot be differentiated reliably on a cytologic basis as both can exhibit marked nuclear atypia. However, nuclear hyperchromasia, high nuclear:cytoplasmic ratio, mitoses and prominent nucleoli raise the level of suspicion for carcinoma.

Oncocytic carcinomas are more likely have direct extrathyroidal spread or metastasis compared to typical follicular carcinomas (5). They metastasize by both hematogenous and lymphatic routes, in contrast to typical follicular carcinomas (75-78). The lungs and bones are the most common sites of metastasis, and metastasis may manifest ten or more years after the primary diagnosis . Both distant and regional lymph node metastasis have adverse prognostic implications (5). Overall five year survival is 50-60% (5,6), largely reflective of the propensity for spread beyond the thyroid. While oncocytic carcinomas are more aggressive than conventional follicular neoplasms in the sense that they are more likely to have extrathyroidal extension or metastasis, stage by stage comparison reveals comparable behavior (79).

Papillary variants

Rare oncocytic neoplasms exhibit papillary architecture throughout. Whether these cases represent a variant of papillary carcinoma or oncocytic carcinoma is controversial. Tumors having nuclei comparable to regular oncocytic neoplasms instead of papillary carcinoma may behave more aggressively (52,53). Neoplasms having papillary architecture, abundant granular eosinophilic cytoplasm and nuclear features typical of papillary carcinoma seem to behave similarly to conventional papillary carcinoma (51). A papillary variant with lymphoid stroma bearing resemblance to Warthin's tumor (papillary cystadenoma lymphomatosum) of the salivary gland was recently reported (80). This variant behaved similar to typical papillary carcinoma.

Particularly vexing is the encapsulated non-invasive variant. Classification options include encapsulated papillary carcinoma with oncocytic features, oncocytic adenoma with papillary features, or the noncommittal encapsulated papillary oncocytic neoplasm (5). While classification is problematic, these encapsulated tumors have behaved in a benign fashion (53).

Poorly Differentiated Carcinoma

The emergence of poorly differentiated carcinoma as a separate category is one of the most significant recent developments in the classification of thyroid tumors. This type of thyroid carcinoma morphologically and clinically bridges the gap between well differentiated and anaplastic carcinomas arising from follicular epithelium. Insular carcinoma is the prototypic form of poorly differentiated carcinoma.

Credit for the first description of insular carcinoma is given to Langhans who used the term wuchernde Struma in his 1907 publication (81). In 1984, Carcangiu, Zampi and Rosai (67) revisited this tumor applying the term insular carcinoma. Their diagnostic criteria were formation of solid clusters ('insulae") of tumor cells, variable numbers of small follicles, tumor cells of uniformly small size, variable but consistently present mitotic activity, capsular and blood vessel invasion, and frequent necrotic foci (Figure 8). Papillary structures were present in a minority of cases but many contained cells with optically clear nuclei. However, the nuclei did not exhibit the degree of overlapping characteristic of papillary carcinoma.

How were these neoplasms been classified prior to 1984? Probably most cases were reported as follicular carcinomas (67) The AFIP second series fascicle published in 1969 (82) notes the range of microscopic patterns of follicular carcinoma and the existence of a microfollicular variant with tightly packed cells sometimes called Langhans' wuchernde struma. The 1988 WHO classification (4) under follicular carcinoma acknowledges a group of poorly differentiated carcinomas which have a worse prognosis and frequent lymph node metastasis in contrast to other follicular carcinomas. Other cases now recognized as poorly differentiated carcinoma had been interpreted previously as papillary, undifferentiated or medullary carcinomas (83).

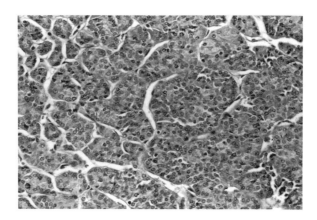

Figure 8. Photomicrograph of poorly differentiated (insular) carcinoma.

The relative incidence of insular carcinoma seems to have regional variation. The highest rates have been reported from northern Italy where insular carcinomas constitute 4-6% of thyroid malignancies (83,84). They appear to be rare in the United States. Whether or not prospective studies or retrospective reclassification will find rates similar to Italy remains to be seen. Patient age ranges from the second to eighth decades with a median in the mid fifties, and the female to male ratio is 2 to 1 (67,83-85).

Insular carcinomas tend to be large (greater than 5 cm), solid masses which range from grayish white to pinkish gray in color. They often exhibit foci of hemorrhage, necrosis or fibrosis. The incidence of extrathyroidal extension at the time of initial diagnosis has been reported in the range of 11 to 59% (67,83,84). One study reported concurrent nodular goiter in 97% of cases (83).

As stated above, insular carcinomas are composed of a homogeneous population of relatively small cells with round nuclei and scant cytoplasm. These cells have been compared to those composing the fetal thyroid (83). Insular carcinomas lack the spindle, giant or large squamoid cells which are characteristically seen in anaplastic carcinoma. The neoplastic cells of insular carcinoma stain positively for thyroglobulin but are negative for calcitonin (67,83-86), thus allowing differentiation from medullary carcinoma. The majority of cases also exhibit cytoplasmic positivity for cytokeratin although the staining is usually focal (67) and limited to low molecular weight cytokeratins (87). Immunoreactivity for p53 in thyroid tumors correlates with the degree of differentiation. Positivity has been reported in 6-14% of papillary and follicular carcinomas, 16-41% of poorly differentiated carcinomas, and in 38-83% of anaplastic thyroid carcinomas (88-90).

Recognition of insular carcinoma is important due to its biologic behavior which is intermediate between indolent well differentiated carcinomas and rapidly fatal anaplastic carcinomas. Nineteen to 74% have nodal, pulmonary or osseous metastasis at the time of initial diagnosis and 48 to 84% experience local or distant recurrence (67,83,84). Approximately 40% of patients die of their disease within the first five years while another 25% or more will be alive with disease (67,83-85).

An important issue regarding poorly differentiated carcinoma is how broadly to define this category. Papotti et al. (83) classified tumors as poorly differentiated carcinoma even if the insular pattern constituted a minor (25-45%) component. In their study, the survival rate of these tumors was comparable to carcinomas with a predominant insular pattern (65-100%), although a significantly higher rate of distant metastasis was observed with predominately insular carcinomas.

Sakamoto et al. (91) defined poorly differentiated carcinomas as those tumors containing solid, trabecular and/or scirrhous patterns but without anaplastic features. They found 5 year survival rates of 65% for poorly differentiated carcinomas compared to 95% for well differentiated carcinomas. Solid, trabecular and/or scirrhous features comprised a minority component of most of the cases classified as poorly differentiated carcinoma. Relative percentages were not quantified, however, and whether or not a very small component of poorly differentiated carcinoma has prognostic significance is unclear. While a threshold for prognostic significance remains to be established, it appears that a poorly differentiated component in an otherwise well differentiated carcinoma indicates a worse prognosis in most cases.

The category of poorly differentiated carcinoma is still in its formative stages and insular carcinoma is the best defined subtype. Studies suggest that this category include other variants of thyroid carcinoma having more aggressive behavior than conventional well differentiated follicular and papillary carcinomas. Histopathologic features shared by these carcinomas include components with insular, solid, trabecular and/or scirrhous growth patterns. Some include columnar cell carcinoma in this general category (92). More studies addressing these issues can be expected in the near future, and the use of cellular and molecular markers may prove to be a valuable adjunct to traditional morphologic methods of classification.

Anaplastic (Undifferentiated) Carcinoma

Anaplastic or undifferentiated carcinoma is a highly malignant neoplasm composed partially or totally by undifferentiated cells. They account for 5 to 10% of malignant thyroid neoplasms (19,93-95). Some evidence suggests that the relative incidence is declining (92). Anaplastic carcinomas generally occur in older individuals who often have a history of a pre-existing goiter or mass. The mean age of patients is usually in the 60-65 year range, and patients less than 50 years of age are rare. Women are affected 3-4 times more often than men. These tumors typically present as large, rapidly growing masses. Total effacement of the gland is frequent. Other common gross findings include extrathyroidal extension and foci of hemorrhage and necrosis. Foci of bone or cartilage are occasionally identifiable.

Microscopic examination reveals one or more of three basic patterns: sarcomatoid, giant cell or squamoid (Figure 9) (5,93,96). The sarcomatoid or spindle cell pattern resembles one or more types of sarcoma including fibrosarcoma, malignant fibrous histiocytoma, hemangiopericytoma or hemangioendothelioma. Occasional cases contain heterologous elements such as cartilage or bone. If a thyroid neoplasm contains a mixture of epithelial and sarcomatoid components, the lesion is still classified as an anaplastic carcinoma as opposed to a carcinosarcoma. Even if an epithelial component is not identifiable, these tumors are usually classified as an anaplastic carcinoma instead of a sarcoma.

The giant cell pattern is characterized by the presence of numerous multinucleated tumor giant cells that are usually quite pleomorphic. Multinucleated giant cells resembling osteoclasts are seen occasionally (96,97). The neoplastic cells usually grow in solid sheets. Pseudoglandular or pseudovascular patterns are seen in some cases. Sometimes abundant neutrophils infiltrate the tumor in a manner similar to inflammatory malignant fibrous histiocytoma. Phagocytosis of neutrophils by tumor giant cells can be seen.

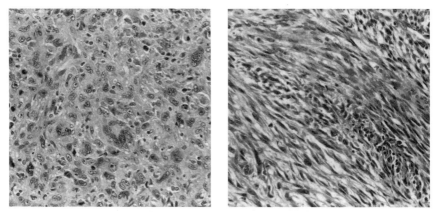

Figure 9. Photomicrographs of anaplastic carcinomas; squamoid (epithelioid) and giant cell patterns (left); sarcomatoid spindle cell pattern (right).

The squamoid, or epithelioid, pattern resembles nonkeratinizing squamous cell carcinoma. The cells contain relatively abundant eosinophilic cytoplasm, are moderately pleomorphic, and often form distinct nests. Admixtures of the three patterns are common, particularly the sarcomatoid and giant cell patterns. All patterns are considered high grade. In the past, a small cell subtype was recognized. This is no longer the case as improved diagnostic techniques have shown most to be lymphomas or medullary carcinomas.

Microscopic findings common to all three patterns are high mitotic rates, foci of necrosis, absence of follicle and colloid formation, intravascular tumor emboli, an invasive intrathyroidal growth pattern, and frequent extrathyroidal extension. Residual well differentiated follicular or papillary neoplasia may be seen.

Immunohistochemical studies usually reveal cytokeratin positivity although it may be only focal (93,98-102). The squamoid foci are usually positive for both high and low molecular weight cytokeratins. Spindle and giant cell components are negative for high molecular weight cytokeratin and variably positive for low molecular weight cytokeratin. Staining for epithelial membrane antigen yields positive results in a minority of cases (96,100,102). Investigators have reported variable results for thyroglobulin (93,96,99-101,103,104). Most cases exhibit little or no positivity, and positivity is usually very focal and weak. Positivity may actually represent entrapped non-neoplastic follicular cells, diffusion of thyroglobulin into tumor cells, or staining of a more differentiated neoplastic component. Immunostaining for thyroglobulin is generally not helpful diagnostically.

Differential diagnosis includes medullary carcinomas and lymphomas. The former is usually distinguishable by calcitonin and chromogranin immunopositivity while the latter shows expression of various lymphoid antigens. Poorly differentiated carcinoma may enter the differential but as discussed in the previous section, poorly differentiated carcinomas lack sarcomatoid, giant cell or squamoid patterns. They have relatively uniform cell populations that lack the pleomorphism of anaplastic carcinomas. Most poorly differentiated carcinomas reportedly express *bcl*-2 while this is unusual in anaplastic carcinomas (87). Differentiation from a true sarcoma may be virtually impossible on a histopathologic basis. However, almost all sarcoma-like tumors that appear to arise in the thyroid are by convention diagnosed as anaplastic carcinomas. The prime exception is angiosarcoma and this tumor will be discussed later in the chapter.

Anaplastic thyroid carcinoma is one of the most aggressive human neoplasms. Rapid enlargement is associated with signs and symptoms reflecting compression or infiltration of adjacent structures in the neck. The vast majority of cases prove fatal within weeks to months, and few patients survive beyond one year (93,94,96).

Medullary Carcinoma

Medullary thyroid carcinoma is a malignant neuroendocrine neoplasm that exhibits C cell differentiation (please see also Chapter 4). The term was first used for thyroid neoplasms by Hazard and colleagues in the 1950's (105,106) although earlier reports seem to have described the same neoplasm (107-109). Origin from the C (parafollicular) cell was first suggested in 1966 (110) and in 1968 calcitonin-like activity was found in an extract from medullary carcinoma (111). Immunofluorescent demonstration of calcitonin within the cells of medullary carcinoma was reported in 1969 (112).

Most cases of medullary carcinoma are sporadic but approximately 25% are hereditary (5,113). The hereditary cases may be a manifestation of MEN 2 (2A) or 3 (2B). Germline mutations of *ret* tyrosine kinase receptor gene have been detected in greater than 90% of hereditary cases while somatic mutations have been found in approximately 45% of sporadic cases (114). Medullary carcinoma may be a single mass or multiple and bilateral. Multiple masses usually indicate a hereditary case, or at least one with a germline mutation.

Medullary carcinomas generally have well defined gross boundaries and are sometimes encapsulated. Color is variable, ranging from white to tan, yellow, pink or gray. Hemorrhage or necrosis are usually absent. Microscopically, medullary carcinomas exhibit a wide range of growth patterns. The classical pattern is rounded nests of cells separated by thin fibrovascular stroma (Figure 10). Trabecular, insular and solid patterns are less common. Follicular, glandular, papillary and tubular patterns have been described but are rare. The cells composing medullary carcinoma also have a wide range of appearances. Most are round to oval with uniformly bland features. Significant numbers of cases contain spindle cells. Uncommon variants are composed of oncocytic, clear, squamous, melanotic, small or giant cells. Stromal amyloid is seen in up to 80% of cases (5,6). C cell hyperplasia, the precursor lesion of medullary carcinoma, can be seen in the surrounding thyroid tissue.

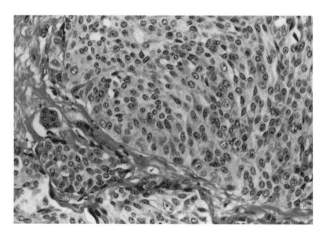

Figure 10. Photomicrograph of medullary carcinoma.

Immunohistochemical studies demonstrate calcitonin and calcitonin gene-related peptide positivity in the vast majority of medullary carcinomas (115-118) Carcinoembryonic antigen (CEA) is evident in most tumors and immunoreactivity for a variety of other polypeptides has been observed (5,115,118). Medullary carcinomas are usually positive for low molecular weight cytokeratins and generic neuroendocrine markers such as chromogranin A, synaptophysin and neuron specific enolase (115,116,118,119). Ultrastructural examination reveals membrane bound neurosecretory granules which correlate with the immunohistochemical findings. Medullary carcinomas are negative for thyroglobulin (120).

Cases of mixed medullary and follicular carcinoma have been reported but their existence is controversial (121-123). True examples are probably very rare. Putative cases may just represent entrapped non-neoplastic thyroid follicles or uptake of thyroglobulin by medullary carcinoma. It is very difficult if not impossible to make a definitive diagnosis based on the primary tumor alone. The WHO criterion for absolute proof is the presence of both types of tumor in a metastasis (4). Two cases of mixed medullary-papillary carcinoma have been reported (124).

Medullary carcinomas spread by both lymphatic and hematogenous routes. The lungs, liver, bone and adrenal glands are the most sites of blood borne metastases. Overall five year survival is reported generally at 65% or higher (5,118,125). Numerous studies have analyzed medullary carcinomas for prognostic features. MEN 2B cases usually behave more aggressively than sporadic cases while familial and MEN 2A cases tend to have more favorable prognoses (125). Reported favorable prognostic indicators include high calcitonin positivity of cells, small size, encapsulation, age < 40 years and female gender while unfavorable indicators are extrathyroidal extension, distant metastasis, mitotic activity, cellular pleomorphism, necrosis, lack of bcl-2 immunoreactivity, and a rising serum calcitonin or CEA level postoperatively (126-130). Amyloid within the tumor has been found to be a favorable indicator by some investigators (125,127) while others have found its presence to be insignificant (118,130). Regional lymph node metastasis has variable prognostic significance (126,129). Two of the most significant unfavorable prognostic indicators appear to be extrathyroidal extension and residual disease following surgical resection (126).

Malignant Lymphoma

Primary thyroid lymphoma is a malignant tumor composed of lymphoid cells with predominant or exclusive involvement of the thyroid gland. Primary thyroid lymphomas constitute from 1 to 8% of all thyroid gland malignancies, with up to 10% in areas of the world where lymphocytic thyroiditis is common (131). The thyroid gland may also be secondary involved by a systemic lymphoma or leukemia. Most patients with primary thyroid lymphoma are women over 50 years of age. Primary thyroid lymphoma arises almost exclusively in thyroid glands affected by lymphocytic or Hashimoto's thyroiditis.

On gross examination, most thyroid lymphomas have homogeneous tan-white (fish flesh) appearance, with extensive effacement of the gland and poor demarcation from the surrounding non-neoplastic thyroid tissue. Extrathyroidal extension is commonly seen. Surrounding thyroid tissue may appear lobular and pale due to thyroiditis.

Microscopically, most of primary thyroid lymphomas are non-Hodgkin lymphomas of B-cell type (more than 95%), 80-90% are diffuse and 10-20% nodular. The most common type is diffuse large cell lymphoma. These tumors demonstrate a diffuse pattern of growth with no germinal centers, effacement of normal follicular architecture, entrapment and invasion of thyroid follicles, and sometimes accumulation of malignant cells within the follicular lumens. Involvement of thyroid capsule and perithyroidal extension is seen in about half of all cases. An additional important diagnostic feature is vascular invasion with infiltration of the vascular wall by neoplastic lymphocytes (132,133). In the AFIP series of 109 primary thyroid lymphomas, diffuse large B-cell lymphoma was found in 51% of cases (134). The other types included extranodal marginal zone B-cell (MALT) lymphoma (28%), follicular center cell lymphoma (13%), high grade B-cell, Burkitt-like (2%), peripheral T-cell (2%), and Hodgkin's lymphoma (1%). Primary plasmacytoma may occasionally develop in the thyroid gland. A case of signet ring cell lymphoma has been reported (135).

Immunohistochemically, thyroid lymphomas are positive for leukocyte common antigen (CD45), pan-B cell markers (or T-cell markers in case of T-cell lymphoma), demonstrate immunoglobulin light-chain restriction, and show no immunoreactivity for cytokeratin, thyroglobulin or calcitonin. This pattern of immunoreactivity is helpful in differential diagnosis of this tumor with anaplastic thyroid carcinoma, poorly-differentiated carcinoma, or medullary carcinoma. In addition, thyroid lymphomas exhibit clonal immunoglobulin or T-cell receptor gene rearrangements, which are not found in benign lymphocytic thyroiditis.

Thyroid lymphomas invade locally and directly extend into surrounding soft tissues, and may involve regional lymph nodes. The tumor recurs locally, but more often distal relapse may be seen. Primary thyroid lymphomas have a tendency to disseminate to the gastrointestinal tract (136,137). Prognostic factors include extrathyroidal extension, cell type (excellent prognosis for MALT lymphomas), and age of patients. In early series, 5-year survival was 50-74% (138,139). Administration of radiation therapy in combination with chemotherapy, with or without surgery, led to a significant increase in survival and decrease in the rate of distant and overall recurrence (140,141).

Rare Primary Tumors

Other types of benign and malignant neoplasia develop rarely within the thyroid gland. A small number of bona fide cases of paraganglioma have been reported (142). Primary paragangliomas are prone to be mistaken for medullary carcinoma or hyalinizing trabecular adenoma, or for an extrathyroidal paraganglioma that has grown adjacent to or extended into the thyroid. Distinction from medullary carcinoma can be very difficult since both are neuroendocrine neoplasms. Positivity for calcitonin, calcitonin gene-related peptide, cytokeratin or CEA supports the diagnosis of medullary carcinoma while the presence of S-100 positive sustentacular cells favors paraganglioma. Unlike hyalinizing trabecular adenoma, paragangliomas are negative for thyroglobulin. Thyroid paragangliomas can be treated with local resection, and no cases of metastasis have been reported (142).

Salivary gland-type neoplasms including pleomorphic adenoma (5) and mucoepidermoid carcinoma (143-145) have been reported. Thyroid mucoepidermoid carcinomas are low grade and behave in an indolent manner (143). A form of mucoepidermoid carcinoma with sclerosis and eosinophilia has been observed in association with Hashimoto's thyroiditis (144,145). Parathyroid tissue is occasionally found within thyroid glands, and development of an adenoma or enlargement due to hyperplasia can simulate a thyroid follicular neoplasm. Hyperplastic or neoplastic parathyroid tissue can be distinguished by positivity for parathormone, absence of thyroglobulin, and clinical evidence of hyperparathyroidism.

Sarcomas are rarely diagnosed as almost all primary thyroid tumors with sarcomatous features are classified as anaplastic carcinomas. The prime exception is epithelioid angiosarcoma (malignant haemangioendothelioma in the WHO classification). This is a rare, highly aggressive tumor which exhibits features of endothelial differentiation. Most cases have occurred in elderly inhabitants of the mountainous regions of central Europe who had long histories of goiter. Distinction from anaplastic carcinoma is not critical as both behave similarly and have dismal prognoses.

Tumors with thymic differentiation occur in or near the thyroid. Chan and Rosai have defined four clinicopathologic entities: ectopic hamartomatous thymoma, ectopic cervical thymoma, spindle epithelial tumor with thymus-like differentiation (SETTLE), and carcinoma showing thymus-like differentiation (CASTLE) (147). Ectopic hamartomatous thymoma is a benign neoplasm that occurs in the soft tissues of the lower neck but has not been reported in the thyroid. Ectopic cervical thymomas have been reported in or immediately adjacent to the thyroid. They are identical histologically to mediastinal thymomas, and most are encapsulated or circumscribed. Complete surgical excision appears to be curative for the majority of patients.

SETTLE is a malignant thyroid tumor composed predominately of relatively uniform spindle cells and foci of cells exhibiting epithelial differentiation. The epithelial cells may exhibit solid growth pattern, tubulopapillary structures or mucinous glands. Grossly, these tumors may have well circumscribed or infiltrative margins. They occur in children or young adults, behave indolently and have the potential to recur locally or metastasize after many years.

CASTLE is a thyroid tumor similar in appearance to lymphoepithelioma-like thymic carcinoma. CASTLE should be distinguished from primary squamous cell carcinoma or metastatic carcinoma since it is an indolent tumor while the latter are aggressive and usually fatal. Distinguishing features of CASTLE are lobulated architecture, expansile growth and low mitotic rate. Primary squamous cell carcinomas of the thyroid are composed of cytological malignant cells with obvious features of squamous differentiation. Since many thyroid tumors may show foci of squamous differentiation, the term squamous cell carcinoma should be reserved for those with exclusive squamous differentiation (4).

Secondary Tumors

Tumors arising elsewhere may involve the thyroid either by direct invasion or metastasis. Squamous cell carcinoma arising in the larynx, pharynx or esophagus is the most common type of neoplasm to invade directly. Metastasis can originate from a variety of sites with kidney, breast and lung being the most common (148). Metastasis may develop even in a primary thyroid neoplasm or hyperplastic nodule (149). Most metastases involving the thyroid are not evident clinically (5).

Distinguishing a metastasis from a primary tumor may be difficult. Metastatic renal cell carcinoma can be particularly challenging as it can resemble a primary tumor with clear cell features. The main primary tumors in the differential diagnosis are follicular neoplasms, oncocytic neoplasms and medullary carcinoma. Immunohistochemical staining for thyroglobulin is helpful in most cases. Staining for calcitonin and/or a general neuroendocrine marker such as chromogranin or synaptophysin distinguishes most cases of medullary carcinoma with clear cell features from renal cell carcinoma.

Tumor-like Lesions

A variety of non-neoplastic conditions can simulate thyroid neoplasms. The most common of these lesions is nodular hyperplasia, which has a variety of alternative names including nodular or multinodular goiter, adenomatous hyperplasia or goiter, and colloid nodule or goiter (please see also Chapter 7). The common mechanisms for hyperplasia of follicular epithelium are increased secretion of thyroid stimulating hormone (TSH) due to increased need for or inadequate production of thyroid hormones, or the presence of autoantibodies with TSH-like activity. Cases associated with increased TSH may be due to inadequate dietary iodine (endemic goiter) or genetic disorders of thyroid metabolism (dyshormonogenetic goiter).

The enlargement of the thyroid gland can range from modest to massive, and be quite asymmetrical. As the follicular epithelium does not respond uniformly to stimulation, the enlargement manifests grossly as one or multiple nodules, some of which may appear encapsulated. Foci of fibrosis, hemorrhage and cyst formation are common. Microscopic examination reveals follicles of varying size within a given specimen. Large follicles containing abundant colloid are seen in most cases. The follicular epithelium may exhibit hyperplastic features characterized by a columnar shape and papillary-like infoldings, or it may appear relatively inactive with low cuboidal morphology. The latter appearance usually predominates as most cases have achieved a euthyroid state. Foci of fresh hemorrhage or hemosiderin deposits, indicative of past hemorrhage, are usually present.

Cases of nodular hyperplasia with multiple nodules generally do not present diagnostic problems. Those with a dominant nodule, however, can be challenging to distinguish from a follicular adenoma or minimally invasive carcinoma. Hyperplastic nodules lack complete encapsulation and usually exhibit a range of follicular growth patterns while follicular neoplasms are encapsulated and have a more uniform growth pattern that differs from the surrounding thyroid tissue. Although a hyperplastic nodule may appear solitary upon gross examination, smaller nodules are usually found in the surrounding tissue when examined microscopically.

A caveat regarding nodular hyperplasia is that malignant neoplasms can arise in this setting. Many pathologists have struggled with cases that have focal features suggestive of follicular variant of papillary carcinoma. In some cases of nodular hyperplasia, extensive papillary architecture is seen in one or more nodules. Distinguishing these hyperplastic lesions from papillary carcinoma is based primarily on the absence of overlapping nuclei and other cytologic features typical of papillary carcinoma.

Graves' disease is associated with diffuse hyperplasia of the thyroid gland. The hyperplastic epithelium can form papillary structures that may be confused with papillary carcinoma, particularly in the absence of pertinent clinical information. Hashimoto's thyroiditis also presents as diffuse, symmetrical enlargement in most cases. Microscopically, this condition is characterized by lymphoid infiltrates with germinal center formations, effacement of the follicular architecture, and oncocytic metaplasia of the follicular epithelium. The metaplastic follicular cells can exhibit significant cytologic atypia and be mistaken for an oncocytic neoplasm, particularly with a limited biopsy or fine needle aspiration. Sometimes follicular cells exhibit nuclear features that are suggestive of papillary carcinoma, and the dense lymphoid infiltrates can simulate lymphoma.

Riedel's struma, or fibrosing thyroiditis, is a rare disorder that can mimic carcinoma. It is probably not a primary inflammatory disease of the thyroid, but instead a fibrosing disorder of the soft tissues that engulfs the gland. The follicular architecture is effaced by dense, keloid-like fibrous tissue and lymphoplasmacytic infiltrates. This condition is distinguished from anaplastic carcinoma by the absence of cytologic atypia, mitoses and necrosis.

References:

1.   Osler W. The Principles and Practice of Medicine. New York: Appelton & Co., 1892.
2.   Warren S, Meissner WA. Tumors of the Thyroid Gland. Washington: Armed Forces Institute of Pathology, 1993.
3.   Hedinger CE, Sobin LH. Histologic typing of Thyroid Tumors, Geneva: World Health Organization, 1974.
4.   Hedinger CE. Histologic Typing of Thyroid Tumors, 2nd ed. Berlin:Springer-Verlag, 1988.

5. Rosai J, Carcangiu ML, DeLellis RA. Tumors of the Thyroid Gland. Washington: Armed Forces Institute of Pathology, 1992.
6. LiVolsi VA. Surgical Pathology of the Thyroid. Philadelphia: W. B. Saunders, 1990.
7. Johannessen JV, Sobrinho-Simoes M. The origin and significance of thyroid psammoma bodies. Lab Invest 1980;43:287-296.
8. Patchefsky AS, Hoch WS. Psammoma bodies in diffuse toxic goiter. Am J Clin Pathol 1972;57:551-556.
9. Dugan JM, Atkinson BF, Avitabile A, Schimmel M, LiVolsi VA. Psammoma bodies in fine needle aspirate of the thyroid in lymphocytic thyroiditis. Acta Cytol 1987;31:330-334.
10. Lee T-K, Myers RT, Marshall RB, Bond MG, Kardon B. The significance of mitotic rate: a retrospective study of 127 thyroid carcinomas. Hum Pathol 1985;16:1042-1046.
11. Carcangiu ML, Zampi G, Pupi A, Castagnoli A, Rosai J. Papillary carcinoma of the thyroid. A clinicopathologic study of 241 cases treated at the University of Florence, Italy. Cancer 1985;55:805-828.
12. Franssila KO. Is the differentiation between papillary and follicular thyroid carcinoma valid? Cancer 1973;32:853-864.
13. Raphael SJ, McKeown-Eyssen G, Asa SL. High-molecular-weight cytokeratin and cytokeratin-19 in the diagnosis of thyroid tumors. Mod Pathol 1994;7:295-300.
14. Schelfhout LJDM, Van Muijen GNP, Fleuren GJ. Expression of keratin 19 distinguishes papillary thyroid carcinoma from follicular carcinoma and follicular thyroid adenoma. Am J Clin Pathol 1989;92:654-658.
15. Figge J, del Rosario AD, Gerasimov G, Dedov I, Bronstein M, Troshina K, Alexandrova G, Kallakury B, Bui HX, Bratslavsky G, Ross JS. Preferential expression of the cell adhesion molecule CD44 in papillary thyroid carcinoma. Exp Mol Pathol 1994;61:203-211.
16. Chhieng DC, Ross JS, Mckenna BJ. CD44 immunostaining of thyroid fine-needle aspirates differentiates thyroid papillary carcinoma from other lesions with nuclear grooves and inclusions. Cancer 1997;81:157-162.
17. Ott RA, McCall AR, McHenry C, Jarosz H, Armin A, Lawrence AM, Paloyan E. The incidence of thyroid carcinoma in Hashimoto's thyroiditis. Am Surg 1987;53:442-445.
18. McConahey WM, Hay ID, Woolner LB, van Heerden JA, Taylor WF. Papillary thyroid cancer treated at the Mayo Clinic, 1946 through 1970: initial manifestations, pathologic findings, therapy and outcome. Mayo Clin Proc 1986;61:978-996.
19. Christensen SB, Ljungberg O, Tibblin S. Thyroid carcinoma in Malmo, 1960-1977: epidemiologic, clinical and prognostic findings in a defined urban population. Cancer 1984;53:1625-1633.
20. Howard RB, Truels WP. Thyroid cancer: 30 year review of 201 cases. Am J Surg 1979;138:934-938.
21. Schindler A-M, van Melle G, Evequoz B, Scazziga B. Prognostic factors in papillary carcinoma of the thyroid. Cancer 1991;68:324-330.
22. Tscholl-Ducommun J, Hedinger CE. Papillary thyroid carcinomas. Morphology and prognosis. Virchows Arch (A) 1982;396:19-39.
23. Lindsay S. Carcinoma of the thyroid gland. A clinical and pathologic study of 293 patients at the University of California Hospital. Springfield, IL. Charles C Thomas, 1960.
24. Chen KT, Rosai J. Follicular variant of thyroid papillary carcinoma: a clinicopathologic study of six cases. Am J Surg Pathol 1977;1:123-130,
25, Rosai J, Zampi G, Carcangiu ML. Papillary carcinoma of the thyroid: a discussion of its several morphologic expressions with particular emphasis on the follicular variant. Am J Surg Pathol 1983;7:809-817.
26. Hawk WA, Hazard JB. The many appearances of papillary carcinoma of the thyroid. Cleveland Clin Quart 1976;43:207-216.
27. Schröder S, Böcker W, Dralle H, Kortman K-B, Stern C. The encapsulated papillary carcinoma of the thyroid. A morphologic subtype of the papillary thyroid carcinoma. Cancer 1984;54:90-93.
28. Evans HL. Encapsulated papillary neoplasms of the thyroid. A study of 14 cases followed for a minimum of 10 years. Am J Surg Pathol 1987;11:592-597.
29. Carcangiu ML, Bianchi S. Diffuse sclerosing variant of papillary thyroid carcinoma. Clinicopathologic study of 15 cases. Am J Surg Pathol 1989;13:1041-1049.
30. Soares J, Limbert E, Sobrinho-Simões M. Diffuse sclerosing variant of papillary thyroid carcinoma. A clinicopathologic study of 10 cases. Pathol Res Pract 1989;185:200-206.

31. Fujimoto Y, Obara T, Ito Y, Kodama T, Aiba M, Yamaguchi K. Diffuse sclerosing variant of papillary carcinoma of the thyroid. Cancer 1990;66:2306-2312.

32. Harach HR, Williams GT, Williams ED. Familial adenomatous polyposis thyroid carcinoma: a distinct type of follicular cell neoplasm. Histopathology 1994;25:549-561.

33. Peters SB, Chatten I, LiVolsi VA. Pediatric papillary thyroid carcinoma. Modern Pathol 1994;7: 55A.

34. Heffess C, Adair C, Thompson L, Wenig B. Morphologic patterns and clinicopathologic features of papillary thyroid carcinoma in children. Modern Pathol 1995;8:53A.

35. Mizukami Y, Noguchi M, Michigishi T, Nonomura A, Hashimoto T, Otake S, Nakamura S, Matsubara F. Papillary thyroid carcinoma in Kanazawa, Japan: prognostic significance of histological subtypes. Histopathology 1992;20:243-250.

36. Nikiforov YE, Gnepp DR. Pediatric thyroid cancer after the Chernobyl disaster: Pathomorphologic study of 84 cases (1991-1992) from the Republic of Belarus. Cancer 1994;74:748-766.

37. Bogdanova T, Bragarnik M, Tronko ND, Harach HR, Thomas GA, Williams ED: Thyroid cancer in the Ukraine post Chernobyl. Thyroid 1995;5,Suppl 1:S-28.

38. Nikiforov YE, Rowland JM, Bove KE, Monforte-Munoz H, Fagin JA. Distinct pattern of ret oncogene rearrangements in morphologic variants of radiation-induced and sporadic thyroid papillary carcinomas in children. Cancer Research 1997;57:1690-1694.

39. Nikiforov YE, Fagin JA, Biddinger P. Association of different ret/PTC rearrangements with behavior and morphology of pediatric papillary carcinoma. Modern Pathol 1998;11:58A.

40. Ostrowski ML, Merino MJ. Tall cell variant of papillary thyroid carcinoma. A reassessment and immunohistochemical study with comparison to the usual type of papillary carcinoma of the thyroid. Am J Surg Pathol 1996;20:964-974.

41. Wenig BM, Heffess CS, Adair CF. Atlas of Endocrine Pathology. Philadelphia: W. B. Saunders, 1997.

42. Johnson TL, Lloyd RV, Thompson NW, Beierwaltes WH, Sisson JC. Prognostic implications of the tall cell variant of papillary thyroid carcinoma. Am J Surg Pathol 1988;12:22-27.

43. Evans HL. Columnar-cell carcinoma of the thyroid. A report of two cases of an aggressive variant of thyroid carcinoma. Am J Clin Pathol 1986;85:77-80.

44. Sobrinho-Simões M, Nesland J, Johannessen J. Columnar-cell carcinoma. Another variant of poorly differentiated carcinoma of the thyroid. Am J Clin Pathol 1988;89:264-267.

45. Berends D. Mouthaan PJ. Columnar-cell carcinoma of the thyroid. Histopathology 1992;20:36-42.

46. Mizukami Y, Nonomura A, Michigishi T, Noguchi M, Nakamura S, Hashimoto T. Columnar cell carcinoma of the thyroid gland: a case report and review of the literature. Hum Pathol 1994;25:1098-1101.

47. Gaertner EM, Davidson M, Wenig BM. The columnar cell variant of papillary carcinoma. Case report and discussion of an unusually aggressive thyroid papillary carcinoma. Am J Surg Pathol 1995;19:940-947.

48. Akslen LA, Varhaug JE. Thyroid carcinoma with mixed tall-cell and columnar-cell features. Am J Clin Pathol 1990;94:442-445.

49. Wenig BM, Thompson LDR, Adair CF, Heffess CS. Columnar cell variant of thyroid papillary carcinoma. Mod Pathol 1995;8:56A.

50. Evans HL. Encapsulated columnar-cell neoplasms of the thyroid. A report of four cases suggesting a favorable prognosis. Am J Surg Pathol 1996;20:1205-1211.

51. Berho M, Suster S. The oncocytic variant of papillary carcinoma of the thyroid: a clinicopathologic study of 15 cases. Hum Pathol 1997;28:47-53.

52. Herrera MF, Hay ID, Wu PS-C, Goellner JR, Ryan JJ, Ebersold JR, Bergstralh EJ, Grant CS. Hürthle cell (oxyphilic) papillary carcinoma of the thyroid: a variant with more aggressive biologic behavior. World J Surg 1992;16:669-675.

53. Barbuto D, Carcangiu ML, Rosai J. Papillary Hürthle cell neoplasms of the thyroid gland. A study of 20 cases. Mod Pathol 1990;3:7A.

54. Joensuu H, Klemi P, Eerola E. DNA aneuploidy in follicular adenomas of the thyroid gland. Am J Pathol 1986;124:373-376.

55. Hostetter AL, Hrafnkelsson J, Wingren SO, Enestrom S, Jordenskjöld B. A comparative study of DNA cytometry methods for benign and malignant thyroid tissue. Am J Clin Pathol 1988;89:760-763.

56. Hruban RH, Huvos AG, Traganos F, Reuter V, Leiberman PH, Melamed MR. Follicular
     neoplasms of the thyroid in men older than 50 years of age. A DNA flow cytometric study. Am J
     Clin Pathol 1990;94:527-532.

57. Carney JA, Ryan J, Goellner JR. Hyalinizing trabecular adenoma of the thyroid gland. Am J Surg
     Pathol 1987;11:583-591.

58. Li M, Carcangiu ML, Rosai J. Abnormal intracellular and extracellular distribution of basement
     membrane material in papillary carcinoma and hyalinizing trabecular tumors of the thyroid:
     implications for deregulation of secretory pathways. Hum Pathol 1997;28:1366-1372.

59. Katoh R, Jasani B, Williams ED. Hyalinizing trabecular adenoma of the thyroid. A report of three
     cases with immunohistochemical and ultrastructural studies. Histopathology 1989;15:211-224.

60. Bronner MP, LiVolsi VA, Jennings TA. Plat: paraganglioma-like adenomas of the thyroid. Surg
     Pathol 1988;1:383-389.

61. Molberg K, Albores-Saavedra J. Hyalinizing trabecular carcinoma of the thyroid gland. Hum
     Pathol 1994;25:192-197.

62. Hazard JB, Kenyon R. Atypical adenoma of the thyroid. Arch Pathol 1954;58:554-563.

63. LiVolsi VA, Asa SL. The demise of follicular carcinoma of the thyroid. Thyroid 1994;4:233-236.

64. Cuello C, Correa P, Eisenberg H. Geographic pathology of thyroid carcinoma. Cancer
     1969;23:230-239.

65. Belfiore A, LaRosa GL, Padova G, Sava L, Ippolito O, Vigneri R. The frequency of cold thyroid
     nodules and thyroid malignancies in patients from an iodine-deficient area. Cancer 1987;60:3096-
     3102.

66. Franssila KO, Ackerman LV, Brown CL, Hedinger CE. Follicular carcinoma. Semin Diagn Pathol
     1985;2:101-122.

67. Carcangiu ML, Zampi G, Rosai J. Poorly differentiated ("insular") thyroid carcinoma: A
     reinterpretation of Langhans' "wuchernde Struma". Am J Surg Pathol 1984;8:655-668.

68. Massin JP, Savoie JC, Garnier H, Guiraudon G, Leger FA, Bacourt F. Pulmonary metastasis in
     differentiated thyroid carcinoma. Study of 58 cases with implications for the primary tumor
     treatment. Cancer 1984;53:982-992.

69. Evans HL. Follicular neoplasms of the thyroid. Cancer 1984;54:535-540.

70. Nagamine Y, Suzuki J, Katakura R, Yoshimoto T, Matoba N, Takaya K. Skull metastasis of
     thyroid carcinoma. Study of 12 cases. J Neurosurg 1985;63:526-531.

71. Lang W, Choritz H, Hundeshagen H. Risk factors in follicular thyroid carcinomas. A retrospective
     follow-up study covering a 14-year period with emphasis on morphological findings. Am J Surg
     Pathol 1986;10:246-255.

72. Simpson WJ, McKinney SE, Carruthers JS, Gospodarowicz MK, Sutcliffe SB, Panzarella T.
     Papillary and follicular thyroid carcinoma. Prognostic factors in 1,578 patients. Am J Med
     1987;83:479-488.

73. Shaha AR, Loree TR, Shah JP. Prognostic factors and risk group analysis in follicular carcinoma
     of the thyroid. Surg 1995;118:1131-1136.

74. Hürthle K. Beitrage zur Kenntiss der Secretionsvorgangs in der Schilddruse. Arch Gesamte
     Physiol 1894;56:1-44.

75. Bronner MP, LiVolsi VA. Oxyphilic (Askanazy/Hürthle cell) tumors of the thyroid: microscopic
     features predict biologic behavior. Surg Pathol 1988;1:137-150.

76. Watson RG, Brennen MD, Goellner JR, van Heerden JA, McConahey WM, Taylor WF. Invasive
     Hürthle cell carcinoma of the thyroid: natural history and management. Mayo Clin Proc
     1984;59:851-855.

77. Carcangiu ML, Bianchi S, Savino D, Voynick IM, Rosai J. Follicular Hürthle cell neoplasms of
     the thyroid gland. A study of 153 cases. Cancer 1991;68:1944-1953.

78. Tollefsen HR, Shah JP, Huvos AG. Hürthle cell carcinoma of the thyroid. Am J Surg
     1975;130:390-394.

79. Evans HL, Vassilopoulou R. Hurthle cell and follicular carcinomas of the thyroid: a comparative
     study. Mod Pathol 1998;11:56A.

80. Apel RL, Asa SL, LiVolsi VA. Papillary Hürthle cell carcinoma with lymphocytic stroma:
     "Warthin-like tumor" of the thyroid. Am J Surg Pathol 1995;19:810-814.

81. Langhans T. Über die epithelialen Formen der malignen Struma. Virchows Arch Pathol Anat
     1907;189:69-188.

82. Meissner WA, Warren S. Tumors of the thyroid gland. Washington: Armed Forces Institute of
     Pathology, 1969.

83. Papotti M, Botto Micca F, Favero A, Palestini N, Bussolati G. Poorly differentiated thyroid carcinomas with primordial cell component. A group of aggressive lesions sharing insular, trabecular, and solid patterns. Am J Surg Pathol 1993;17:291-301.

84. Pilotti S, Collini P, Mariani L, Placucci M, Bongarzone I, Vigneri P, Cipriani S, Falcetta F, Miceli R, Pierotti MA, Rilke F. Insular carcinoma. A distinct de novo entity among follicular carcinomas of the thyroid gland. Am J Surg Pathol 1997;21:1466-1473.

85. Flynn SD, Forman BH, Stewart AF, Kinder BK. Poorly differentiated ("insular") carcinoma of the thyroid gland: an aggressive subset of differentiated thyroid neoplasms. Surgery 1988;104:963-970.

86. Killeen RM, Barnes L, Watson CG, Marsh WL, Chase DW, Schuller DE. Poorly differentiated ('insular') thyroid carcinoma. Arch Otolaryngol Head Neck Surg 1990;116:1082-1086.

87. Pilotti S, Collini P, Del Bo R, Cattoretti G, Pierotti MA, Rilke F. A novel panel of antibodies that segregates immunocytochemically poorly differentiated carcinoma from undifferentiated carcinoma of the thyroid gland. Am J Surg Pathol 1994;18:1054-1064.

88. Carr K, Heffess C, Jin L, Lloyd R. Immunohistochemical analysis of thyroid carcinomas utilizing antibodies to p53 and Ki-67. Applied Immunohistochemistry 1993; 1:201-207.

89. Dobashi Y, Sakamoto A, Sugimura H, Mernyei M, Mori M, Oyama T, Machinami R. Overexpression of p53 as a possible prognostic factor in human thyroid carcinoma. Am J Surg Pathol 1993;17:375-381.

90. Soares P, Cameselle-Teijeiro J, Sobrinho-Simoes M. Immunohistochemical detection of p53 in differentiated, poorly differentiated and undifferentiated carcinomas of the thyroid. Histopathology 1994;24:205-210.

91. Sakamoto A, Kasai N, Sugano H. Poorly differentiated carcinoma of the thyroid. A clinicopathologic entity for a high-risk group of papillary and follicular carcinomas. Cancer 1983;52:1849-1855.

92. Sobrinho-Simões M. Tumours of thyroid: a brief overview with emphasis on the most controversial issues. Curr Diag Pathol 1995;2:15-22.

93. Carcangiu ML, Steeper T, Zampi G, Rosai J. Anaplastic thyroid carcinoma. A study of 70 cases. Am J Clin Pathol 1985;83:135-158.

94. Nel CJC, van Heerden JA, Goellner JR, Gharib H, McConahey WM, Taylor WM, Grant CS. Anaplastic carcinoma of the thyroid: a clinicopathologic study of 82 cases. Mayo Clin Proc 1985;60:51-58.

95. Rosai J, Saxen EA, Woolner L. Undifferentiated and poorly differentiated carcinoma. Sem Diag Pathol 1985;2:123-136.

96. Venkatesh YSS, Ordonez NG, Schultz PN, Hickey RC, Goefert H, Samaan NA. Anaplastic carcinoma of the thyroid. A clinicopathologic study of 121 cases. Cancer 1990;66:321-330.

97. Gaffey MJ, Lack EE, Christ ML, Weiss LM. Anaplastic thyroid carcinoma with osteoclast-like giant cells. A clinicopathologic, immunohistochemical, and ultrastructural study. Am J Surg Pathol 1991;15:160-168.

98. Miettinen M, Franssila K, Lehto V-P, Paasivuo R, Virtanen I. Expression of intermediate filament proteins in thyroid gland and thyroid tumors. Lab Invest 1984;50:262-270.

99. Hurlimann J, Gardiol D, Scazziga B. Immunohistology of anaplastic thyroid carcinoma. A study of 43 cases. Histopathology 1987;11:567-580.

100. Ordóñez NG, el-Naggar AK, Hickey RC, Samaan NA. Anaplastic thyroid carcinoma. Immunocytochemical study of 32 cases. Am J Clin Pathol 1991;96:15-24.

101. LiVolsi VA, Brooks JJ, Arendash-Durand B. Anaplastic thyroid tumors: immunohistology. Am J Clin Pathol 1987;87:434-442.

102. Wilson NW, Pambakian H, Richardson TC, Stokoe MR, Makin CA, Heyderman E. Epithelial markers in thyroid carcinoma: an immunoperoxidase study. Histopathology 1986;10:815-829.

103. Albores-Saavedra J, Nadji M, Civantos F, Morales AR. Thyroglobulin in carcinoma of the thyroid: an immunohistochemical study. Hum Pathol 1983;14:62-66.

104. Ryff-de Leche A, Staub JJ, Kohler-Faden R, Muller-Brand J, Heitz PU. Thyroglobulin production by malignant thyroid tumors. An immunocytochemical and radioimmunoassay study. Cancer 1986;57:1145-1153.

105. Hazard JB, Crile G Jr, Dinsmore RS, Hawk WA, Kenyon R. Neoplasms of the thyroid; classification, morphology, and treatment. Arch Pathol 1955;59:502-513.

106. Hazard JB, Hawk WA, Crile G Jr. Medullary (solid) carcinoma of the thyroid - a clinicopathologic entity. J Clin Endocrinol Metab 1959;19:152-161.

107. Jaquet J. Ein Fall von metastasierenden Amyloidtumoren (Lymphosarkom). Virchows Arch Pathol Anat 1906;185:251-268.
108. Stoffel E. Lokales Amyloid der Schilddrüse. Virchows Arch Pathol Anat 1910;210:245-252.
109. Horn RC Jr. Carcinoma of the thyroid. Description of a distinctive morphological variant and report of seven cases. Cancer 1951;4:697-707.
110. Williams ED. Histogenesis of medullary carcinoma of the thyroid. J Clin Path 1966;19:114-118.
111. Meyer JS, Abdel-Bari W. Granules and thyrocalcitonin like activity in medullary carcinoma of the thyroid gland. N Engl J Med 1968;278:523-529.
112. Bussolati G, Foster GV, Clark MB, Pearse AGE. Immunofluorescent localisation of calcitonin in medullary (c cell) thyroid carcinoma, using antibody to the pure porcine hormone. Virchows Arch Abt Zellpath 1969;2:234-238.
113. Ledger GA, Khosla S, Lindor NM, Thibodeau, Gharib H. Genetic testing in the diagnosis and management of multiple endocrine neoplasia type II. Ann Intern Med 1995;122:118-124.
114. Eng C, Clayton D, Schuffenecker I, Lenoir G, Cote G, Gagel RF, van Amstel HKP, Lips CJM, Nishisho I, Takai S-I, Marsh DJ, Robinson BG, Frank-Raue K, Raue F, Xue F, Noll WW, Romei C, Pacini F, Fink M, Niederle B, Zedenius J, Nordenskjöld M, Komminoth P, Hendy GN, Gharib H, Thibodeau SN, Lacroix A, Frilling A, Ponder BAJ, Mulligan LM. The relationship between specific RET proto-oncogene mutations and disease phenotype in multiple endocrine neoplasia type 2. JAMA 1996;276:1575-1579.
115. Uribe M, Grimes M, Fenoglio-Preiser CM, Feind C. Medullary carcinoma of the thyroid gland. Clinical, pathological, and immunocytochemical features with review of the literature. Am J Surg Pathol 1985;9:577-594.
116. Sikri KL, Varndell IM, Hamib QA, Wilson BS, Kameya T, Ponder BAJ, Lloyd RV, Bloom SR, Polak JM. Medullary carcinoma of the thyroid. An immunocytochemical and histochemical study of 25 cases using eight separate markers. Cancer 1985;56:2481-2491.
117. Steenbergh PH, Höppener JW, Zandberg J, van de Ven WJ, Jansz HS, Lips CJ. Calcitonin gene related peptide coding sequence is conserved in the human genome and is expressed in medullary thyroid carcinoma. J Clin Endocrinol Metab 1984;59:358-360.
118. Schröder S, Böcker W, Baisch H, Bürk CG, Arps H, Meiners I, Kastendieck H, Heitz PU, Klöppel G. Prognostic factors in medullary thyroid carcinoma. Survival in relation to age, sex, stage, histology, immunocytochemistry, and DNA content. Cancer 1988;61:806-816.
119. Santa G. Carcangiu ML, Rosai J. The biochemical and immunohistochemical profile of thyroid neoplasia. Pathol Annu 1988;23:129-157.
120. de Micco C, Chapel F, Dor A-M, Garcia S, Ruf J, Carayon P, Henry J-F, Lebreuil G. Thyroglobulin in medullary carcinoma: immunohistochemical study with polyclonal and monoclonal antibodies. Hum Pathol 1993;24:256-262.
121. Hales M, Rosenau W, Okerlund MD, Galante M. Carcinoma of the thyroid with a mixed medullary and follicular pattern: morphologic, immunohistochemical and clinical laboratory studies. Cancer 1982;50:1352-1359.
122. Pflatz M, Hedinger CH, Muhlethaler JP. Mixed medullary and follicular carcinoma of the thyroid. Virchows Arch (A) 1983;400:53-59.
123. Ljungberg O, Bondeson L, Bondeson A-G. Differentiated thyroid carcinoma, intermediate type: a new tumor entity with features of follicular and parafollicular cell carcinoma. Hum Pathol 1984;15:218-228.
124. Albores-Saavedra J, Gorraez de la Mora T, de la Torre-Rendon F, Gould E. Mixed medullary-papillary carcinoma of the thyroid: a previously unrecognized variant of thyroid carcinoma. Hum Pathol 1990;21:1151-1155.
125. Heshmati HM, Gharib H, van Heerden JA, Sizemore GW. Advances and controversies in the diagnosis and management of medullary thyroid carcinoma. Am J Med 1997;103:60-69.
126. Brierly J, Tsang R, Simpson WJ, Gospadarowicz M, Sutcliffe S, Panzarella T. Medullary thyroid carcinoma: analyses of survival and prognostic factors and the role of radiation therapy in local control. Thyroid 1996;6:305-310.
127. Bergholm V, Adami H-O, Auer G, Bergström R, Bäckdahl M, Grimelius L, Hansson G, Ljungberg O, Wilander E. Histopathologic characteristics and nuclear DNA content as prognostic factors in medullary thyroid carcinoma. A nationwide study in Sweden. Cancer 1989;64:135-142.
128. Viale G, Roncalli M, Grimelius L, Graziani D, Wilander E, Johansson H, Bergholm U, Coggi G. Prognostic value of Bcl-2 immunoreactivity in medullary thyroid carcinoma. Hum Pathol 1995;26:945-950.

129. Saad MF, Ordonez NG, Rashid RK, Guido JJ, Hill CS Jr, Hickey RC, Samaar NA. Medullary carcinoma of the thyroid: a study of the clinical features and prognostic factors in 161 patients. Medicine 1984;63:319-342.

130. Dottorini ME, Assi A, Sironi M, Sangalli G, Spreafico G, Columbo L. Multivariate analysis of patients with medullary thyroid carcinoma. Prognostic significance and impact on treatment of clinical and pathologic variables. Cancer 1996;77:1556-1565.

131. Heimann R, Vannineuse A, De Sloover C, Dor P. Malignant lymphomas and undifferentiated small carcinomas of the thyroid: a clinicopathologic review in the light of the Kiel classification for malignant lymphomas. Histopathology 1978;2:201-213.

132. Compagno J, Oertel JE. Malignant lymphoma and other lymphoproliferative disorders of the thyroid gland. A clinicopathologic study of 245 cases. Am J Clin Pathol 1980;74:1-11.

133. Oertel JE. Heffess CS. Lymphoma of the thyroid and related disorders. Semin Oncol 1987;14:333-342.

134. Thompson LDR, Derringer GA, Abbondanzo SI, Heffess CS. Primary malignant lymphomas of the thyroid gland: A clinicopathologic study of 109 cases. Modern Pathol 1998;11:59A.

135. Allevato PA, Kini SR, Rebuck JW, Miller JM, Hamburger JI. Signet ring cell lymphoma of the thyroid: a case report. Hum Pathol 1985;16:1066-1068.

136. McDermott EWM, Cassidy N, Heffernan SJ. Perforation through undiagnosed small bowel involvement in primary thyroid lymphoma during chemotherapy. Cancer 1992;69:572-573.

137. Stone CW, Slease RB, Brubaker D, Fabian C, Grozea PN. Thyroid lymphoma with gastrointestinal involvement: report of three cases. Am J Hematol 1986;21:357-365.

138. Devine RM, Edis AJ, Banks PM. Primary lymphoma of the thyroid: a review of the Mayo Clinic experience through 1978. World J Surg 1981;5:33-38.

139. Aozasa K, Inoue A, Tajima K, Miyauchi A, Matsuzuka F, Kuma K. Malignant lymphoma of the thyroid gland. Analysis of 79 patients with emphasis on histologic prognostic factors. Cancer 1986;58:100-104.

140. Matsuzuka F, Miyauchi A, Katayama S, Norabayashi I, Ikeda H, Kuma K, Sugawara M. Clinical aspects of primary thyroid lymphoma: diagnosis and treatment based on our experience of 119 cases. Thyroid 1993;3:93-99.

141. Doria R, Jekel JF, Cooper D. The case for combined modality therapy. Cancer 1994;73:200-206.

142. LaGuette J, Matias-Guiu X, Rosai J. Thyroid paraganglioma: a clinicopathologic and immunohistochemical study of three cases. Am J Surg Pathol 1997;21:748-753.

143. Wenig BM, Adair CF, Heffess CS. Primary mucoepidermoid carcinoma of the thyroid gland: a report of six cases and a review of the literature of a follicular epithelial-derived tumor. Hum Pathol 1995;26:1099-1108.

144. Chan JKC, Albores-Saavedra J, Battifora H, Carcangiu ML, Rosai J. Sclerosing mucoepidermoid thyroid carcinoma with eosinophilia. A distinctive low-grade malignancy arising from the metaplastic follicles of Hashimoto's thyroiditis. Am J Surg Pathol 1991;15:438-448.

145. Sim SJ, Ro JY, Ordonez NG, Cleary KR, Ayala AG. Sclerosing mucoepidermoid carcinoma with eosinophilia of the thyroid: report of two patients, one with distant metastasis, and review of the literature. Hum Pathol 1997;28:1091-1096.

146. Hedinger CE. Geographic pathology of thyroid diseases. Pathol Res Pract 1981;171:285-292.

147. Chan JKC, Rosai J. Tumors of the neck showing thymic or related branchial pouch differentiation: a unifying concept. Hum Pathol 1991;22:349-367.

148. Ivy HK, Cancer metastatic to the thyroid: a diagnostic problem. Mayo Clin Proc 1984;59:856-859.

149. Ro JY, Guerrieri C, el-Naggar AK, Ordonez NG, Sorge JG, Ayala AG. Carcinomas metastatic to follicular adenomas of the thyroid gland. Report of two cases. Arch Pathol Lab Med 1994;118:551-556.

6 THYROID NODULES: APPROACHES TO DIAGNOSIS AND MANAGEMENT

Yogish C. Kudva, M.D., M.R.C.P. (U.K.)
Hossein Gharib, M.D., F.A.C.P., F.A.C.E.
Mayo Clinic, Rochester, Minnesota

Introduction

Nodules frequently occur in classic endocrine organs such as the thyroid, adrenal, and pituitary. Evaluation of unrelated clinical problems with increasing use of ever-improving imaging techniques has led to recognition of incidental nodules in most endocrine glands, including the thyroid. Most nodules are benign. The prevalence of nodules is highest in the thyroid gland. Thyroid nodules constitute a common, significant, and evolving part of clinical endocrine practice, with continuing controversies. Over the years, the approach to thyroid nodules has become more effective, with acceptance and increased appropriate use of fine-needle aspiration (FNA) cytology. Furthermore, randomized clinical trials of levothyroxine (T4) suppression therapy, with careful documentation of adverse effects, have ensured appropriate use of this option. We describe the prevalence, clinical evaluation, and diagnostic testing of thyroid nodules and review management guidelines, including percutaneous alcohol injection. Also, we discuss thyroid incidentalomas, pediatric thyroid nodules, and management of irradiated thyroid.

Clinical Importance

Prevalence Studies

The prevalence of thyroid nodules depends on the demography of the population studied, iodine sufficiency in the diet, exposure to ionizing irradiation, and the method of detection (1-3). The prevalence of thyroid nodules increases with age, and in the adult United States population, the prevalence of palpable thyroid nodules is 4% to 7% (4). The annual incidence of such nodules is 0.1% (4). Irradiation of the thyroid, especially in the pediatric population, results in an annual incidence of thyroid nodules of 2% (5). The peak incidence of thyroid nodules is 15 to 25 years after exposure to ionizing radiation (5). Nodules are detected with a several-fold increased frequency by high-resolution ultrasonography (6), during surgery (7), or at autopsy (8). Indeed, thyroid nodules were present at autopsy in 50% of patients with no clinically significant nodules (8). Of clinically solitary thyroid nodules, 50% represent a dominant nodule in a multinodular goiter (9). Therefore, "nodular thyroid disease" is an appropriate term to address this common clinical problem.

Clinical Evaluation

Most thyroid nodules are asymptomatic and discovered by the patient or by a physician during neck palpation. They also may be detected during imaging or surgery for an unrelated clinical problem. Important questions at initial evaluation include the thyroid status of the patient and the risk of malignancy. Thyroid nodules are more likely to be malignant in men and children (1,2). Exposure to ionizing irradiation increases the risk of benign and malignant thyroid nodules (1). Rapid growth of the nodule and hoarseness related to recurrent laryngeal nerve infiltration suggest malignancy. Both features are uncommon in thyroid cancer. Physical examination should document the location, size, consistency, and mobility of the nodule and the presence of lymphadenopathy.

Diagnostic Tests

FNA

FNA cytology is the most important step in the management of thyroid nodules and has increasingly been practiced in the last 2 decades (2,10,11). It reliably distinguishes benign from malignant nodules. Satisfactory results from this procedure are dependent on performance and interpretation by experienced personnel. FNA has resulted in a decrease in the number of operations performed for benign thyroid disease and an increase in appropriate identification of malignant thyroid lesions requiring surgery (see also Chapter 10).

Technique. The best quality specimens are obtained by physicians who palpate the thyroid and perform FNA regularly. Traditionally, clinical endocrinologists and surgeons have performed this procedure. It is an office procedure performed with the patient supine. Maximal exposure is ensured by extending the patient's neck and resting the area between the shoulder blades on a sandbag or similar device. The area to be aspirated is identified by palpation, and the skin cleansed with alcohol wipes. Local anesthesia is unnecessary. A 1.5-inch 25-gauge needle attached to a 10-mL plastic syringe is used. Placing the syringe in a pistol-grip syringe holder is an option that our medical center has practiced to advantage. This practice allows the free hand to be used to palpate and fix the nodule. When the needle tip is in the nodule, suction is applied and the needle is moved gently up and down to sample the nodule extensively. The syringe may be detached from the needle so the aspirate can be visualized before the needle is withdrawn. The syringe is reattached to the needle, and the aspirate is gently forced out through the needle onto two to four slides. The slides are either placed immediately in 95% alcohol and prepared with a modified Papanicolaou stain or they are air dried and stained by the May-Grünwald technique. The aspiration may be repeated twice, providing the thyroid cytopathologist with 8 to 12 slides per procedure. After the procedure has been completed, local pressure is applied to the biopsy area with alcohol wipes or cotton pads. The patient is dismissed after a few minutes. Complications related to the procedure are exceedingly rare. Mild pain and a hematoma may occur but are self-limiting.

FNA Results. Optimal interpretation of cytologic specimens requires training in thyroid cytopathology. Specimens are classified as diagnostic or nondiagnostic. Even for experienced personnel, 10% of aspirations yield nondiagnostic specimens. Currently, the criteria for defining an adequate specimen have not been standardized (please see also Chapter 8). At most medical centers, diagnostic specimens are defined as two to three groups of 15 to 30 cells per slide on two to five slides. Diagnostic specimens may be benign (approximately 75% of specimens), suspicious (20%), or malignant (5%). The sensitivity, specificity, and accuracy of FNA in identifying malignancy have been confirmed by several series (12-14). A recent review reported combined data from two institutions (15). Of 16,576 FNA specimens, 15.7% were nondiagnostic. Of the 84.3% diagnostic specimens, 68.5% were benign, 3.5% were malignant, and the other 28% were indeterminate, and 2,577 nodules were excised. The sensitivity, specificity, and accuracy were 98%, 99%, and 98%, respectively. Different cytologic diagnostic categories of thyroid FNA results are illustrated in Table 1.

Table 1. Cytopathologic Diagnostic Categories for Thyroid
Fine-Needle Aspiration Biopsy Specimens

Category	Examples
Diagnostic (satisfactory)	
Benign (negative)	Colloid nodule
	Hashimoto's thyroiditis
	Subacute thyroiditis
	Cyst
Suspicious (indeterminate)	Follicular neoplasm
	Hürthle cell neoplasm
	Other findings suggestive but not
	diagnostic of malignant lesion
Malignant (positive)	Papillary carcinoma
	Medullary carcinoma
	Anaplastic carcinoma
	Lymphoma
	Metastatic carcinoma
Nondiagnostic (unsatisfactory)	Foam cells only
	Cyst fluid only
	Too few follicular cells
	Excessive air drying
	Too much blood

Modified from Gharib (4). By permission of GEM Communications.

Special Considerations

Follicular Neoplasms. Follicular neoplasms pose a problem because malignancy in such neoplasms cannot be diagnosed on cytology. If the nodule is hyperfunctioning on thyroid scanning and serum thyroid-stimulating hormone (TSH) is suppressed, observation or lumpectomy is appropriate (see Management, below) (Fig. 1). When the serum concentration of TSH is normal, patients with follicular neoplasms should have surgery. Malignancy is found in only 10% to 15% of these nodules. Therefore, up to 85% of such patients may undergo an unnecessary operation. Risk factors for carcinoma in this subgroup of patients include younger age, nodule size greater than 4 cm, and fixed primary nodule (16). Of benign follicular adenomas, 80% stain positively for thyroid peroxidase, whereas less than 75% of follicular thyroid carcinomas are positive (17).

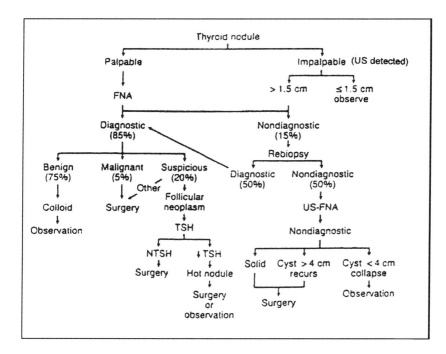

Fig. 1. Algorithm for management of nodular thyroid disease based on fine-needle aspiration (FNA). FNA is the test of choice. Additional management is based on FNA results. NTSH, normal TSH; TSH, thyroid-stimulating hormone; US-FNA, ultrasonographic FNA. (From Gharib [4]. By permission of GEM Communications.)

Probability of Malignancy. The probability of malignancy with each of the four interpretations of FNA is shown in Table 2. Benign cytology on FNA carries a 2% probability of malignancy. When the specimen is adequate for diagnosis, 12% ultimately shows carcinoma, consisting of 2% false-negative results (mentioned above), 5% to 6% malignant among those considered suspicious, and 4% to 5% malignant. The probability of carcinoma in suspicious nodules is 29%. When Hürthle cell or follicular neoplasia is suspected on FNA, the probability of such neoplasms is 13% and 14%, respectively. The probability of malignancy in smears interpreted as malignant is 95% to 100%. Of nondiagnostic smears, 50% provide satisfactory specimens on a second biopsy. At our medical center, 7% of nodules persistently nondiagnostic on FNA underwent surgery. The probability of malignancy in such patients is 12%. Therefore, it is prudent to evaluate further, to follow carefully, and to treat nondiagnostic nodules and to avoid labeling these nodules as "negative for malignancy" and concluding that they are likely benign.

Table 2. The Probability of Malignancy Based on Fine-Needle
Aspiration Cytology[*]

Cytology	Probability of malignancy, %	
Benign	2	
Nondiagnostic	12	
Diagnostic	12	
Suspicious	29	
Hürthle cell neoplasm		13
Follicular neoplasm		14
Papillary carcinoma		60
Malignant	99	

[*]Unpublished personal data based on 16,000 fine-needle aspiration results.

Medullary Thyroid Carcinoma.   The true prevalence of medullary thyroid carcinoma (MTC), cancer of the calcitonin-secreting C cells, is unknown. MTC may be sporadic (80%) or familial (20%). FNA is not a sensitive technique to diagnose MTC at an early stage when cure is possible (18). Sporadic MTC (SMTC) is diagnosed more often than not at surgery for suspicious FNA. Because MTC is more malignant than differentiated thyroid cancer, it is important to diagnose the disorder early (19). The approach to this clinical issue may be addressed by asking several questions: 1) What is the prevalence of SMTC among thyroidectomized patients? 2) How useful is the serum concentration of calcitonin in the preoperative diagnosis of SMTC? 3) How does one further evaluate patients with nondiagnostic increases in calcitonin concentration? 4) Is screening for SMTC cost-effective? Recent studies have addressed some of these questions.

In the only study to evaluate the prevalence of SMTC among patients undergoing thyroidectomy, 1.37% of 1,167 patients who had surgery for nodular thyroid disease (including euthyroid multinodular goiter, toxic multinodular goiter, and solitary nodules in euthyroid patients) has SMTC (20).   Tests to diagnose SMTC preoperatively include basal serum concentration of calcitonin, pentagastrin stimulation, and screening for mutations of the *RET* proto-oncogene. These tests have been studied by four different groups of investigators (20-23). The specificity of the assay used to estimate calcitonin concentration is an extremely important consideration when interpreting such studies.   Two of the four studies that addressed this issue used radioimmunoassay (21,23).   Rieu et al. (22) used radioimmunoassay for the first year, followed by immunoradiometric assay for the subsequent 4 years.   Pacini et al. (21) reported increased concentrations of calcitonin and MTC in 8 of 1,385 patients. Rieu et al. (22) reported similar findings in 4 of 469 patients. Neither study addressed the relevance of minimal increases in serum concentrations of calcitonin. Furthermore, the true prevalence of MTC was not determined, because thyroid exploration was undertaken only in patients with abnormal concentrations of calcitonin, FNA cytology, or both.

Niccoli et al. (20) used a two-site immunoradiometric assay and reported increased basal concentrations of calcitonin in 34 patients. At thyroidectomy, 41% of these patients showed foci of MTC. Serum concentrations of calcitonin that were increased to the extent diagnostic for MTC (> 200 pg/mL) were present in only five (35%) patients with MTC. Mild increases in the serum concentration of calcitonin were present in patients with autoimmune thyroid disease and differentiated thyroid cancer. Vierhapper et al. (23) described increased basal concentrations in serum calcitonin (> 6 pg/mL) in 55 patients. Basal levels greater than 100 pg/mL were described in three patients. Although a pentagastrin-induced increase above 100 pg/mL was present in 1 of 21 patients with basal concentrations of 6 to 10 pg/mL, 10 of 31 patients with basal concentrations of 10 to 100 pg/mL demonstrated a peak concentration greater than 100 pg/mL. Of these 14 patients, 12 underwent surgery and 6 of them had C-cell hyperplasia. Vierhapper et al. (23) recommended that measurements of the basal concentration of calcitonin be supplemented with pentagastrin testing in all patients with nodular thyroid disease and basal concentrations of calcitonin greater than 10 pg/mL.

Another solution to the problem of nodular thyroid disease, increased serum concentration of calcitonin, and benign FNA cytology is molecular testing for *RET* proto-oncogene mutations that cause hereditary MTC. However, because only 5% to 7% of patients with apparent SMTC have such germ-line mutations (24), *RET* proto-oncogene mutation testing probably is not cost-effective. Also, because prognosis in MTC is dependent on early diagnosis, additional studies are needed to answer the question of whether routine estimation of serum concentration of calcitonin in thyroid nodule evaluation is cost-effective in the long term.

Limitations of FNA

The limitations of FNA include nondiagnostic results, indeterminate or suspicious cytology, and false-negative results with malignant nodules.
Nondiagnostic results may occur in 10% to 15% of aspirations and depend on the nature of the nodules and the expertise of the clinician and cytologist (2,10). Predominantly cystic lesions are the most common cause of the nondiagnostic interpretation. Such lesions should be reaspirated, with or without ultrasonographic guidance. Experienced clinicians may repeat the procedure before resorting to ultrasonographically directed FNA. Persistently nondiagnostic results may warrant surgical excision. Surgery is also recommended for cysts larger than 4 cm and for recurrent cysts (25). Nodules with varied pathologic features may yield indeterminate results (10,26,27). Follicular neoplasia (see below), Hürthle cell neoplasia, and papillary carcinoma compose this group. Also, 20% to 30% of results may be indeterminate, and 20% of such lesions may ultimately prove to be malignant (10).

Radioisotope Thyroid Scan

Previously, thyroid scanning with radioiodine (^{123}I) and technetium (^{99m}Tc) isotopes was widely used in the evaluation of nodules but has been replaced by FNA. With scanning, nodules may be classified as hypofunctioning (cold), hyperfunctioning (hot), or indeterminate. Approximately 80% to 85% of nodules are cold, 5% are hot, and the rest are indeterminate (1). Malignancy occurs in only 5% to 15% of cold nodules. Therefore, a large proportion of positive scans (cold nodules) will be falsely positive. Hyperfunctioning (hot) nodules are often solitary in otherwise normal glands and are seldom malignant, but they may be clinically toxic (Fig. 2). Serum concentrations of TSH are commonly suppressed. Hot nodules are more common in women and are more likely to become toxic if greater than 3.0 cm in diameter (15). Thyroid scans have high sensitivity but very low specificity. The scan may help in the decision-making process of how to treat follicular neoplasms (see above). Thyroid scans are also useful in postoperative evaluation of differentiated thyroid cancer.

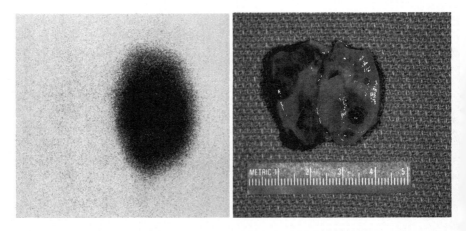

Fig. 2. *Left,* Technetium-99m pertechnetate scan in a 32-year-old woman with an autonomously functioning left lobe nodule, complete suppression of right lobe, and serum TSH 0.06 mIU/L. *Right,* Left lobectomy revealed a benign, 4 x 2.5-cm follicular adenoma. Postoperatively, serum TSH was 5.7 mIU/L.

Ultrasonography

Current ultrasonographic technology produces high-resolution thyroid images by using sound frequencies between 5 and 10 MHz. High-frequency sound waves are emitted by a transmitter that also acts as a receiver for returning echoes. Spatial resolution is outstanding for solid nodules as small as 3 mm in size and for cystic nodules as small as 2 mm, with high-resolution sonography (15,28). However, current sonography does not regularly and reliably differentiate benign from malignant nodules. Well-defined nodule margins, hyperechogenicity in comparison with surrounding thyroid tissue, and a peripheral eggshell pattern of calcification are characteristic features of benign nodules (Fig. 3) (5). Irregular nodule margins, hypoechoic changes, and microcalcifications suggest malignancy. High-resolution ultrasonography has documented solid components in all cystic lesions (Fig. 4). Therefore, according to current opinion, a "pure" cyst does not exist (15).

If FNA biopsy with direct palpation is unsuccessful, ultrasonographic-guided FNA may be used to aspirate nodules. Ultrasonography is extremely useful in the management of thyroid cancer. Early recurrence of cancer may be detected in the thyroid bed, and the number, size, and location of cervical nodes can be identified precisely and aspirated for cytology.

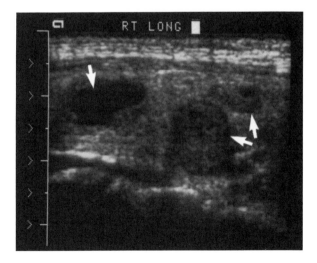

Fig. 3. Sonogram of the thyroid region in sagittal projection. Images demonstrate a 1.4-cm mass composed of equal amounts of solid and cystic tissue in the superior pole and two solid masses less than 1 cm in the inferior pole of the right thyroid lobe (*arrows*). US-FNA of solid lesions showed benign cytology. The combination of nodules suggests a multinodular gland.

Management

Single Nodule

Our approach to diagnosis and management of solitary thyroid nodules is summarized in the algorithm in Figure 1. When FNA cytology is benign, follow-up after 6 months and annually thereafter is recommended. Enlarging, recurrent cystic, and clinically suspicious nodules require reaspiration. Surgery is advised for patients with cytologically suspicious or malignant nodules. The type of thyroid surgery is decided on the basis of the subtype of thyroid cancer.

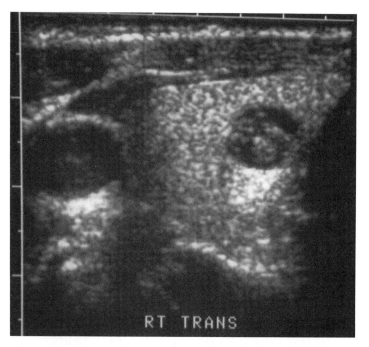

Fig. 4. Transverse sonogram of right thyroid lobe showing a 2-cm nodule with cystic and solid components. Fine-needle aspiration biopsy demonstrated benign follicular cells and colloid ("colloid nodule").

Some experts believe that routine frozen section may not avoid a second operation. Also, overreliance on the results of frozen sections in decision making may lead to unnecessary cancer surgery (29). On the basis of two studies, Hamburger et al. (29,30) recommended frozen sections only in patients with unsatisfactory FNA results or suspected malignancy. Frozen section is routinely used in all thyroid operations at the Mayo Clinic. The benefits of the procedure depend on the expertise of the pathologist and the resources available at the medical center (31). Routine use of frozen section may not be cost-effective at all medical centers. A solitary benign nodule is best treated with complete lobectomy. Optimal treatment for a multinodular goiter is subtotal thyroidectomy. Papillary and follicular thyroid carcinoma should be treated with total or near-total thyroidectomy, defined as ipsilateral total lobectomy and subtotal contralateral lobectomy. Total thyroidectomy with central node dissection is optimal for both types of MTC.

Multinodular Gland

The risk of malignancy in a multinodular gland is 5% to 10% (15). Dominant, enlarging, and otherwise clinically suspicious nodules should be aspirated. Thereafter, the management is not different from that for a solitary nodule. Patients with large glands and symptoms from pressure on surrounding structures should have surgical treatment unless they are a poor surgical risk. Asymptomatic patients with displacement of the airway should be evaluated further with flow volume loop testing to determine further management.

T4 Suppression

Several factors need to be considered when addressing the question of suppressive therapy for thyroid nodules (4).
1. Benign thyroid nodules represent a spectrum of pathologic entities (Table 3), each of which presumably has a different pathogenesis and natural history. Spontaneous decrease in the size or disappearance of nodules has been well documented in several studies. Kuma et al. (32) followed 134 patients with cytologically benign thyroid nodules for 9 to 11 years, and thyroid carcinoma (papillary) developed in only 1 patient. Also, 30% of nodules disappeared completely and 13% decreased in size, and 23% of solitary nodules increased in size and 33% remained stable.
2. Nodules with constitutive activation of the TSH receptor system do not respond to suppressive therapy.
3. Previous studies of suppression therapy with T_4 had several methodologic flaws, including 1) failure to characterize the number, size, and pathologic type of nodule; 2) failure to document TSH suppression; 3) lack of adequate controls; and 4) inadequate assessment of risk factors such as iodine deficiency and exposure to ionizing radiation.
4. TSH suppression causes significant cardiac and skeletal morbidity.

Several studies have considered the issues mentioned above (Table 3) (4). Although all eight studies were controlled (33-40), only four were placebo-controlled. Nodule type was determined by FNA, and nodule size was documented by ultrasonography. On combining data from these studies, 246 patients were treated with T_4 suppression and 209 served as controls. Study duration varied from 6 to 21 months. Second-generation TSH assays confirmed the success of T_4 therapy in most of these studies. Five studies showed no significant difference in nodule size between T_4-treated and control groups. However, three other studies showed a 31% to 58% reduction in nodule size.

Thyroidologists disagree about suppression therapy. Some (27) suggest T_4 therapy for 6 to 12 months, with target TSH concentrations between 0.1 and 0.5 mIU/L, and others (41) recommend a conservative approach for older patients and nodules smaller than 1.5 cm in size and suppressive therapy for other patients. Cooper (42) suppresses TSH below 0.1 mIU/L for 1 year in men and premenopausal women. Treatment is continued with a goal TSH near normal or management is conservative if the nodule shows response.

Table 3. Comparison of Response Rate in Eight Randomized Controlled Trials
of Thyroxine Suppressive Therapy for Nodular Thyroid Disease

| Study | Site | Patients, no. | | Nodule | Nodule Shrinkage, %[*] | Duration of Rx, mo |
		LT$_4$ Rx	Controls			
Gharib et al. (33)	USA	28	25 (P)	S	NS	6
Cheung et al. (34)	Hong Kong	37	37	S & M	NS	18
Berghout et al. (35)	Netherlands	26	26 (P)	M	58	9
Diacinti et al. (36)	Italy	16	19	S & M	31	9
Reverter et al. (37)	Spain	20	20	S	NS	11
Papini et al. (38)	Italy	51	50 (P)	S	NS	12
La Rosa et al. (39)	Italy	23	22 (P)	S	39	12
Mainini et al. (40)	Italy	45	10	S	NS	21

LT$_4$, levothyroxine; M, multiple; NS, not significant; P, placebo treatment in controls; Rx, therapy; S, single.

[*]Nodule shrinkage defined as > 50% decrease in nodule size or volume.
From Gharib (4). By permission of GEM Communications.

In general, patients with benign nodules benefit little from T_4 therapy. Spontaneous decrease in nodule size or even nodule disappearance is not uncommon, although most nodules remain unchanged when followed without therapy (43). Only a small group of patients (< 20%) with benign thyroid nodules may respond to suppression therapy. Because reliable predictive factors are not yet known, our approach is to avoid T_4 suppression and instead to follow patients who have benign nodular thyroid disease with neck palpation at 6 months and annually thereafter.

Adverse Effects of Suppressive Therapy. Bone mineral loss and cardiac effects are well-documented side effects of biochemical hyperthyroidism. Recently, studies have documented similar side effects with T_4 suppression (15,27,44). Bone mineral loss has been reported in postmenopausal women but not in premenopausal women or in men (15,27,44-46). Atrial fibrillation in the elderly may be increased threefold when TSH is suppressed (47). In postmenopausal women treated with the goal of TSH suppression, antiosteoporotic measures, including estrogen replacement, supplemental calcium, and occasionally bisphosphonates, may be strongly considered (41,48).

Percutaneous Alcohol Injection for Thyroid Nodules

Recently, percutaneous alcohol injection under ultrasonographic guidance has been used to treat solid and cystic thyroid nodules (49). Currently, this procedure is reserved for patients who are not candidates for conventional treatment because of medical reasons. No long-term follow-up is yet available for this new treatment.

This new treatment involves injection of 95% ethanol under ultrasonographic guidance with a 22- to 25-gauge needle. The injection may be performed once or twice weekly, with some patients requiring several injections. The disadvantages of this procedure include complications (local pain, fever, and recurrent laryngeal nerve trauma) and inconvenience.

Other Considerations

Thyroid Incidentalomas

An incidentaloma is defined as a mass lesion identified serendipitously in the absence of symptoms attributable to the lesion. Increasingly, thyroid incidentalomas are being diagnosed because of better imaging techniques and more frequent use of imaging. Thyroid incidentalomas are detected during imaging of the parathyroid glands and carotid arteries. Incidentalomas are impalpable and commonly smaller than 1.5 cm in diameter. Such lesions are present in at least 35% of healthy women and 20% of healthy men 20 to 50 years old (28). The low frequency of thyroid malignancy reassures us that most thyroid incidentalomas have little clinical significance and justifies conservative management. Nodules larger than 1.5 cm in size, nodules with ultrasonographic characteristics suspicious for malignancy, or patients with a history of thyroid irradiation require FNA. In the absence of such risk factors for thyroid carcinoma, follow-up palpation is recommended (28).

Thyroid Nodules in Children

The prevalence of thyroid nodules in children and adolescents (up to age 20) is considerably less than in adults. When nodules are present, they are more likely to be malignant, but this has been questioned recently. Recently, Gharib et al. (50) reported a series of 47 children who had FNA for thyroid nodules: 66% of the nodules were benign, 15% were malignant, 6% were suspicious, and 13% were nondiagnostic. Although some authors have recommended surgical excision of all thyroid nodules in children, this recent study confirms the reliability of FNA in children and suggests management based on cytologic results. Suppressive therapy is not recommended in children because of the obvious problems of long-term treatment and related lack of compliance.

Management of the Irradiated Thyroid

A low dose of irradiation to the thyroid increases the incidence of benign and malignant nodules. Lesions that develop in these patients show two peaks of incidence, at 3 to 5 years and at 15 to 30 years after exposure (2,5). Practical guidelines have been suggested by DeGroot (5). Management of patients with impalpable nodules after radiation exposure was reviewed in a decision analysis, with the conclusion that simple observation without additional studies or therapy is preferred (51). FNA biopsy and management based on cytology is appropriate for patients with palpable solitary nodules. Multinodular glands in these patients are best treated by near-total thyroidectomy. Suppressive therapy does not prevent development of nodules in people with previous irradiation of the thyroid (51). However, it may prevent the recurrence of nodules after partial thyroid resection in these patients (52).

Conclusions

Thyroid nodules are extremely common and show an age-dependent prevalence, ranging from 1% to 7%. Prevalence increases with age. High-resolution ultrasonography and neck surgery detect several-fold more nodules than palpation. FNA cytology performed by an experienced physician in combination with interpretation by an expert cytopathologist is the most appropriate diagnostic test. Most thyroid nodules are benign. Only 4% of nodules may be malignant, and most of these are papillary thyroid carcinomas. Thyroid scanning is useful if a nodule is associated with suppressed serum TSH (question of hot nodule) or if the size of the gland is important in management. High-resolution ultrasonography has limited application in nodule diagnosis but is widely used in cancer management. Currently, T_4 suppression is not considered useful in preventing nodule enlargement or in inducing nodule regression.

References

1.   Rojeski MT, Gharib H. Nodular thyroid disease. Evaluation and management. N Engl J Med 1985; 313:428.
2.   Mazzaferri EL. Management of a solitary thyroid nodule. N Engl J Med 1993; 328:553
3.   Gharib H. Fine-needle aspiration biopsy of thyroid nodules: advantages, limitations, and effect. Mayo Clin Proc 1994;69:44.
4.   Gharib H. Management of thyroid nodules: another look. Thyroid Today 1997; 20:1.
5.   DeGroot LJ. Diagnostic approach and management of patients exposed to irradiation to the thyroid. J Clin Endocrinol Metab 1989; 69:925.
6.   Brander A, Viikinkoski P, Nickels J, Kivisaari L. Thyroid gland: US screening in a random adult population. Radiology 1991; 181:683.
7.   Lever EG, Refetoff S, Straus FH II, Nguyen M, Kaplan EL. Coexisting thyroid and parathyroid disease—are they related? Surgery 1983; 94:893.
8.   Mortensen JD, Woolner LB, Bennett WA. Gross and microscopic findings in clinically normal thyroid glands. J Clin Endocrinol Metab 1955; 15:1270.

9.   Tan GH, Gharib H, Reading CC. Solitary thyroid nodule. Comparison between palpation and ultrasonography. Arch Intern Med 1995; 155:2418.

10. Gharib H, Goellner JR . Fine-needle aspiration biopsy of the thyroid: an appraisal. Ann Intern Med 1993; 118:282.

11. Solomon D. Fine needle aspiration of the thyroid: an update. Thyroid Today 1993; 16:1.

12. Merchant WJ, Thomas SM, Coppen MJ, Prentice MG. The role of thyroid fine needle aspiration (FNA) cytology in a District General Hospital setting. Cytopathology 1995;6:409.

13. Agrawal S. Diagnostic accuracy and role of fine needle aspiration cytology in management of thyroid nodules. J Surg Oncol 1995; 58:168.

14. Holleman F, Hoekstra JB, Ruitenberg HM. Evaluation of fine needle aspiration (FNA) cytology in the diagnosis of thyroid nodules. Cytopathology 1995; 6:168.

15. Giuffrida D, Gharib H. Controversies in the management of cold, hot, and occult thyroid nodules. Am J Med 1995; 99:642.

16. Schlinkert RT, van Heerden JA, Goellner JR, Gharib H, Smith SL, Rosales RF, Weaver AL. Factors that predict malignant thyroid lesions when fine-needle aspiration is "suspicious for follicular neoplasm." Mayo Clin Proc 1997; 72:913.

17. Henry JF, Denizot A, Porcelli A, Villafane M, Zoro P, Garcia S, De Micco C. Thyroperoxidase immunodetection for the diagnosis of malignancy on fine-needle aspiration of thyroid nodules. World J Surg 1994; 18:529.

18. Horvit PK, Gagel RF. The goitrous patient with an elevated serum calcitonin—what to do? (Editorial.) J Clin Endocrinol Metab 1997; 82:335.

19. Dunn JT. When is a thyroid nodule a sporadic medullary carcinoma? (Editorial.) J Clin Endocrinol Metab 1994; 78:824.

20. Niccoli P, Wion-Barbot N, Caron P, Henry JF, de Micco C, Saint Andre JP, Bigorgne JC, Modigliani E, Conte-Devolx B and the French Medullary Study Group. Interest of routine measurement of serum calcitonin: study in a large series of thyroidectomized patients. J Clin Endocrinol Metab 1997; 82:338.

21. Pacini F, Fonatanelli M, Fugazzola L, Elisei R, Romei C, Di Coscio G, Miccoli P, Pinchera A. Routine measurement of serum calcitonin in nodular thyroid diseases allows the preoperative diagnosis of unsuspected sporadic medullary thyroid carcinoma. J Clin Endocrinol Metab 1994; 78:826.

22. Rieu M, Lame MC, Richard A, Lissak B, Sambort B, Vuong-Ngoc P, Berrod JL, Fombeur JP. Prevalence of sporadic medullary thyroid carcinoma: the importance of routine measurement of serum calcitonin in the diagnostic evaluation of thyroid nodules. Clin Endocrinol (Oxf) 1995; 42:453

23. Vierhapper H, Raber W, Bieglmayer C, Kaserer K, Weinhausl A, Niederle B. Routine measurement of plasma calcitonin in nodular thyroid diseases. J Clin Endocrinol Metab 1997; 82: 1589.

24. Wohllk N, Cote GJ, Bugalho MM, Ordonex N, Evans DB, Goepfert H, Khorana S, Schultz P, Richards CS, Gagel RF. Relevance of RET proto-oncogene mutations in sporadic medullary thyroid carcinoma. J Clin Endocrinol Metab 1996; 81:3740.

25. McHenry CR, Walfish PG, Rosen IB. Non-diagnostic fine needle aspiration biopsy: a dilemma in management of nodular thyroid disease. Am Surg 1993; 59:415.

26. Gharib H, Goellner JR, Johnson DA. Fine-needle aspiration cytology of the thyroid. A 12-year experience with 11,000 biopsies. Clin Lab Med 1993; 13:699.

27. Burch HB. Evaluation and management of the solid thyroid nodule. Endocrinol Metab Clin North Am 1995; 24:663.

28. Tan GH, Gharib H. Thyroid incidentalomas: management approaches to nonpalpable nodules discovered incidentally on thyroid imaging. Ann Intern Med 1997; 126:226.

29. Hamburger JI, Husain M. Contribution of intraoperative pathology evaluation to surgical management of thyroid nodules. Endocrinol Metab Clin North Am 1990; 19:509.

30. Hamburger JI, Hamburger SW. Declining role of frozen section in surgical planning for thyroid nodules. Surgery 1985; 98:307.

31. Aguilar-Diosdado M, Contreras A, Gavilan I, Escobar-Jimenez L, Giron JA, Escribano JC, Beltran M, Garcia-Curiel A, Vazquez JM. Thyroid nodules. Role of fine needle aspiration and intraoperative frozen section examination. Acta Cytol 1997; 41:677.

32. Kuma K, Matsuzuka F, Yokozawa T, Miyauchi A, Sugawara M. Fate of untreated benign thyroid nodules: results of long-term follow-up. World J Surg 1994; 18:495.

33. Gharib H, James EM, Charboneau JW, Naessens JM, Offord KP, Gorman CA. Suppressive therapy with levothyroxine for solitary thyroid nodules. A double-blind controlled clinical study. N Engl J Med 1987; 317:70.

34. Cheung PS, Lee JM, Boey JH. Thyroxine suppressive therapy of benign solitary thyroid nodules: a prospective randomized study. World J Surg 1989; 13:818.

35. Berghout A, Wiersinga WM, Drexhage HA, Smits NJ, Touber JL. Comparison of placebo with L-thyroxine alone or with carbimazole for treatment of sporadic non-toxic goitre. Lancet 1990; 336:193.

36. Diacinti D, Salabe GB, Olivieri A, D'Erasmo E, Tomei E, Lotz-Salabe H, De Martinis C. Efficacy of L-thyroxine (L-T4) therapy on the volume of the thyroid gland and nodules in patients with euthyroid nodular goiter (ENG) [Italian]. Minerva Med 1992; 83:745.

37. Reverter JL, Lucas A, Salinas I, Audi L, Foz M, Sanmarti A. Suppressive therapy with levothyroxine for solitary thyroid nodules. Clin Endocrinol (Oxf) 1992; 36:25.

38. Papini E, Bacci V, Panunzi C, Pacella CM, Fabbrini R, Bizzarri G, Petrucci L, Giammarco V, La Medica P, Masala M, Pitaro M, Nardi F. A prospective randomized trial of levothyroxine suppressive therapy for solitary thyroid nodules. Clin Endocrinol (Oxf) 1993; 38:507.

39. La Rosa GL, Lupo L, Giuffrida D, Gullo D, Vigneri R, Belfiore A. Levothyroxine and potassium iodide are both effective in treating benign solitary solid cold nodules of the thyroid. Ann Intern Med 1995; 122:1.

40. Mainini E, Martinelli I, Morandi G, Villa S, Stefani I, Mazzi C. Levothyroxine suppressive therapy for solitary thyroid nodule. J Endocrinol Invest 1995; 18:796.

41. Daniels GH Thyroid nodules and nodular thyroids: a clinical overview. Compr Ther 1996; 22:239.

42. Cooper DS. Thyroxine suppression therapy for benign nodular disease. J Clin Endocrinol Metab 1995; 80:331.

43. Gharib H, Mazzaferri EL. Thyroxine suppressive therapy in patients with nodular thyroid disease. Ann Intern Med 1998; 128:_____.

44. Faber J, Galloe AM. Changes in bone mass during prolonged subclinical hyperthyroidism due to L-thyroxine treatment: a meta-analysis. Eur J Endocrinol 1994; 130:350.

45. Schneider DL, Barrett-Connor EL, Morton DJ. Thyroid hormone use and bone mineral density in elderly women. Effects of estrogen. JAMA 1994; 271:1245.

46. Stall GM, Harris S, Sokoll LJ, Dawson-Hughes B. Accelerated bone loss in hypothyroid patients overtreated with L-thyroxine. Ann Intern Med 1990; 113:265.

47. Sawin CT, Geller A, Wolf PA, Belanger AJ, Baker E, Bacharach P, Wilson PW, Benjamin EJ, D'Agostino RB. Low serum thyrotropin concentrations as a risk factor for atrial fibrillation in older persons. N Engl J Med 1994; 331:1249.

48. Wartofsky L. Levothyroxine therapy and osteoporosis. An end to the controversy? Arch Intern Med 1995; 155:1130.

49. Goletti O, Monzani F, Lenziardi M, Lippolis PV, De Negri F, Caraccio N, Cavina E, Baschieri L. Cold thyroid nodules: a new application of percutaneous ethanol injection treatment. J Clin Ultrasound 1994; 22:175.

50. Gharib H, Zimmerman D, Goellner JR, Bridley SM, LeBlanc SM. Fine-needle aspiration biopsy: use in diagnosis and management of pediatric thyroid diseases. Endocr Pract 1995; 1:9.

51. Stockwell RM, Barry M, Davidoff F Managing thyroid abnormalities in adults exposed to upper body irradiation in childhood: a decision analysis. Should patients without palpable nodules be scanned and those with scan defects be subjected to subtotal thyroidectomy? J Clin Endocrinol Metab 1984; 58:804.

52. Fogelfeld L, Wiviott MB, Shore-Freedman E, Blend M, Bekerman C, Pinsky S, Schneider AB. Recurrence of thyroid nodules after surgical removal in patients irradiated in childhood for benign conditions. N Engl J Med 1989; 320:835.

7 PATHOGENESIS AND TREATMENT OF MULTINODULAR GOITER

Michael Derwahl
University Clinics of Bochum
Germany

Hugo Studer
Bern, Switzerland

Introduction

It may not be altogether evident, why a chapter on multinodular goiter is included in this book on thyroid *cancer,* since the transformation of the thyroid gland into a multinodular goiter has been considered during a whole century to result from a non-neoplastic, adaptive process triggered and maintained by iodine deficiency. However, within the past two decades, multinodular goiter and, in particular, goiter nodules have gradually been moved into the list of true thyroid neoplasias. This chapter will therefore focus on the events that entailed this shift of paradigm[1].

Definition of multinodular goiter (MNG)

MNG is an enlargement of the thyroid gland due to multifocal, clonal or polyclonal proliferation of thyrocytes that produce functionally and morphologically widely heterogeneous cohorts of new follicles or follicle-like structures.

The newly generated tissue either forms one of two types of sharply delimitated lesions (i.e. adenomas and thyroid nodules), but more often, the new follicles are embedded within normal thyroid tissue without recognizable boundaries between the two structures.

---

[1] Exhaustive reviews of the experimental data discussed in the eight first sections of this chapter are presented in references 1, 2, 3 and 4.

Definitions of »adenoma«, »thyroid nodule« and »pseudonodule«

3 Components of Multinodular Goiters

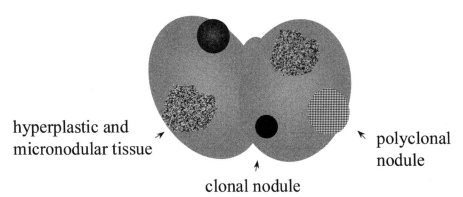

hyperplastic and
micronodular tissue

polyclonal
nodule

clonal nodule

Figure 1. The 3 components of multinodular goiter: clonal nodules or adenomas, polyclonal nodules and hyperplastic and micronodular tissues.

According to WHO criteria, a thyroid adenoma is defined as a well circumscribed, phenotypically uniform thyroid lesion (5). However, since the time this definition has been coined, two important findings have revealed a) that adenomas as defined by WHO criteria are usually clonal tumors (6-10) and b) that phenotypical uniformity is by no means an invariable feature of these clonal tumors (11). Accordingly, the term »adenoma« is used here to describe a *sharply delimitated, clonal* thyroid tumor, whose morphological structure is strictly distinct from that of the surrounding tissue. The term »clonal« refers to the progeny of a single mother cell. Moreover, we restrict the term »adenoma« to *functionally homogeneous* - i.e. either »cold« or »hot« - lesions.

The term »**thyroid nodule**« as used in this chapter, applies to a *sharply delimitated, clonal or polyclonal* thyroid lesion of *heterogeneous structure and function*. The anatomical structure of a »thyroid nodule« is clearly different from that of normal thyroid tissue, but may be identical to that of the surrounding goitrous tissue proliferating in a non-nodular fashion. The term »polyclonal« refers to the progeny of an unknown number of different mother cells.

The term »**pseudonodule**« describes a *macroscopically nodular* lesion which is, however, *poorly or only partially* (i.e. in only part of its circumference) *delimitated from the surrounding, identically structured goiter* tissue. Pseudonodules arise from the proliferation of morphologically and functionally heterogeneous follicles squeezed into the spiderlike meshes of inextensible strands of connective tissue, which results from scarring of the invariable necroses occurring within expanding goiters (1).

The role of iodine deficiency in the pathogenesis of MNG: A critical reappraisal

Due to the spectacular success of preventive medicine in eradicating *endemic* MNG by eliminating iodine deficiency, nearly all efforts of the research community interested in MNG has been funneled - during many past decades - into the mechanisms enabling the thyroid gland to adapt to iodine deficiency. The few critical minds drawing attention to a number of facets of MNG that cannot be simple consequences of iodine deficiency, went mostly unheard. The following is a list of some characteristics of MNG that cannot be explained by iodine deficiency (ref. 12 and later sections of this chapter):

- MNG goiter is a frequent thyroid disease in areas never exposed to iodine deficiency. This type of goiter is called *sporadic* MNG.
- Iodine deficiency - through subtle, chronic enhancement of TSH secretion - may well produce a *diffuse* enlargement of the thyroid gland, but cannot account by itself for the invariable *nodular transformation* of any long persisting goiter.
- Many goiter nodules are embedded within entirely normal, i.e. unstimulated thyroid tissue.
- Individual nodules within MNG may produce excessive amounts of hormones, thus suppressing TSH production and - at the extreme end of a large spectrum - causing thyrotoxicosis. This may even occur in children. Goiter growth may nevertheless continue.
- The incidence of thyrotoxicosis increases as well with the length of time a MNG persists as with its size.
- MNG are characterized by a tremendous heterogeneity of structure and function between goiters as well as within an individual goiter. »Cold« versus »hot« nodules — or macrofollicular, colloid-rich versus solid nodules — are but two pairs of examples.
- A low intrathyroidal iodine concentration may as well be *consequence*, rather than a *cause* of MNG growth. Moreover, some MNG contain high amounts of iodine.
- Nodules within MNG may be clonal as well as polyclonal and both types of nodules may coexist within the same MNG.

What, then, is the undeniable role of iodine deficiency in the pathogenesis of MNG? — Chronic (but not acute (13)) iodine deficiency - through the action of the classical feed-back mechanism - entails a subtle enhancement of endogenous TSH secretion. All normal thyrocytes and the large majority of all cells of benign neoplasias possess receptors for TSH, which is the main exogenous stimulatory agent of thyroid function and. - in synergism with growth factors and growth factor-dependent signaling pathways - also of thyroid growth (see also Chapter 3). Thus, iodine deficiency enhances function in all normal thyrocytes and growth in those cells with intact, receptor-dependent networks of pathways involved in the control of proliferation, but - due to constitutive heterogeneity between the individual cells - the result is not the same in all cells: e. g. some thyrocytes have such a high innate growth potential that they will, in the long range, outgrow their fellow cells regardless of iodine supply. These cells will inevitably form nodules with time. The process is, however, amplified and accelerated, but not fundamentally changed, by superimposed iodine deficiency. Or, as another example, a fraction of normal cells lack significant iodide transport or iodine organification capacity (14,15) while still having a higher than average replication potency. In this case, TSH will not stimulate iodine metabolism, but may still play a part in the constitutively activated growth machinery of a cold nodule that would anyway have formed later in a lifetime.

Thus, the ultimate causes of MNG are to be sought within the thyrocytes themselves, in analogy to most other benign neoplasias (2,3,4). Iodine deficiency is not a prerequisite to the growth of a MNG, but its presence may dramatically change the clinical course of the disease. *Sporadic* and *endemic* MNG are fundamentally the same disease of the thyroid gland, except for the higher incidence, the higher prevalence and the younger mean age of patients from areas afflicted by severe iodine deficiency.

In vitro studies relevant to the pathogenesis of MNG

The following sections will review some fundamental biological properties of thyroid cells in culture that may help understanding the bizarre heterogeneity of the clinical appearance of MNG.

In vitro cultured, two dimensionally growing thyroid follicular cells

A current opinion holds that the progeny of a single cell consists of cells with strictly identical functional and morphological qualities. However, there are mechanisms that create a new diversity within the offspring of a single cell. This has been demonstrated for a number of tissues including those derived from thyroid follicular cells. To cite but two examples: Griffin (16) showed the emergence of enzymatic variability in subclones of human skin fibroblasts and Davies (17) produced subclones of thyrocytes with widely varying growth dependency on TSH from cloned FRTL 5 cells. Taking up these and other leads, we have studied heterogeneity of growth and of a number of functions in two-dimensional cultures of cloned und wild-type thyrocytes from rat, cat and human glands. Every single function studied turned out to be unequally expressed and individually regulated among the members of a cell progeny. This was true for thyroglobulin production, iodide transport and organification, endocytosis (reviewed in ref. 2), inhibition of proliferation by TGFβ (18) and by pharmacological doses of iodide (19) and - most relevant in the present context - spontaneous and TSH-stimulated growth (20-25). Moreover, the highly individual replication rates of each subclone of FRTL 5 cells proved to be stable over many generations, with, however, always a small fraction of cells escaping this general rule (26). The high variability of growth patterns between the progeny of single cells and its stability over subsequent generations was first established by Absher et al. (27) and by Martin et al (28) and later confirmed by many others (reviewed in 3).

The second most striking phenomenon emerging from studies on two-dimensional cell cultures was the non-random distribution of cells with similar functional and proliferative qualities. Be it thyroglobulin synthesis, iodide transport and organic binding (studied in tissue fragments, not in cell cultures (15)), endocytosis or growth: Cells with similar functional qualities were not randomly scattered all over the tissue, but invariably tended to occur in clusters, just as they do in intact thyroids and in MNG (14,15,21)

A further potentially interesting observation in respect to the pathogenesis of autonomous growth in MNG is the entirely TSH-independent (i.e. autonomous) in vitro replication of human embryonic - in contrast to adult - thyrocytes (23) (see also section on experimental evidence for autonomous growth)

In vitro cultured, three-dimensionally growing thyroid follicular cells

Single, dispersed thyrocytes grow into three-dimensional clusters when embedded in gels containing appropriate culture medium. Using this technique, the essential findings observed in two-dimensional cultures (above) are faithfully reproduced.

Most importantly, each cell generates a progeny of a different size - just as in two-dimensional cultures - and there is again no correlation whatever between the number of cells in a clonal colony and the fraction of its ^{3}H-thymidine labeled cells. This finding - puzzling at first glance - is probably paramount to the understanding of MNG growth. It is indeed reproduced in human goiter tissue. It demonstrates that the growth of the thyroid gland proceeds in a non-random fashion by bursts of active replication - followed by irregularly spaced intervals - within cohorts of coordinated cells (14,20,21,29).

Experimental *in vivo* studies relevant to the pathogenesis of MNG

Cell transplants growing in nude mice retain the heterogeneity seen in slide-flask cultures

One way to exclude the possibility that heterogeneity of growth and function observed with any type of thyrocytes cultured in vitro may be artificially influenced by the unnatural medium was opened when transplantation onto nude mice became available. Extensive experiments with this model - using cloned FRTL5 cells as well as human and feline cells and whole tissue fragments - have confirmed the essential conclusions drawn from culture experiments and they have, in addition, produced valuable insight into the mechanisms of autonomous growth (14,20,22). Just as in culture, the transplants of fragments of goiter tissue grow by episodic replication of regionally dispersed clusters of coordinated cells. Identical growth patterns characterize growth of the MNG in situ (Fig 2). The ultimate size of a colony depends on the mean length of the quiet intervals between the growth spurts (21,29).

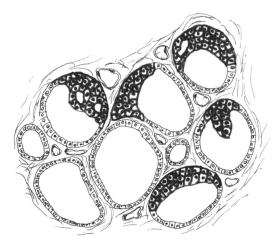

Figure 2. Type I of MNG growth: Countless foci of proliferating cells (grey background), alternating with quiescent cell patches, are scattered all over many follicles in all or in several spatially separated areas of a goiter. The schematic drawing is based on immunohistochemical staining (see fig. 3) of multiple serial sections of human MNG (11,14,29).The polyfocal proliferation of countless cell patches is the prevailing growth pattern in MNG, even in clonal nodules. The foci of actively growing tissue widely vary in size. They may, on the one hand, involve the entire gland, or else, they may be scattered in spatially separated regions of a goiter, often forming pseudonodules by compression of the surrounding normal tissue (1).

It must be realized that the regulation of cell growth in the intact thyroid is very different from that of any in vitro or in vivo model based on cultured cells (19,20) . To cite but one striking example, the serum concentration of iodide that inhibits growth of a normal mouse thyroid is 175 times higher than that producing the same effect in a transplant (19). Thus, conclusive answers as to the regulation of cell growth have to come from studies on the intact gland, be it in situ or in transplants.

Follicular epithelia of the normal thyroid gland may contain clonogenic cells

As suggested by in vitro experiments, a small fraction of the normal follicular cells may have the intrinsic propensity to divide at a faster rate than the bulk of all other cells. This can indeed be demonstrated in the intact thyroid gland. For example, when slowly growing mouse thyroids are labeled with a single injection of ^{3}H-thymidine, about 1 of 1000 follicular cells will be labeled after two hours and all labeled cells are single. However, three weeks later, only 50 % of labeled cells will still be single or in pairs, while the remaining 50 % have divided several times, forming coherent colonies of up to 12 cells (30). Other authors (31) have produced evidence suggesting that the rat thyroid contains a small fraction (probably less than 1 $^0/_{00}$) of clonogenic cells.

The most striking evidence for the excessive growth potential of a small subset of normal thyrocytes comes from the time-honored observation that chronic stimulation of the thyroid gland will invariably produce a number of nodules, often termed »adenomas«. While most stimulated thyrocytes are endowed with mechanisms that prevent further replication after a few rounds of cell division (32), some cells escape this physiological growth restriction. ^{3}H-thymidine labeling experiments in goitrogen treated mice demonstrate the persistently excessive growth rate of this tiny fraction of thyrocytes which form morphologically distinct »adenomas« within a few weeks of ongoing stimulation (2,3,20).

Serendipitous observations in human thyroids provide examples of what is probably the equivalent of clonogenic cells by revealing   tiny buds of actively growing cells protruding into the lumen of *normal* follicles (Fig 3) (3).

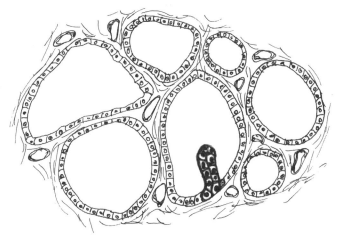

Figure 3. Type II of MNG growth: Very early stage of a single, actively growing, focal thyroid lesion (grey background). This schematic drawing is based on a serendipitous finding in the macroscopically normal thyroid tissue of a 26 years old female patient operated for a papillary carcinoma. The original, 1μ thin serial sections were immunohistochemically stained for p21 ras, IGF, EGF-r and the proliferating cells nuclear antigen PCNA (Fig 2 in ref. 3). Actual proliferation of the tiny bud originating from the hull of a normal follicle and protruding into its lumen was demonstrated by a layer of PCNA-positive cells and by heavy expression of p21ras, IGF and - to a lesser extent - EGF-r. Similar observations are described in ref. 11 and 29. It cannot be decided whether the bud illustrated in the figure originated from a single cell or from small cohorts of adjacent cells. It is, therefore, conceivable that single, well-delimited *polyclonal* thyroid nodules or *clonal* adenomas eventually evolve from a single, highly proliferating cell family such as that shown in the figure. However, only rarely are they embedded within *entirely normal* follicular epithelia. Much more often, they occur *within diffusely or multifocally proliferating* multinodular goiters (see fig. 2), thus forming cold or hot adenomas or true thyroid nodules within diffusely goitrous glands.

New follicles are generated from single cells or from small families of mother cells and these progenitor cells are of polyclonal origin: Two fundamental facts in MN-goitrogenesis

Follicular cells newly generated in a growing thyroid gland are used in one of two ways: Either they will enlarge the hull of new follicles, thus producing macrofollicular structures containing some ten thousand times more cells than the original microfollicle. On the other hand, a newly generated follicle may produce a second daughter follicle as soon as it forms a bud consisting of a few cells, and the offspring follicles, having inherited the same growth propensity, may do the same. The result is new solid or microfollicular tissue. Whether the structure of the newly formed tissue is entirely dependent on the constitutive traits of the mother cells or, if it is, additionally, modified by other factors - such as the amount of colloid produced per cell - is unknown (4).

The two most fundamental facts in the pathogenesis of MNG are, on the one hand, the exact mechanism by which a progeny of follicles is generated from the hull of a mother follicle and, on the other hand, the natural polyclonality of the progenitor tissue:

- As for folliculogenesis, it is theoretically conceivable that daughter follicles arise from tied-off segments of mother follicles. However, experimental evidence demonstrates that new daughter follicles grow out from *single* cells or from *small families* of predestined cells within the hull of a mother follicle (14,15). They may, thus, be clonal as well as polyclonal (see corresponding section).
- All normal tissues, including the thyroid and its individual follicles (33), consist of cells of *polyclonal* origin. From these two premises, it must be inferred that goiter nodules within the same goiter may be of clonal as well as of polyclonal composition and, moreover, that two clonal lesions can be derived from different mother cells (2,3). This has indeed been confirmed in human MNG (10).

If some cells have a higher intrinsic growth propensity than others and if, moreover, this trait is heritable, the offspring of these privileged cells will gradually outgrow their fellow cells. The late result may be the growth of a nodule. Moreover, growth may become dissociated from many functional properties in proliferating follicular cells (see section on functional heterogeneity). Thus, the degree of sodium iodide symporter activity and/or of the iodine organifying system in the mother cells will determine whether its progeny forms a »cold« or a »hot« nodule (2,3,14,15)

It should be added that descendence from polyclonal and, thus, unequally equipped mother cells, is no longer considered to be the sole mechanism responsible for creating heterogeneity within an offspring of cells. Rather, polymorphism may be acquired, and it may secondarily arise even in a clonal progeny (2,11).

Experimental evidence for autonomous growth

While non-neoplastic endocrine hyperplasia requires the continuous impact of a growth-stimulating agent - such as TSH in endemic goiter - true neoplastic growth proceeds by intracellular mechanisms independent of any exogenous stimuli. This is indeed the case in human MNG.

Experimental evidence for the autonomy of the growth process in MNG cannot be derived solely from in vitro experiments, since the growth regulation of intact glands is profoundly different from that in any tissue obtained by cell cultures (19,20).

A very high, entirely TSH-independent growth rate is a hallmark of the fetal thyroid gland. In newborn rats, the rapid natural thyroid growth goes on unabated even if TSH secretion is suppressed (34). Human fetal thyroids also contain a high fraction of proliferating cells, whose growth rate remains unaltered when transplanted to thyroxine-treated nude mice (23). In the mouse thyroid, the fraction of these autonomously growing cells falls from some 30 % in the fetal gland to 1 % (but never to 0) in the adult gland (15). It is thus tempting to speculate that the few clonogenic cells in normal thyroids have failed to switch from the fetal to the adult type of growth regulation. This view has recently been supported by experiments with autonomously proliferating embryonic smooth muscle cells, whose excessive growth rate is normally suppressed by molecules produced only in adult cells: Failure of this process is conceivably responsible for atherosclerotic lesions (35).

One mechanism possibly involved in the pathogenesis of growth heterogeneity is the naturally occurring or acquired resistance of some subsets of follicular cells toward the growth inhibiting action of TGFß (18). This phenomenon has not only been shown in cloned FRTL5 cells, but also in primary cultures of human goiter cells (18).

Autonomous growth is the single most impressive *clinical* trait that MNG's share with any other type of benign neoplasias. The aggressive, TSH-independent proliferation of MNG tissue can also be documented *experimentally*. Indeed, when fragments of human or cat MNG are transplanted to TSH-suppressed nude mice, a high fraction of all cells continue to divide unabated . In contrast, normal thyroid tissue - just as any thyroid cell transplant - only grows if endogenous TSH production is maintained at high levels (2,3,14,20,22).

Lessons from naturally occurring MNG in old cats

Nature has provided at least one easily accessible counterpart of human MNG. Indeed, thyrotoxicosis is not an infrequent diagnosis in aging cats brought to veterinary hospitals because of signs and symptoms akin to those of hyperthyroidism in man. Thyroid hormones are elevated and TSH is suppressed. The disease is caused by the growth of multiple hyperplastic nodules with scintigraphically demonstrable excessive iodine turnover within otherwise *normal* thyroid tissue. The size of the nodules ranges from very large, macroscopic lesions down to tiny proliferative foci consisting of but a few cells. Some glands are literally studded with a multitude of micro- and macronodules (22).

Numerous attempts at identifying a thyroid stimulating agent akin to the circulating immunoglobulins in Graves' disease have failed to produce convincing results. This was to be expected, since - in sharp contrast to the universally hyperplastic gland in Graves' disease and in hyperthyroidism due to germ-line mutations of the TSH receptor gene - the large majority of all follicles outside the nodules do not show any sign of stimulation. Thus, a circulating thyroid stimulating agent cannot possibly account for the growth of nodules within a *normal* thyroid. Rather, the nodules must be considered to be true autonomously proliferating neoplastic lesions. In support of this interpretation, fragments of nodular tissue fully maintain their high growth rate when transplanted onto nude mice with suppressed endogenous TSH secretion (22). Furthermore, individual follicles, enzymatically isolated from the hyperplastic, hyperfunctioning nodules and cultivated in a chemically defined, TSH-free serum, still grow at a fast rate and metabolize iodine almost as in vivo (24).

Thus, MNG in aging cats is - at least in those aspects investigated so far - comparable to the human disease. The analogy includes the amazing heterogeneity of intercellular and interfollicular morphology and function (22). It remains to be investigated whether cat goiter nodules are clonal or polyclonal, and we do not know if they contain any of the activating mutations described for human goiter nodules and adenomas (see section on molecular aspects).

A rather impressive additional documentation of the degree of intercellular heterogeneity in feline MNG comes from a comparison of 5 different cell lines cultivated from isolated follicles of adenomatous tissue: While all 5 cell lines produced thyroglobulin, they profoundly differed in their morphogenetic potential as well as in their response to TSH, EGF, retinoic acid and iodide (25).

The three most characteristic hallmarks of human MNG: Heterogeneity of structure and of function and TSH-independent growth

Structural heterogeneity

The relative amount of the main structural components of human MNG - i.e. follicles, stroma and blood vessels - varies within a very wide range. The same nearly infinite range of pleomorphism of the form and the size characterizes the *follicles* as well as the *thyrocytes* themselves that aggregate to build the monolayered follicular epithelium (1, 2). The countless intermingled structural variations not only occur in *different goiters*, but no less so in *different regions within the same goiter* (2,14,15). Typical pictures have appeared in many publications (reviewed in ref. 1).

The basic structures that are found in the individual nodules of MNG's occur in their most pure form in the rare »adenomas« that appear - with or without hyperthyroidism - in children and young adults (36,37). These structures are (Fig 4):

1. Macrofollicular nodules
2. Microfollicular and/ or solid nodules
3. Nodules with excessive stromal components (usually associated with microfollicular or solid epithelial components).

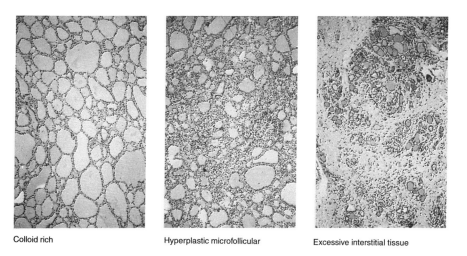

Colloid rich   Hyperplastic microfollicular   Excessive interstitial tissue

Figure 4. The three basic morphological variations of MNG tissue: A) Macrofollicular structure. B) Microfollicular or solid tissue C) Predominance of connective tissue.

Most thyroid nodules appearing at a young age are sharply delimitated from the normal tissue, most often surrounded by some kind of a capsule, and they have a strikingly individual structure. Their architecture is usually monomorphic, although locally restricted aberrations from the dominant structure are frequent (36). Thus, these nodules fulfill the criteria of true adenomas. Surprisingly, even this type of thyroid tumor may be of polyclonal origin (37).

The same well circumscribed, more or less *monomorphic* nodules also occur in MNG's of adult patients. In this case, they are usually *clonal* adenomas (10,11). However, much more often, adult goiters contain numerous *heterogeneously built foci of proliferating follicular* cells that may or may not be well-delimited from the surrounding tissue, thus fulfilling the criteria either of true nodules or, alternatively, forming diffusely proliferating tissue or pseudonodules (see definitions and Fig. 1).

Functional heterogeneity

The most familiar aspect of functional heterogeneity of MNG is the patchy pattern that usually appears on iodine or technetium scintiscans. Except for the comparably rare cases of only one or two sharply circumscribed »hot« nodules within an otherwise normal gland (called »toxic adenomas« on purely clinical grounds), the scan of a MNG usually shows irregular, regionally widely differing uptake without strict correlation to particular structures. The underlying mechanisms clearly appear on ^{125}I autoradiographs: Any follicle - irrespective of its size and shape and of the volume of the individual thyrocytes - may have a high or a low iodine turnover, or even no iodine metabolism at all (2,14,15). Two adjacent follicles in a MNG may be »cold« because iodide transport is deficient in the one and iodine organification in the other (38,39). The overall conclusions are, firstly, that there is a very wide spectrum of the intensity of iodine metabolism between different follicles within a single goiter and, secondly, that there is no way to predict an individual follicle's metabolic activity from any of its morphological characteristics (14,15). A typical autoradiograph illustrating this claim is given in fig. 5.

Regional heterogeneity of function in MNG is by no means restricted to iodine metabolism. For example, the orderly function of the TSH-dependent Gs-adenylate-cyclase cascade - the most important pathway regulating growth and function in the *normal* thyroid - is severely disrupted in MNG. While basal and TSH-stimulated adenylate cyclase activity are closely correlated and evenly distributed throughout the *normal* thyroid, this correlation is totally lost in MNG and, moreover, the basal activity of the enzyme varies erratically within a wide range in different regions of the same goiter (40). As another example, in nonfunctioning thyroid nodules $G_{s\alpha}$ expression is neither correlated to the basal or TSH-stimulated AC activity nor to the proliferation rate of these tumors (41). Still other examples of the functional heterogeneity of MNG are regional differences in thyroglobulin synthesis and endocytotic response or the dissociation between iodine metabolism and iodotyrosine deiodinase activity (2,42)

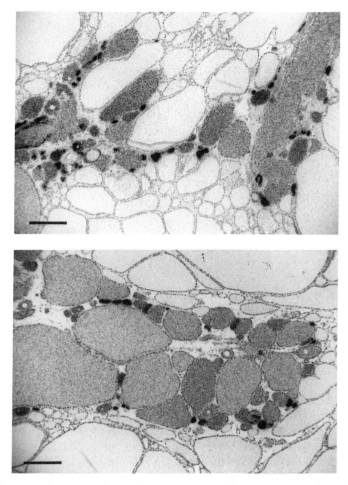

Figure 5. Two autoradiographs of a large multinodular goiter in a 68-yr.-old female patient with normal serum concentration of thyroid hormones but suppressed TSH secretion (not raising after TRH). [125]I was given 17 hr before surgery (44). Cohorts of follicles with high autonomous iodine turnover alternate with entirely »cold« follicles, while the anatomical structure of both types of follicles is identical. Thus, there is no correlation whatever between structure and iodine turnover and - since all follicles were part of a diffusely growing goiter - the same lack of correlation probably holds for growth and function (reproduced from Fig. 4 of ref. 3 with permission of the Editors). Bar = 200μm.

Clinical evidence for TSH-independent, i.e. autonomous goiter growth

An MNG may cease growing at any stage of its evolution and at any age of the patient. At the other end of the spectrum, thyroid nodules may suddenly appear to enlarge at a fast pace. This is not necessarily a sign of malignant growth or of a change in cell division rates, but the mere *clinical* counterpart of the curvilinear relation between cell number and tumor mass (3,43). In between the two ends of the spectrum are the slowly growing goiters that enlarge their volume almost imperceptibly over many years by generating new follicles, some of them with high intrinsic iodine turnover (4,44). Thus, as the goiter mass increases, so does TSH-independent hormone production. At an early stage, thyroid hormone concentration in the blood remains within normal ranges, while TSH is already suppressed, a condition termed »preclinical hyperthyroidism« (45). Later in life, overt thyrotoxicosis may appear (44). There is indeed an direct relationship between the size of a goiter and its autonomous hormone production (46-48). Thus, MNG may grow autonomously, i.e. in the absence of measurable serum TSH levels. Of course, this is not to say that *normal* TSH levels in truly euthyroid MNG do not help maintaining growth. Under these conditions, TSH suppression may indeed retard MNG growth, as discussed in the section on therapy of MNG.

Autonomous growth of MNG's - clinically apparent in patients and experimentally in transplant-bearing, TSH-suppressed mice as well as in goiter follicles cultured in a TSH-free medium (see above) - is the single most characteristic hallmark that this thyroid disease shares with every other benign tumor (3).

Clonal and polyclonal nodules in MNG

Any investigation into the clonality of MNG-tissue requires careful consideration of the fact that only one of the two fundamentally different types of goiter tissue is amenable to clonal analysis, and this only in female individuals. Indeed, meaningful sampling is only possible in clear-cut and well circumscribed nodules, where several spatially distinct samples within the same nodule must yield identical results in order to establish clonality (3). In contrast, no data are available - for want of an adequate *in situ* methodology - on the microclonal composition of the most typical and, sometimes, the only existing tissue in MNG, which consists of the diffusely proliferating thyrocytes. These cells produce the widely heterogeneous follicles that are embedded without clear borders between the normal follicles. Thus, the size and the number of the single microclones that have grown out in MNG to form the diffusely hyperplastic tissue - often arranged in pseudonodules (1, Fig. 1) - remains totally unknown at the present time.

A number of studies have been devoted to unraveling the clonal or polyclonal nature of thyroid nodules.(6,7,9,10,37). The overall result of these studies is unequivocal: The nodules in MNG' s may be of clonal as well of polyclonal nature. Some MNG's contain only polyclonal nodules, while others are studded with exclusively clonal lesions. If multiple clonal nodules are present, they appear to be derived either from the same ancestor cell - surprisingly so even when scattered over widely spaced regions - or else, they may represent more than one unrelated clone(10,49). Occasionally, such multiclonal MNG may even contain a malignant lesion (10).

Of particular interest is the unexpected finding that 10 out of 14 nodules within MNG, which had regrown in relatively young patients after subtotal thyroidectomy, were polyclonal rather than clonal (50). These lesions must either be generated by de novo proliferation of residual clusters of differing thyrocytes sharing the common trait of an exceedingly high intrinsic growth rate, or - alternatively - a few remaining cohorts of follicular cells derived from different ancestor cells have responded in a common way to unknown growth-stimulating molecular events.

The coexistence of polyclonal nodules with multiple clonal lesions derived from different parental cells is an important finding on the way of unraveling the pathogenesis of MNG (10). It has recently been expanded by the demonstration that the same goiter may harbor toxic adenomas with two different mutations of the TSH receptor (ref. 49, and section on molecular aspects). Like in other tumors, such as Hodgkin's disease (51,52), these findings may be taken to indicate an early polyclonal lesion preceding the appearance of clonally expanding nodules.

Heterogeneity of clonal nodules

It is widely believed that clonal tissue - generated by the progeny of a single cell - is necessarily monophenotypical in respect to structure and homogeneous in respect to function. This stringent view is certainly incorrect, since intercellular heterogeneity and - more recently - intraclonal mutations (51, 52) are common and widely known phenomena (2, 3 with ref. list, 11)

Clonal thyroid nodules provide a most impressive illustration of this fact. It is true that an uniform histomorphological structure of a well circumscribed thyroid nodule usually predicts its monoclonality. In contrast, even a high degree of structural and functional heterogeneity does not exclude the clonal origin of a thyroid lesion. In our own series of 24 clonal nodules embedded within MNG's, only 3 had a histomorphologically uniform structure, while 21 were heterogeneous and indistinguishable from polyclonal neoplasias (11)). Even growth is not an evenly and randomly distributed event among the cells of a clonal nodule. Rather, the microfocal, multicentric pattern of actively growing cell cohorts alternating with patches of resting cells (fig. 2)- first described in polyclonal nodules (6) - is faithfully reproduced within clonal neoplasias (11).

While the generation of heterogeneity of structure and function is easily understood in polyclonal neoplasms, the mechanisms that create diversity among the offspring of a single cell are different. Ongoing mutations within a clonal neoplasm are a well established mechanism (51,52), but other events, such as propagation of epigenetically acquired traits, are undoubtedly involved (2,3,47).

Molecular aspects of the pathogenesis of goiter nodules and adenomas

When considering investigations into the molecular events underlying the pathogenesis of benign thyroid lesions, one must be aware of one fundamental restriction: All reports published so far deal almost exclusively with only one of the two types of MNG tissue, which are the clearly circumscribed and easily recognizable nodules and (in the case of structural homogeneity) adenomas (see figure 1). On the contrary, the often predominant, diffusely proliferating tissue devoid of recognizable boundaries toward the normal thyroid structures have so far been virtually excluded from investigations into aberrations of their molecular machinery. The following considerations make no exception to this fact.

The cytogenetic and molecular mechanisms that stimulate abnormal thyroid cell growth and cause clonal expansion of a single cell or autonomous replication of cohorts of cells are still poorly understood (3). In principal there are three different types of alterations that reflect the transformed state of benign thyroid tumors.
  1. Overexpression of growth factors and their related receptors.
  2. Overexpression and mutational activation of signaling proteins.
  3. Alterations within the TSH receptor-dependent signaling pathway.

Overexpression of growth factors, their related receptors and of signaling proteins

In the normal thyroid gland - as in any other organ and tissue - the cell number is maintained constant by a balance between cell proliferation and apoptosis (53). In each cell, growth-related protooncogenes, growth-factors and their receptors and apoptosis-related proteins are expressed at only low levels (3, 54). To cite just one example, in a normal, resting thyroid gland less than 1 in 1000 cells constitutively overexpress the growth-associated ras gene product p 21 (29). Thus in most cells, growth-promoting proteins are probably present in amounts insufficient to promote cell replication. However, if the thyroid is stimulated by the trophic hormone TSH, e.g. under the conditions of iodine deficiency, the resting state is disrupted and hyperplasia will develop (3). As shown in rats, the stimulation is associated with a marked expression of growth factors and their receptors and of protooncogenes such as IGF-1, EGF receptor, ras gene product p21 and Gs-alpha protein (29,41,55). These experimental findings closely resemble those observed in nodular goiters (overview in ref. 3). Overexpression of IGF-1 (56), IGF-1 receptor (57), EGF receptor (58, 59), bFGF (60), the growth inhibitory TGFß (61), the signaling proteins ras (11) and Gsα (41, 62) has indeed been described in nodular goiters and in benign thyroid adenomas and nodules. However, one of the most striking hallmarks of nodular goiters is the markedly heterogeneous expression of these growth-associated proteins not only in different goiters, but also in different regions of the same nodules and even in different cells of the same follicle (2,3). This finding points to an unexpected complexity of growth regulation within these tumors. (3).

Nodular transformation of a primarily diffuse goiter and the incidence of thyroid tumors increase markedly with age (3). Aging is associated, on the one hand, with a slowdown of cell proliferation and, on the other hand, with an increase in the likelihood of genomic instability and neoplastic transformation (63). The higher incidence of transforming events is commonly related to the large increase in the frequency of chromosomal aberrations (64). Besides loss of chromosomes, translocation of chromosomal parts or other major deletions, chromosomal aberrations include amplifications of genes, alterations in regulatory gene regions or altered interaction between different transcription factors. All these mechanisms are known to cause overexpression of genes coding for signaling proteins, growth factors or growth factor receptors (65). With the exception of ras gene mutations in a few nonfunctioning adenomas (66) and Gsα and TSHr gene mutations in some toxic adenomas and toxic goiter nodules (see next paragraph), no other mutations and alterations have so far been revealed in the large majority of all thyroid nodules and carcinomas.

The pathogenesis of goiter nodules and adenomas is much more complex. It involves not only overexpression of protooncogenes, growth factors or growth factor receptors but also locally operating growth-promoting mutations and regulatory abnormalities which may precede, follow and / or interact with the primary events. In addition, epigenetic and environmental factors such as iodine deficiency contribute to the pathogenesis of goiter nodules by amplifying growth promoting processes.

Major questions remain to be answered. For example, the molecular basis for the dissociation between growth and function - a very common phenomenon in most MNG - is as obscure at the present time as are the mechanisms governing the interregionally highly heterogeneous overexpression of growth-related proteins.

The concept of constitutive intercellular heterogeneity of growth regulating mechanisms is still the most attractive one to explain why some cohorts of cells grow out to form nodules, whereas others do not (cf. above). The molecular basis for the heterogeneity is, however, unknown. Due to an individually different intrinsic growth potential and an equally individual proliferation rate in response to stimulation with growth factors, overexpression of growth-related proteins may cause the outgrowth of those cells endowed with a high growth propensity (2). In turn, proliferation will favor other mutational events that finally lead to tumor formation.

TSH and growth of multinodular goiter

In the normal thyroid gland, TSH is the main regulator of differentiated functions and of all thyroid-specific genes (67). However, in patients with nodular goiters, TSH is often suppressed as a consequence of functional autonomy with increased local production of thyroid hormones and subsequent inhibition of pituitary TSH secretion (68). Thus. many nodular goiters function and grow in the absence of biologically relevant TSH levels. However, since differentiated functions are maintained, although at a variable level (4), TSH-dependent signaling still appears to be involved in the cellular control of the diseased tissue. This apparent contradiction has recently, at least in part, been unraveled. Indeed, in some toxic adenomas and toxic goiter nodules, the cAMP signaling cascade may still be highly active, despite suppression of TSH secretion. In this case, nodules may be activated by mutations in the TSHr or the Gsα gene. These mutations have indeed been shown to constitutively activate the TSHr dependent adenylate cyclase signaling. Thus they mimic the stimulatory effect of TSH (see next paragraph).

However, the large majority of all goiter nodules - whether proliferating diffusely or as nodules and adenomas - are not hyperfunctioning but - on the contrary - poorly functioning (in terms of iodine metabolism) or nonfunctioning at all. In patients harboring such nodular goiters, TSH secretion is usually also within the normal range. At first glance this seems to argue against the concept that TSH is a major growth factor in this type of goiter. However, such a straightforward conclusion neglects the unexpected complexity of TSH-dependent signaling as part of a network of interactive positive and negative signals.

There is no doubt that TSH not only controls differentiated function, including expression of all thyroid specific genes and many housekeeping genes, but also regulates the expression of growth factors and their receptors (67). This has been demonstrated for the expression of EGF receptors (69) and for IGF-I / insulin signaling. Indeed, TSH affects insulin / IGF-I growth factor system by three different mechanisms: TSH enhances expression of IGF-I messenger RNA (70) and insulin receptor messenger RNA (71) and decreases protein levels of different IGF-I binding proteins (72), thereby raising the availability of free IGF-I. There is some evidence that IGF-I dependent signaling is of eminent importance for growth of the human thyroid gland. E. g. in patients with acromegaly goiters may be caused by high intrathyroidal IGF-I levels (73) and growth of toxic thyroid adenomas (see next paragraph) is most likely modulated by IGF-I (74). Thus, even TSH levels in the normal range may, at least in some thyroid diseases, enhance growth via growth-promoting pathways other than the cyclic AMP cascade.

In a subset of nonfunctioning thyroid adenomas and goiter nodules, other, TSH-independent mechanisms, including overexpression of normal Gs-α protein, may activate the cAMP cascade. In fact, Gsα overexpression has been detected in a substantial number of nonfunctioning thyroid adenomas (41). Therefore, it is conceivable that despite normal TSH or even suppressed TSH secretion TSH-dependent signaling may still be maintained by Gs-α overexpression. Other molecular, still unknown mechanisms may as well activate the cAMP cascade to an extent appropriate to maintain and to regulate differentiated function and control expression of growth factors and their receptors. Of particular interest in this context is the observation that both basal and TSH-dependent adenylate cyclase activity may greatly vary in different regions of the same goiter despite exposure to undoubtedly exactly identical TSH levels at every single point in time (40).

Alterations within TSHr dependent signaling pathways

Due to the dual role of TSH that synergizes thyroid function with regulation of growth factor-dependent pathways (67,71), hyperfunctioning thyroid tumors were altogether expected to bear molecular alterations of the TSHr- and Gsα-adenylate cyclase signaling pathways. Such alterations have indeed been detected in the TSHr and in the Gsα genes in some toxic adenomas and goiter nodules and very rarely in thyroid carcinomas (Overview: 75,76,62,77). The frequency of these mutations that constitutively activate the adenylate cyclase cascade in toxic adenomas is still controversial. However, there is no doubt that in regions with iodine deficiency activating mutations are much more frequent, whereas in countries with a high iodide supply such as Japan or the United States, these mutations are very rare or even absent (75). Even in regions with iodine-deficiency, a substantial number of toxic adenomas do not harbor TSHr of Gsα mutations. This may conceivably be explained by still undetected activating mutations in the two genes or else, by mutations in other signaling proteins of the TSHr-dependent pathways. Alternatively, the TSH-dependent cascade in toxic adenomas may be constitutively activated by overexpression (not mutations) of elements of the signaling pathway. Indeed, we have recently reported on the overexpression of functional Gsα in more than 90% of all toxic adenomas (62).

In order to put into perspective the role of the presently known activating mutations in the pathogenesis of MNG, it must be emphasized that this type of TSHr and Gsα mutations is mainly restricted to hyperfunctioning tumors, i.e. toxic adenomas and goiter nodules and hyperthyroid carcinomas, with the exception of some nonfunctioning thyroid carcinomas that harbor Gsα mutations (78). In contrast, the bulk of all goitrous tissue - be it nodular of diffuse - is not hyperfunctioning but very often even poorly functioning.

It has been postulated that activating TSH and Gsα gene mutations - if present - are the sole cause of toxic adenomas (79). However, there is an increasing body of evidence that these mutations are not sufficient to generate tumors. Doubts about this hypothesis are supported by the recent finding that in primary cultures of human thyrocytes overexpression of Gsα under the control of a retroviral vector does not promote thyroid growth (80). In these experiments, the cells transfected with the Gsα retroviral vector did not grow out to form colonies, while thyrocytes overexpressing the p21ras protein showed the expected effect. At first glance the data seem to be contradictory to results recently obtained by expression of Gsα or TSHr gene mutants in FRTL-5 cells which showed a higher proliferation rate in response to the expression of activating mutants (81,82). However, a highly selected, clonogenic and immortalized cell line such as FRTL 5 cells may already have been altered by several mutational events and, thus may be not representative for this particular aspect of human pathology. Evidence against a direct growth-promoting effect of TSHr and Gsα mutations also comes from different transgenic mice expressing cAMP-stimulating genes, whose thyroids primarily develop hyperthyroidism and only secondarily - most often exclusively in old animals - undergo nodular transformation (83,84).

There is also some clinical evidence that activation of the cAMP cascade primarily stimulates thyroid function while secondary events are necessary to promote tumor growth. Support for this claim comes from the clinical courses of a number of thyroid diseases, including Graves' disease caused by chronic TSHr antibody mediated stimulation of the TSHr (85), and the recently described autosomal-dominant hyperthyroidism due to TSHr germline mutations with subsequent stimulation of the entire population of polyclonal thyrocytes (86). In both diseases nodular transformation of primarily diffuse goiters evolves with time (85,86,87). The same process has been observed in the rare goiters caused by TSH-secreting pituitary adenomas (88) and in selective pituitary resistance to thyroid hormones (89). Finally, nodular growth invariably occurs in long-standing TSH-triggered iodine deficiency goiter (2,3). In all these diseases, diffuse goiters develop at first but secondarily and as late event, often taking years or even decades, nodular transformation occurs. Yet, focal nodular growth cannot be explained by the sole activation by TSH, TSHr antibodies or mutations within the TSHr dependent signaling.

Thus, the molecular mechanisms that ultimately cause toxic adenomas and nodules that do not harbor TSH or Gsα mutations remain to be unraveled. It seems reasonable to assume that in these adenomas activating events have to be expected along the TSHr-dependent signaling or, alternatively, within the regulatory circuit of this pathway, since otherwise hyperfunction would not occur. Equally unanswered is the question as to the nature of the secondary processes that stimulate a hyperfunctioning thyrocyte to grow out into an adenoma. Some speculations go as follows. Since activating mutations of the TSHr of Gsα gene mimic the effect of TSH and thereby may enhance the expression of IGF-I mRNA, the dependent signaling is likely to be augmented in those toxic adenomas that bear such mutations. Indeed, enhanced expression of IGF-1 mRNA and stimulation of the corresponding receptor by autocrine secretion of IGF-1 were demonstrated in some toxic adenomas (74). This is of particular interest, since the growth-promoting effect of TSH depends on or may even be mediated by IGF-1- signaling (cf. above). Indirect support for this concept comes from experiments with thyrocytes derived from toxic adenomas. In culture, these cells grew in response to TSH in the absence of exogenous IGF-1 suggesting that IGF-1-dependent signaling is already maximally activated (90). In another recent report, TSH has been demonstrated to decrease steady state levels of IGF binding proteins 3 and 5 and, to a lesser extent, IGF binding protein 4 (72). Thus, in toxic adenomas mutational activation of the adenylate cyclase cascade may not only upregulate IGF-1 and insulin receptor mRNA, whose expression is also enhanced by TSH (71), but also increase the availability of unbound IGF-1. In summary, in a subset of toxic thyroid nodules mutations in the TSHr or the Gsα gene represent an important and possibly the initial step within an array of other pathogenic events that promote clonal expansion of the affected hyperfunctioning thyroid cells and finally the outgrow of clonal tumors. Additional alterations include increased expression of EGF receptors (58), IGF-I receptors (57), basic fibroblast growth factor (bFGF) (60), decreased synthesis of growth inhibitory transforming growth factor ß (TGFß) (61) and enhanced synthesis of ras (11) and Gsα protein (41,62). Moreover, it has recently been shown that a subset of cloned thyrocytes may be constitutively resistant to the growth inhibitory effect of TGFß and that resistance to TGFß may be acquired through chronic exposure to the compound (18). Interestingly, TGFß resistance is very common in thyrocytes derived from human thyroid nodules (18).

The rarity of toxic thyroid adenomas in regions with ample iodine supply points to an important pathogenetic role of iodine deficiency - most likely a consequence of subtle, long-standing stimulation of TSHr dependent-signaling (91,75). Iodide itself and different organic iodine compounds - albeit at supraphysiological concentrations - inhibit signaling of growth-promoting pathways such as those depending on EGF receptors (92). It is still an open question whether the lack of an inhibitory effect of iodide may lead to a relative higher activity of growth-stimulatory pathways, thereby contributing to the higher prevalence of goiter nodules and adenomas in iodine deficiency areas.

It might be surprising that a chapter on molecular biology of MNG allots such a large space to the discussion of data on toxic adenomas, since this type of thyroid nodules is a rare byproduct arising in the course of goitrous transformation of a thyroid gland. The explanation comes from the simple fact that toxic adenomas are the thyroid lesions that have attracted most interest of molecular biologists, whereas there is scant data are available on molecular alterations in the much more common types of goiter structures, such as non-nodular goiter tissue, eufunctioning nodules and so-called "cold" nodules.

Therapy of multinodular goiter

Treatment of multinodular goiter nodules with levothyroxine and / or iodide

Since therapeutic approaches and treatment of single benign nodules are dealt with in chapter 6, the following discussion focuses on management of multinodular goiters. However, the two diseases are often - perhaps most often - inseparable, since close pathological workup and systematic ultrasonographic studies on thyroids presenting with clinically uninodular disease commonly show multiple additional nodules (93,94). Although apparently single nodules are often called "adenomas"[2], the true nature of any thyroid nodule (see definition) cannot be defined by clinical means. Moreover, there are no fundamental differences in the response of nodular and multinodular goiter tissue to TSH-suppressive therapy. Therefore, although most studies on the efficacy of thyroid hormone treatment focus on the more easily measurable volume reduction of single nodules rather than on the whole gland, the two variants of the same disease are discussed conjointly.

Treatment of multinodular goiter either with levothyroxine or, in regions with iodine deficiency, with levothyroxine and / or iodine remains unsatisfactory. Whereas some studies demonstrated efficacy of levothyroxine suppressive therapy of thyroid nodules, others could not find a significant volume reduction in comparison to untreated patients (Table 1).

The term "adenomas" is used in this section strictly in its clinical sense.

In Table 1, an overview of studies that showed a substantial reduction of at least 50% of nodule volume in response to levothyroxine and / or iodine treatment is shown. On average, only one third of patients (range 14-56%) with a solitary benign thyroid nodule responded to a TSH-suppressive therapy with a significant reduction of nodule volume. It is noteworthy that in two studies a similar reduction of nodule volume was observed in treated and untreated patients indicating a spontaneous regression of nodules (97,99).

Table 1 Changes of thyroid nodule size during treatment with levothyroxine and / or iodide as evaluated by ultrasonography.

Authors	No. of pat.	Duration [months]	Treatment	% pat. with ≥ 50% reduction of nodule vol.
Morita et al. 1989 (95)	49	3	T4 100μg	37
Celani et al. 1990 (96)	122	6-12	T4 100-200μg	56
Gharib et al. 1987 (97)	53	6	T4 3μg/kg bw Placebo	14 20
Papini et al. 1993 (98)	101	12	T4 2μg/kg bw Placebo	20 6
Cheung et al. 1989 (99)	74	18	T4 Control	16 14
Celani et al. 1993[1] (100)	104	6	T4 2.2. μg/kg bw Control	27 10
La Rosa et al. 1995 (101)	48	12	T4 suppr. dose KI 2mg/2 weeks	39 20
Lima et al. 1997 (102)	54	12	T4 200 μg Control	37 5
	47[2]	12	T4 200 μg Control	30 0

T4, levothyroxine; KI, potassium iodid; bw, body weight
[1] multinodular goiter; volume of each nodule was evaluated.
[2] In this part of the study total volume of multinodular goiter was assessed.

Treatment of multinodular goiter with potassium iodide may also reduce nodule volume, albeit to a lower extent in comparison to levothyroxine treatment. In a recent study, treatment of patients with non-functioning nodules resulted in reduction of nodule volume of 50% or more in 40% of levothyroxine-treated patients but only in 23% of patients receiving potassium iodide (101). Whether treatment of patients with iodide is more effective in reducing nodule volume in patients from iodine deficiency areas is still unknown.

It has often been speculated that the response of thyroid nodules to levothyroxine therapy may depend on their histological characteristics. Indeed, a recent study demonstrates that the cytological features of thyroid nodules may, a least in part, determine the efficacy of a TSH-suppressive therapy (103). The authors of this study investigated the cytological patterns of nodules by fine-needle aspiration prior to levothyroxine treatment. Although only 33% of all nodules shrank, 62% of colloid nodules and 57% of small degenerative nodules showed a significant volume reduction ($\geq$ 50%), whereas hyperplastic and fibrotic nodules did not respond.

The volume of thyroid nodules is another factor that determines the efficacy of levothyroxine treatment. In one study, only nodules with a volume of less than 10 ml shrank, with maximum therapeutic effect in nodules less than 5 ml, whereas nodules of more than 10 ml did not respond (101). Other pretreatment variables such as patients' age, duration of goiter and TRH-induced TSH response cannot predict responsiveness to levothyroxine treatment (99). Moreover, as outlined above, different thyroid nodules and the non-nodular goiter tissues within the same gland may have profoundly differing structure and function. Thus, a uniform response of the whole goiter and of all its nodules to levothyroxine treatment cannot be expected.

There are only a few studies on the efficacy of levothyroxine suppressive therapy on the total volume of nontoxic multinodular goiter (102, 104, 105). In most investigations the responsiveness is very low. A somewhat more favorable result was obtained in a very recent study that demonstrated regression of glandular volume of 50% or more in one third of patients with multinodular goiter treated with 200 µg levothyroxine daily for 12 months (102). Again, the poor response in most studies may be explained by the heterogeneity of multinodular goiters that contain autonomously growing and functioning components not affected by TSH-suppressive therapy (2,3). Indeed, even the non-nodular tissue may grow and function autonomously. If so, levothyroxine treatment is likely to be useless. It may even be fraught with side-effects.

A prerequisite for adequate treatment of multinodular goiter and apparently single goiter nodules is the exclusion of malignancy in fine-needle aspirates and of autonomous function by measurement of TSH. If TSH is suppressed, a technetium pertechnetate scintigram is advisable. On average, levothyroxine doses of 1.5 to 2.0 µg per KG body weight (total dose of 100 to 150µg/d) are sufficient for TSH suppression. Foremost in patients with a history of cardiac disease and in postmenopausal women with higher risk for development of osteoporosis higher levothyroxine doses should be avoided. In these patients, the levothyroxine dose should be adjusted to reduce TSH concentration only into the lower normal range. From most prospective studies, it can be concluded that levothyroxine suppressive therapy should be continued for at least one year. However, optimal duration of therapy cannot be predicted and regrowth of levothyroxine-sensitive goiter nodules to their original size after stopping treatment is a common phenomenon. Therefore, a further prerequisite for medical goiter treatment is a high degree of compliance of the patient and his or her willingness to accept regular follow-up. Should goiter growth resume or continue under treatment, a definitive form of therapy - most likely surgery - is mandatory. While many clinicians consider a 50% or even a

30% reduction of goiter or nodular volume as a success, a note of caution is in order. Indeed, any remaining nodule - particularly in younger patients - remains a problem (not only for fear of cancer) and requires regular controls unless definitive arrest of growth is established.

Radioiodine treatment for nontoxic multinodular goiter

Although surgery is considered standard therapy for nontoxic multinodular goiter, radioiodine treatment may be an alternative with a low risk for elderly patients, especially those with cardiopulmonary diseases (106-109). A mean volume reduction of 40% after 1 year and 50-60% after 3-5 years can be achieved by this mode of therapy (106,108). Side-effects include mild radiation thyroiditis as an early event and hypo- and hyperthyroidism (106-108). In a very recent study, development of autoimmune hyperthyroidism was seen in 3 of 80 patients treated with radioiodine for volume reduction of multinodular goiter (109). Thyrotoxicosis developed in these patients 3, 6, or 10 months after 131-I therapy, respectively. A more serious risk is the occurrence of cancer, with a life-time risk in people of 65 years or older of approximately 0.5% (107). It should also be born in mind that "cold" nodules and "cold" areas within a goiter are either not accessible or only partly accessible to radioiodine treatment. Thus, since clinical experience is still limited and long-term follow-up is limited, radioiodine treatment should be restricted to selected cases of multinodular goiter in elderly patients.

Alternative treatment of toxic, nonfunctioning and cystic goiter nodules with percutaneous ethanol injection

Percutaneous ethanol injection (PEI) therapy under sonographic guidance was first proposed by Livraghi in 1990 as possible treatment for autonomously functioning thyroid nodules (110). Since that time several prospective studies with pretoxic and toxic "adenomas" and nodules have been performed and PEI therapy has been extended to treatment of solid nonfunctioning and cystic thyroid nodules (111-117). In a recent multicenter study with 242 patients with toxic "adenomas" and 187 pretoxic "adenomas", successful treatment, defined by normal TSH and normal free thyroid hormone levels and recovery of tracer uptake in extranodular tissue, was achieved in 66.5% of patients with toxic "adenomas" and in 83.4% of patients with pretoxic "adenomas" after a 12 months follow-up (113). In another follow-up study of up to 5 years (median 2.5) PEI treatment resulted in a complete cure in all patients with pretoxic thyroid "adenomas" (n=40) and in 60 (77.9%) patients with toxic "adenomas" (115).

PEI treatment was also effective in cystic thyroid nodules (111, 114). In a more recent study 85% of patients with cystic thyroid nodules (n=17) had a volume reduction of more than 90% of the initial lesion after 6 months (114). In solid nonfunctioning nodules PEI therapy decreased mean pretreatment nodule volume from 21.0 ml (range 5.4-54.6 ml) to 7.7 + 5.7 ml at the end of treatment and to 4.4 + 3.8 ml at 1 year follow-up (116). All studies published so far suggest that PEI is a safe and efficient therapeutic tool. Yet, prospective randomized clinical trials that compare PEI with radioiodine treatment and surgery are missing. Furthermore, only the short-term effect of ethanol, that appears to cause coagulative necrosis and local small vessels thrombosis (reviewed in 117), but not long-term morphological changes are known. Therefore PEI therapy still remains an experimental procedure.

Surgical treatment of thyroid nodules and multinodular goiter and recurrence rate

For nonfunctioning thyroid nodules, with and without suspicion of malignancy, for large toxic multinodular goiter and large toxic nodules, surgery remains standard therapy (118), although in selected cases an alternative mode of treatment may be chosen (cf. above). A surgical approach is undisputed if fine-needle aspirates yield positive or suspicious material, if there is compression of structures of the neck and sometimes for cosmetic concerns (118).

Between 4 and 7% of individuals in the United States have thyroid nodules, with 5:1 female/male sex ratio (119). In large population studies the frequency of cancer in patients with cold nodules were 6.4% and 5.3% in iodine-sufficient areas and 2.7% in iodine-deficient areas with an overall higher incidence of thyroid nodules in the latter regions (120,121). Furthermore, the frequency of thyroid cancer in patients with solitary nodules and multiple goiter nodules was not different (120). A different picture emerged in children and in adolescents with solitary thyroid nodules in whom up to 25.5% of nodules were reported to be malignant (122). Thus, the younger a patient, the more likely is surgical removal of a nodule the treatment of choice. In patients with solitary nodules and negative results in fine-needle aspirates long-term clinical monitoring including ultrasonographic controls are acceptable alternatives (see also above).

The single most important characteristic of multinodular goiter that directs the therapeutic approach toward surgery is recent growth of the whole goiter or some of its nodules. Although active growth is not to be confounded with malignant transformation (see above), it indicates an autonomous, neoplastic process that is best controlled by surgical resection of all diseased tissue. Several studies have shown that for patients operated on for multinodular goiter in a department specialized for thyroid surgery, the frequency of serious side-effects is relatively low, with permanent recurrent laryngeal palsy rate about 1% or even less and permanent hypocalcaemia less than 1% (123,124). (see also Chapter 10). If surgery is chosen as the therapeutical approach, the relatively high rate of recurrent goiter is of major concern. A high incidence of recurrent goiters in patients undergoing surgery for nontoxic nodular goiter irrespective of treatment with levothyroxine is commonly observed (125-128). In a long-term follow-up study of 143 patients who underwent subtotal thyroidectomy for multinodular goiter some 30 years ago goiters regrew in about 40% of patients, independently of treatment with levothyroxine. In a recent study, a more favorable outcome, albeit after a mean follow-up of only 6.4 years, was seen in 104 patients from an iodine-deficient region with recurrent goiter in 28% of untreated and 8.9% of treated patients (126). In any case these studies clearly demonstrate that there is a higher rate of goiter recurrence years and decades after surgery. Whether this argues in favor of more or less total thyroidectomy has to be proven in clinical studies.

Concluding remarks

Multinodular goiter: A particular form of a benign neoplastic process

Most investigations on tumor pathogenesis do not specifically consider the possibility that the tissue they analyze may be heterogeneous in many respects. MNG is a prominent example of an extremely heterogeneous tissue, whose abnormal growth is driven, as in any other neoplastic process, by mechanisms operating within and between the diseased thyrocytes themselves. There is probably no other organ where pathological growth can be studied concomitantly with so many different aspects of function and structure. A number of striking conclusions have emerged from such studies. The most important ones are:

- Excessive growth may be entirely dissociated from any of the functional, structural and metabolic characteristics of a tissue sample. The most striking example is the cold nodule.
- Growth and function (and their coordination or dissociation) may not only widely differ in distant regions of the same goiter, but even between adjacent follicles or between the neighboring cells of a single follicle.
- Not all thyrocytes within a goiter proliferate at the same pace and at the same time. Rather, growth proceeds at irregular intervals within small cohorts of coordinated cells. This holds true even for clonal adenomas.
- While gain-of-function mutations of the TSH receptor gene and the gene encoding the $G_{s\alpha}$ subunit have been demonstrated in a subset of those goiter nodules that produce excessive amounts of hormones, other mutations - if present - await to be detected in the large majority of all other, non-hyperfunctioning goitrous lesions, be it nodular or diffusely proliferating tissue.
- The high frequency of nodular growth within a goitrous gland is altogether amazing. It indicates that some subsets of thyrocytes have a higher growth propensity - be it constitutive or acquired - than the bulk of the diffusely proliferating follicular cells of the surrounding tissue.
- Sharply circumscribed goiter nodules may be clonal as well as polyclonal, and the two types of nodules may coexist within the same MNG. Moreover, two clonal adenomas may be derived from different mother cells. These findings are compatible with an early polyclonal stage of a later clonal tumor.

TSH is but one factor within the growth-promoting network of a MNG. However, goiter growth may as well proceed in the absence of TSH. Activating events - a few of them known and certainly not all of them depending on mutations - may affect the TSH-dependent pathways, but a probably large number of additional events must undoubtedly occur at countless points within the intricate network of interplaying growth-driving mechanisms.

These are some of the main facts that have removed MNG from the time-honored list of purely secondary, hyperplastic thyroid diseases caused by iodine deficiency. Most components of multinodular goiters are true neoplastic tissues. Their tremendous structural and functional heterogeneity - down to the single cells - suggests that any attempt to unravel the mystery of abnormal growth must consider the highly individual way a follicular cell behaves within a growing goiter.

References

1. Studer H, Ramelli F. Simple goiter and its variants: Euthyroid and hyperthyroid multinodular goiter. Endocr Rev 1982; 3 :40-62.
2. Studer H, Peter HJ, Gerber H. Natural heterogeneity of thyroid cells: The basis for understanding thyroid function and nodular goiter growth. Endocr Rev 1989; 10:125-135.
3. Studer H, Derwahl M. Mechanisms of nonneoplastic endocrine hyperplasia — A changing concept: A review focused on the thyroid gland. Endocr Rev 1995; 16:411-426.
4. Studer H, Gerber H. Multinodular goiter. In: DeGroot L (ed) Endocrinology, ed. 3 Saunders Philadelphia, 1995; 769-782.
5. Hedinger C, Williams ED, Sobin LH. Histological typing of thyroid tumors. WHO, international histological classification of tumors, ed. 2, Springer, Berlin, 5-6, 1989.
6. Namba H, Matsuo K, Fagin JA. Clonal composition of benign and malignant human thyroid tumors. J Clin Invest 1990; 86:120-125.
7. Fey MF, Peter HJ, Hinds HI, Zimmermann A, Liechti-Gallati S, Gerber H, Studer H, Tobler A. Clonal anlaysis of human tumors with M27ß, a highly informative polymorphic X chromosomal probe. J Clin Invest 1991; 89:1438-1444.
8. Hicks DG, LiVolsi, VA, Neldich JA, Puck JM, Kant JA. Clonal analysis of solitary follicular nodules in the thyroid. Am J Path 1990; 137:553-562.
9. Kopp P, Jaggi R, Tobler A, Borisch B, Oestreicher M, Sbacan L, Jameson JL, Fey M. Clonal X-inactivation analysis of human tumors using the human androgen receptor gene (HUMARA) polymorphism: a nonradioactive and semiquantitative strategy applicable to fresh and archival tissue. Mol Cell Probes 1997; 11:217-228.
10. Kopp P, Aeschimann S, Asmis L, Tobler A, Fey MF, Studer H. Polyclonal and clonal nodules may coexist within multinodular goiters. J Clin Endocrinol Metab 1994; 79:134-139.
11. Aeschimann S, Kopp PA, Kimura ET, Zbaeren J, Tobler A, Fey MF, Studer H. Morphological and functional polymorphism within clonal thyroid nodules. J Clin Endocrinol Metab 1993; 77:846-851.
12. Aeschimann S, Buergi U, Wagner HE, Kaempf J, Lauber K, Studer H. Low intrathyroidal iodine concentration in non-endemic human goiters: a consequence rather than a cause of autonomous goiter growth. J Endocrinol 1994; 140:155-164.
13. Brabant G, Bergmann P, Kirsch CM, Köhrle J, Hesch RD, von zur Mühlen A. Early adaptation of thyrotropin and thyroglobulin secretion to experimentally decreased iodine supply in man. Metabolism 1992 ; 41: 1093-1096.
14. Peter HJ, Gerber H, Studer H, Smeds S. Pathogenesis of heterogeneity in human multinodular goiter. A study of growth and function of thyroid tissue transplanted onto nude mice. J Clin Invest 1985; 76:1992-2002.
15. Peter HJ, Studer H, Forster R, Gerber H. The pathogenesis of hot and cold follicles in multinodular goiters. J Clin Endocrinol Metab 1982; 55: 941-946.
16. Griffin JE, Allman DR, Durrant JL, Wilson JD. Variation in 5α-reductase activity in cloned human fibroblasts. J Biol Chem 1981; 256:3662-3666.
17. Davies TF, Yang C, Platzer M. Cloning the Fisher rat thyroid cell line FRTL5. Endocrinology 1987; 121:78-83.
18. Asmis LM, Kaempf J, von Grünigen C, Kimura ET, Wagner HE, Studer H. Acquired and naturally occurring resistance of thyroid follicular cells to the growth inhibitory action of

transforming growth factor β1(TGF β1). J Endocrinol 1996; 149:485-496.

19.   Aeschimann S, Gerber H, von Gruenigen C, Oestreicher M, Studer H. The degree of inhibition of thyroid follicular cell proliferation by iodine is a highly individual characteristic of each cell and profoundly differs in *vitro* and *in vivo*. Eur J Endorinol 1994; 130:595-600.

20.   Peter HJ, Gerber H, Studer H, Groscurth P, Zakarija M. Comparison of FRTL-5 growth in vitro with that of xenotransplanted cells and the thyroid of the recipient mouse. Endocrinology 1991; 128:211-219.

21.   Derwahl M, Studer H, Huber G, Gerber H, Peter HJ. Intercellular propagation of individually programmed growth bursts in FRTL-5 cells. Implications for interpreting growth factor actions. Endocrinology 1990; 127:2104-2110.

22.   Peter HJ, Gerber H, Studer H, Becker DV, Peterson ME. Autonomy of growth and of iodine metabolism in hyperthyroid feline goiters transplanted onto nude mice. J Clin Invest 1987; 80:491-498.

23.   Peter HJ, Studer H, Groscurth P. Autonomous growth, but not autonomous function, in embryonic human thyroids. A clue to understanding autonomous goiter growth? J Clin Endocrinol Metab 1988; 66:968-973.

24.   Peter HJ, Gerber H, Studer H, Peterson ME, Becker DV,Groscurth P. Autnonomous growth and function of cultured thyroid follicles from cats with spontaneous hyperthyroidism. Thyroid 1991; 1:331-338.

25.   Gerber H, Peter HJ, Bösiger J, Studer H, Drews R, Ferguson DC, Becker DV. Different continuous cell lines from adenomatous feline goiters widely differ in morphological, functional and growth aspects. In: Gordon A, Gross J, Hennemann G (eds.) Progress in Thyroid Research, Balkema, Rotterdam, 1991; 541-544.

26.   Huber G, Derwahl M, Kaempf J, Peter HJ, Gerber H, Studer H. Generation of intercellular heterogeneity of growth and function in cloned rat thyroid cells (FRTL5). Endocrinology 1990; 126:1639-1645.

27.   Absher PM, Absher RG, Barnes WD. Genealogies of clones of diploid fibroblasts. Cinematographic observations of cell division patterns in relation to population age. Exp Cell Res 1974; 88:95-104.

28.   Martin GM, Sprague CA, Norwood TH, Pendergrass WR. Clonal selection, attenuation and differentiation in an *in vitro* model of hyperplasia. Am J Path 1974; 74:137-154.

29.   Studer H, Gerber H, Zbaeren J, Peter HJ. Histomorphological and immunohistochemical evidence that human nodular goiters grow by episodic replication of multiple clusters of thyroid follicular cells. J Clin Endocrinol Metab 1992; 75:1151-1158.

30.   Smeds S, Peter HJ, Jörtsö E, Gerber H, Studer H. Naturally occurring clusters of rapidly replicating follicular cells in mouse thyroid glands. Cancer Res 1987; 47:1646-1651.

31.   Groch KM, Clifton KH. The effects of goitrogenesis, involution and goitrogenic rechallenge on the clonogenic cell content of the rat thyroid. Acta Endocrinol (Copenh) 1992; 126:515-523.

32.   Smith P, Wynford-Thomas D. Control of thyroid follicular cell proliferation - cellular aspects. In: Wynford-Thomas D, Williams ED (eds) Thyroid Tumours. Churchill Livingstone, London, 1989; 66-90.

33.   Feder N. Solitary cells and enzyme exchange in tertaparental mice. Nature 1976; 263:67-69.

34.   Logothetopoulos J. Growth and function of the thyroid gland in rats injected with L-thyroxine from birth to maturity. Endocrinology 1963; 73:349-352.

35.   Majack RJ. Extinction of autonomous growth potential in embryonic: adult vascular smooth muscle cells heterokaryons. J Clin Invest 1995; 95: 464-468.

36.   Aebi U, Gerber H, Studer H. Thyroid adenomas: a morphologically and functionally heterogeneous thyroid disease. In: Gordon A, Gross J, Hennemann G (eds) Progress in Thyroid Research, Balkema, Rotterdam, 1991; pp. 679-682.

37.   Namba H, Ross JL, Goodman D, Fagin JA. Solitary polyclonal autonomous thyroid nodule: a rare cause of childhood hyperthyroidism. J Clin Endocrinol Metab 1991; 72:1108-1112.

38.   Schürch M, Peter HJ, Gerber HJ, Studer H. Cold follicles in a multinodular human goiter arise partly from a failing iodide pump or and partly from deficient iodine organification. J Clin Endocrinol Metab 1990;71:1224-1229.

39.   Spitzweg C, Job AW, Heufelder AE . Analysis of human iodide symporter gene expression in patients with thyroid diseases. 79th Meeting Endocrine Soc, 1997; Abstract 30-1, p. 108.

40.   Rentsch HP, Studer H, Frauchiger B, Siebenhüner L. Topographical heterogeneity of basal and thyrotropin-stimulated adenosine 3',5'-monophosphate in human nodular goiter. J Clin Endocrinol Metab 1981; 53:514-521.

41. Hamacher Ch, Studer H, Zbaeren J, Schatz H, Derwahl M. Expression of functional stimulatory guanine nucleotide binding protein in nonfunctioning thyroid adenomas is not correlated to adenylate cyclase activity and growth of these tumors. J Clin Endocrinol Metab 1995; 80:1724-1732.

42. Conti A, Kneubuehl, F, Studer H, Kohler H, Buergi H. Increased iodotyrosine deiodinase in human goiters and in rats treated with perchlorate. In: Robbins J, Braverman LE (eds) Thyroid Research, Excerpta Medica, Amsterdam 1975; 166-168.

43. Gullino PM. Natural history of breast cancer. Progression from hyperplasia to neoplasia as predicted by angiogenesis. Cancer 1977; 39:2697-2703.

44. Studer H, Hunziker HR, Ruchti C. Morphologic and functional substrate of thyrotoxicosis caused by nodular goiters. Am J Med 1978; 65:272-234.

45. Gemsenjäger E, Staub JJ, Girard J, Heitz PH. Preclinical hyperthyroidism in multinodular goiter. J Clin Endocrinol Metab 1967; 43:810-816.

46. Laurberg P, Pederssen KM, Vestergard H, Sigurdsson G. High incidence of multinodular toxic goiter in the elderly population in a low iodine intake area vs. high incodence of Graves' disease in the young in a high iodine intake area. J Int Med 1991; 229:415-420.

47. Fenzi GF, Ceccarelli C, Macchia E. Residents of a moderate endemic goiter area Clin Endocrin (Oxf) 1985; 23:115-122.

48. Rieu M, Bekka S, Sambor B, Berrod JL, Fombeur JL. Prevalence of subclinical hyperthyroidism and relationship between thyroid hormonal status and thyroid ultrasonsographic parameters in patients with non-toxic nodular goiters. Clin Endocrinol (Oxf) 1993; 39:67-71.

49. Duprez L, Hermans J, van Sande J, Dumont J, Vassart G, Parma J. Two autonomous nodules of a patient with multinodular goiter harbor different activating mutations of the thyrotropin receptor gene. J Clin Endocrinol Metab 1997; 82:306-308.

50. Harrer P, Broecker M, Zint A, Zumtobel V, Derwahl M. Thyroid nodules in recurrent multinodular goiters are predominantly polyclonal J Endocrinol Invest 1998; (in press)

51. Ohno T, Stribley JA, Wu G, Hinrichs SH, Weisenburger DD, Chan WC. Clonality in nodular lymphocyte-predominant Hodgkin's disease. N Engl J Med 1997; 337:459-465.

52. Gutierrez MI, Bhatia K, Cherney B, Capello D, Gaidano G, Magrath I. Intraclonal molecular heterogeneity suggests a hierarchy of pathogenetic events in Burkitt's lymphoma. Ann Oncol 1997; 8:987-994.

53. Schwartzman RA, Cidlowski JA. Apoptosis: the biochemistry and molecular biology of programmed cell death. Endocr Rev 1993; 14:133-151.

54. Bröcker M, de Buhr I, Papageorgiou G, Schatz H, Derwahl M. Expression of apoptosis-related proteins in thyroid tumors and thyroid carcinoma cell lines. Exp Clin Endocrinol Diabetes 1996; 104: 20-23.

55. Gerber H, Zbaeren J, Kopp P, Aeschimann S, Maciel R, Studer H. Human nodular goiters grow by episodic replication of disseminated cell cohorts expressing several growth factors at the same time. J Endocr Invest 1992; 15 [Suppl 2]:Abstract 95.

56. Minuto F, Barreca A, Del Monte P, Cariola G, Torre GC, Giordano G. Immunoreactive insulin-like growth factor I (IGF-1) and IGF-binding protein content in human thyroid tissue. J Clin Endocrinol Metab 1989; 68:621-626.

57. Vanelli GB, Barni T, Modigliani U, Paulin I, Serio M, Maggi M, Fiorelli G, Balboni GC. Insulin-like growth factor-I receptors in nonfunctioning thyroid nodules. J Clin Endocrinol Metab 1990; 71:1175-1182.

58. Di Carlo A, Mariano A, Pisano G, Parmeggiani U, Beguinot L, Macchia V. Epidermal growth factor and thyrotropin response in human thyroid tissues. J Endocrinol Invest 1990; 13:293 - 299.

59. Westermark, K, Lundqvist M, Wallin G, Dahlman T, Hacker GW, Heldin NE, Grimelius L. EGF-receptors in human normal and pathological thyroid tissue. Histopathology 1996; 28:221-227.

60. Gärtner R, Veitenhansl M, Atkas J, Schophol D. Role of basis fibroblast growth factor in the pathogenesis of nodular goiter. Exp Clin Endocrinol Diabetes 1996; 104:36-38.

61. Morosini PP; Taccaliti A, Montironi R, Scarpelli M, Diamanti L, Simonella G, Mancini V, Petrelli MD, Mantero F. TGF-beta 1 immunohistochemistry in goiter: comparison of patients with recurrence or no recuurence. Thyroid 1996; 6:417-422.

62. Derwahl M, Hamacher Ch, Russo D et al. Constitutive activation of the Gsα-protein-adenylate cyclase pathway may not be sufficient to generate toxic thyroid. J Clin Endocrinol Metab 1996; 81:1898-1904.

63. Rubin H, Chow M, Yao A. Cellular aging, destabilization, and cancer. Proc. Natl. Acad. Sci.

USA 1991; 93:1825-1830.

64. Chow M, Rubin H. Irreversibility of cellular aging and neoplastic transformation: a clonal analysis. Proc. Natl. Acad. Sci. USA 1996; 93:9793-9798.

65. Bishop JM. Molecular themes in oncogenesis. Cell 1991; 64:235-248.

66. Namba H, Gutman RA, Matsuo K, Alvarez A, Fagin JA. H-ras protooncogene mutations in human thyroid neoplasms. J Clin Endocrinol Metab 1990; 71:223-229.

67. Dumont JE, Lamy F, Roger P, Maenhaut C. Physiological and pathological regulation of thyoid cell proliferation and differentiation by thyrotropin and other factors. Physiol Rev 1992; 72:667-679.

68. Studer H, Gerber H. Toxic multinodular goiter. In: Braverman LE, Utiger RE (eds.) The Thyroid, ed. 6 Lippincott, Philadelphia, 1991; pp 692-697, 1107-1117.

69. Westermark K, Karlsson FA, Westermark B. Thyrotropin modulates EGF receptor function in porcine thyroid follicle cells. Mol Cell Endocrinol 1985; 40:17-23.

70. Hofbauer LC, Rafferzeder M, Janssen OE, Gärtner R. Insulin-like growth factor I messenger ribonucleic acid expression in porcine thyroid follicles is regulated by thyrotropin and iodine. Eur J Endocrinol, 1995; 132(5):605-610.

71. Burikhanov R, Coulonval K, Pirson I, Lamy F, Dumont JE, Roger PP. Thyrotropin via cyclic AMP induces insulin receptor expression and insulin co-stimulation of growth and amplifies insulin and insulin-like growth factor signaling pathways in dog thyroid epithelial cells. J Biol Chem, 1996; 271 (46):29400-29406.

72. Eggo MC, King WJ, Black EG, Sheppard MC. Functional human thyroid cells and their insulin-like growth factor-binding proteins: regulation by thyrotropin cyclic 3',5' adenosine monophosphate, and growth factors. J Clin Endocrinol Metab 1996; 81:3056-3062.

73. Cheung NW, Boyages SC. The thyroid gland in acromegaly: an ultrasonographic study. Clin Endocrinol (Oxf), 1997; 46:545-549.

74. Williams DW, Williams ED, Wynford-Thomas D. Evidence for autocrine production of IGF-1 in human thyroid adenomas. Mol Cell Endocrinol 1989; 61:139-143.

75. Derwahl M. Editorial: TSH receptor and Gs-alpha gene mutations in the pathogenesis of toxic thyroid adenomas: a note of caution. J Clin Endocrinol Metab 1996; 81:1-3.

76. Russo D, Arturi F, Schlumberger M, Caillou B, Monier R, Filetti S, Suarez HG. Activating muations of the TSH receptor in differentiated thyroid carcinomas. Oncogene 1995; 11:1907-1911.

77. Holzapfel HP, Fuhrer D, Wonerow P, Weinland G, Scherbaum WA, Paschke R. Identification of constitutively activating somatic thyrotropin receptor mutations in a subset of toxic multinodular goiters. J Clin Endocrinol Metab 1997; 82: 4229-4233.

78. Suarez HG, du Villard JA, Caillou B, Schlumberger M, Parmentier C, Monier R. gsp mutations in human thyroid tumours. Oncogene 1991; 6:677-679.

79. Parma J, van Sande J, Swillens S, Tonacchera M, Dumont J, Vassart G. Somatic mutations causing constitutive activity of the thyrotropin receptor are the major cause of hyperfunctioning thyroid adenomas; identification of additional mutations activating both the cyclic adenosine 3'5'-monophosphate and inositol phosphate-Ca2+ cascades. Mol Endocrinol 1995; 9:725-733.

80. Ivan M, Ludgate M, Gire V, Bond JA, Wynford-Thomas D. An amphotropic retroviral vector expressing a mutant gsp oncogene: effects on human thyroid cells in vitro. J Clin Endocrinol Metab 1997; 82:2702-2708.

81. Muca C, Vallar L. Expression of mutationally activated G alpha stimulates growth and differentiation of thyroid FRTL5 cells. Oncogene, 1994; 9:3647-3653.

82. Porcellini A, Ruggiano G, Pannain S, Ciullo I, Amabile G, Fenzi G, Avvedimento EV. Mutations of thyrotropin receptor isolated from thyroid autonomous functioning adenomas confer TSH-independent growth to thyroid cells. Oncogene 1997; 15:781-179.

83. Michiels FM, Caillou B, Talbot M, Dessaps-Freichey F, Maunoury MT, Schlumberger M, Mercken L, Monier R, Feunteun J. Oncogenic potential of guanine nucleotide stimulatory factor alpha subunit in thyroid glands of transgenic mice. Proc Natl Acad Sci USA 1994; 91:10488-10492.

84. Zeiger MA, Saji M, Gusev, Y, Westra WH, Takiyama Y, Dooley WC, Kohn LD, Levine MA. Thyroid-specific expression of cholera toxin A1 subunit causes thyroid hyperplasia and hyperthyroidism in transgenic mice. Endocrinology 1997; 138:3133-3140.

85. Studer H, Huber G, Derwahl M, Frey P. Die Umwandlung von Basedowstrumen in Knotenkröpfe: ein Grund des Hyperthyreoserezidivs. Schweiz med Wschr 1989; 119:203-208.

86. Kopp P, van Sande J, Parma J et al. Brief report: congenital hyperthyroidism caused by a

mutation in the thyrotropin-receptor gene. N Engl J Med 1995; 332:150 - 154.

87.   Duprez L, Parma J, Van Sande J et al. Germline mutations in the thyrotropin receptor gene cause non-autoimmune autosomal dominant hyperthyroidism. Nature Genet 1994; 7:396 - 401.

88.   Abs R, Stevenaert A, Beckers A. Autonomously functioning thyroid nodules in a patient with thyrotropin-secreting pituitary adenoma: possible cause-effect relationship. Eur J Endocrinol 1994; 131:355-358.

89.   Vesely DI. Selective pituitary resistance to thyroid hormones after treatment of a toxic multinodular goiter. South Med J 1988; 81:1173-1176.

90.   Williams DW, Williams ED, Wynford-Thomas D. Loss of independence on IGF-I for proliferation of human thyroid adenoma cells. Br J Cancer 1988; 57:535-359.

91.   Hintze G, Emrich D, Köbberling J. Treatment of endemic goitre due to iodine deficiency with iodine, levothyroxine or both: results of a multicentre trial. Europ J Clin Invest 1989; 19:527-534.

92.   Gärtner R, Dugrillon A, Bechtner G. Evidence that iodolactones are the mediators of growth inhibition by iodine on the thyroid. Acta Med Austriaca, 1996; 23:47-51.

93.   Hay ID, Reading CC, Carbonau JW. High-resolution realtime ultrasonography and unsuspected micronodular thyroid disease [letter]. Lancet 1984; 1:916.

94.   Mortensen JD, Woolner LB, Bennet WA. Gross and microscopic findings in clinically normal thyroid glands. J Clin Endocrinol Metab 1955; 15:1270-1276.

95.   Morita T, Tamai H, Ohshima A, Komaki G, Matsubayashi S, Kuma K, Nakagawa T. Changes in serum thyroid hormone, thyrotropin and thyroglobulin concentration during thyroxine therapy in patients with solitary thyroid nodules. J Clin Endocrinol Metab 1989; 69:227-230.

96.   Celani MF, Mariani M, Mariani G. On the usefulness of levothyroxine suppressive therapy in the medical treatment of benign solitary, solid or predominantly solid, thyroid nodules. Acta Endocrinol (Copenh) 1990; 123:603-608.

97.   Gharib H, James EM, Charboneau JW, Naesens JM, Offord KP, Gorman CA. Suppressive therapy with levothyroxine for solitary thyroid nodules. A double-blind controlled clinical study. N Engl J Med 1987; 317:70-75.

98.   Papini, Bacci V, Panunzi C, Pacella CM, Fabbrini R, Bizzarri G, Petrucci L, Giammarco V, La Medica P, Masala M et al. A prospective randomized trial of levothyroxine suppressive therapy for solitary thyroid nodules. Clin Endocrinol (Oxf) 1993; 38:507-513.

99.   Cheung PS, Lee JM, Boey JH. Thyroxine suppressive therapy of benign solitary thyroid nodules: a prospective randomized study. World J Surg 1989; 13:818-822.

100. Celani MF. Levothyroxine suppressive therapy in the medical management of nontoxic benign multinodular goiter. Exp Clin Endocrinol 1993; 101:326-332.

101. La Rosa GL, Lupo L, Giuffrida D, Gullo d, Vigneri R, Belfiore A. Levothyroxine and potassium iodide are both effective in treating benign solid cold nodules of the thyroid. Ann Intern Med 1995; 122:1-8.

102. Lima N, Knobel M, Cavaliere H, Sztejnsznajd C, Tomimori E, Medeiros-Neto G. Levothyroxine suppressive therapy is partially effective in treating patients with benign, solid thyroid nodules and multinodular goiters. Thyroid 1997; 7:691-697.

103. La Rosa GL, Ippolito AM, Lupo L, Cercabene G, Santonocito MG, Vigneri R, Belfiore A. Cold thyroid nodule reduction with L-thyroxine can be predicted by initial nodule volume and cytological characteristics. Clin Endocrinol Metab 1996; 81:4385-4387.

104. Badillo J, Shimaoka K, Lessmann EM, Marchetta FC, Sokal JE. Treatment of nontoxic goiter with sodium liothyronine. JAMA 1963; 184:151-158.

105. Berghout A, Wiersinga WM, Drexhage HA, Smits NJ, Touber JL. Comparison of placebo with L-thyroxine alone or with carbimazole for treatment of sporadic non-toxic goitre. Lancet 1990; 336:193-197.

106. Nygaard B, Hegedus L, Gervil M, Hjalgrim H, Soe-Jensen P, Hansen JM. Radioiodine treatment of multinodular non-toxic goitre. BMJ 1993; 307:828-832.

107. Huysmans DA, Buijs WC, van den Ven MT, van den Broek WJ, Kloppenburg PW, Hermus AR, Corstens FH. Dosimetry and risk estimates of radioiodine therapy for large, multinodular goiters. J Nuc Med 1996; 37:2072-2079.

108. Huysmans D, Hermus A, Edelbroek M, Barentsz J, Corstens F, Kloppenburg P. Radioiodine for nontoxic multinodular goiter. Thyroid 1997; 7:235-239.

109. Huysmans AK, Hermus RM, Edelbroek MA, Tjabbes T, Oostdijk A, Ross HA, Corstens FH, Kloppenburg PW. Autoimmune hyperthyroidism occurring late after radioiodine treatment for volume reduction of large multinodular goiters. Thyroid 1997; 7:535-539.

110. Livraghi T, Paracchi A, Ferrari C, Bergonzi M, Grarvaglia G, Ranieri P, Vetorri C. Treatment of

autonomous thyroid nodules with percutaneous ethanol injection: preliminary results. Work in progress. Radiology 1990; 175:827-829.

111. Verde G, Papini E, Pacell CM, Gallotti S, Strada S, Fabbrini R, Bizzarri G, Rinaldi R, Panunzi C et al. Ultrasound guided percutaneous ethanol injection in the treatment of cystic thyroid nodules. Clin Endocrinol (Oxf) 1994; 41:719-724.

112. Papini E, Pacella CM, Verde G. Percutaneous ethanol injection (PEI): what is the role in the treatment of benign thyroid nodules? Thyroid 1995; 5:147-150.

113. Lippi F, Ferrari C, Manetti L, Rago T, Santini F, Monzani F, Bellitti P, Papini E, Busnardo B, Angelini F, Pinchera A. Treatment of solitary autonomous thyroid nodules by percutaneous ethanol injection: results of an Italian multicenter study. The Multicenter study group. J Clin Endocrinol Metab 1996; 81:3261-3264.

114. Ferrari C, Reschini E, Paacchi A. Treatment of the autonomous thyroid nodule: a review. Eur J Endocrinol 1996; 135:383-390.

115. Monzani F, Caraccio N, Goletti O, Lippolis PV, Casolaro A, Del Guerra P, Cavina E, Miccoli P. Five-year follow-up of percutaneous ethanol injection for the treatment of hyperfunctioning thyroid nodules: a study of 117 patients. Clin Endocrinol (Oxf) 1997; 46:9-15.

116. Caraccio N, Goletti O, Lippolis PV, Casolaro A, Cavina E, Miccoli P, Monzani F. Is percutaneous ethanol injection a useful alternative for the treatment of the cold benign thyroid nodule? Five years' experience. Thyroid 1997; 7:699-704.

117. Bennedbaek FN, Karstrup S, Hegedus L. Percutaneous ethanol injection therapy in the treatment of thyroid and parathyroid diseases. Eur J Endocrinol 1997; 136:240-250.

118. Singer PA, Cooper DS, Daniels GH, Ladenson PW, Greenspan FS, Levy EG, Braverman LE, Clark OH, McDougall IR, Ain KV, Dorfman SG. Treatment guidelines for patients with thyroid nodules and well-differentiated thyroid cancer. American Thyroid Association. Arch Intern Med 1996; 156:2165-2172.

119. Mazzaferri EL. Management of a solitary thyroid nodule. N Engl J Med 1993; 328:553-559.

120. Belfiore A, La Rosa GL, La Porta GA, Giuffrida D, Milazzo G, Lupo L, Regalbuto C, Vigneri R. Cancer risk in patients with cold thyroid nodules: relevance of iodide intake, sex, age and multinodularity. Am J Med 1992; 93:363-369.

121. Kuma K, Matsuzuka F, Kobayashi A, Hirai K, Morita S, Miyauchi A, Katayama S, Sugawara M. Outcome of long standing solitary thyroid nodules. World J Surg 1992; 16:583-587.

122. Hung W, Anderson KD, Chandra RS, Kapur SP, Patterson K, Randolph JG, August GP. Solitary thyroid nodules in 71 children and adolescents. J Pediatr Surg 1992; 27:1407-1409.

123. Pelizzo MR, Bernante P, Toniato A, Fassina A. Frequency of thyroid carcinoma in a recent series of 539 consecutive thyroidectomies for multinodular goiter. Tumori 1997; 83:653-655.

124. al-Suliman NN, Ryttov NF, Qvist N, Blichert-Toft M, Graversen HP. Experience in a specialist thyroid surgery unit: a demographic study, surgical complications, and outcome. Eur J Surg 1997; 163:13-20.

125. Bistrup C, Nielsen JD, Gregersen G, Franch P. Preventive effect of levothyroxine in patients operated for non-toxic goitre: a randomized trial of one hundred patients with nine years follow-up. Clin. Endocrinol.Oxf. 1994; 40:323-327.

126. Rzepka AH, Cissewski K, Olbricht T, Reinwein D. Effectiveness of prophylactic therapy on goiter recurrence in an area with low iodine intake - a sonographic follow-up study. Clin. Investig. 1994; 72:967-970.

127. Rojdmark J, Jarhult J. High long term recurrence rate after subtotal thyroidectomy for nodular goitre. Eur. J. Surg. 1995; 161:725-727.

128. Zelmanovitz T, Zelmanovitz F, Genro S, Gus P, de Azevedo MJ, Gross JL. Analysis of the factors associated with recurrence of post-thyroidectomy goiter. Rev. Assoc. Med. Bras. 1995; 41:86-90.

8 CYTOPATHOLOGY OF THYROID NODULES:

Yolanda C. Oertel, M.D.
George Washington University
Washington, D.C.

Introduction

The value of fine needle aspiration (FNA) in the diagnosis and management of thyroid nodules has been well established (1-5). We share the opinion of Hayes et al. (6) that FNA should be the first test ordered when evaluating any palpable thyroid lesion. In this era of cost containment, FNA can be used even more effectively if attention is paid to the fundamentals. According to Kaplan, "The main current limitations are the inability of even skilled operators to obtain an adequate specimen in up to 20% of the cases......(this) problem probably is beyond remedy."(7) I disagree. Based on over 20 years experience at a university medical center, I believe that more emphasis must be placed on the technique employed to obtain the sample (8-10). A discussion of technique is beyond the scope of the present chapter. Although the procedure is simple, it is not simple-minded. It can be taught or perfected in a relatively short time. I cannot overemphasize that a good sample is the cornerstone of diagnosis. A pathologist is only as good as the sample obtained or received.

Aspirates (FNA) should not be confused with needle biopsies (Tru-cut, Vim-Silverman, etc.) that require a local anesthetic and yield tissue fragments that are processed and embedded in paraffin for histologic diagnosis. FNA does not require injection of a local anesthetic, but application of an ice cube to the site is helpful.

Assessing thyroid aspirates

The pathologist's responsibility is to determine whether the sample is representative of the lesion in question and adequate in quantity. This task is easier if the pathologist is the one performing the aspiration. Otherwise, the physician performing the procedure must provide the information necessary to make this assessment. Briefly, if the pathologist has to count the number of cells per smear, it is my opinion that the sample is not adequate (11,12). When interpreting aspirates, I try to answer two questions: If this is a sample of a lesion in my thyroid, do I consider it diagnostic? Can my treatment (be it medical or surgical) be based upon this sample?

All cytologic descriptions in this chapter are from smears stained with Diff-Quik, a commercially available variant of the May-Grünwald-Giemsa hematological stain.

Background of the smears

Often colloid is present in the background. Its appearance is markedly varied, from thin and homogeneous to geometric, crumbled, cracked, dense, etc. (8)

Number of cells

The number of cells will vary with the prowess of the aspirator. Very cellular specimens may represent "tumor cellularity," or they may be a cell-rich sample expertly obtained from a non-neoplastic nodule. Also, hypocellular specimens, diluted by blood, may represent poor samples from a follicular neoplasm obtained by a vigorous aspirator.

Arrangement of cells

The arrangement of the cells is of great value in determining the type of lesion. If the cells are forming spherules (Fig. 8.1) and honeycomb-like sheets (Fig. 8.2), the lesion is most likely non-neoplastic. If rosettes and tubules (Fig. 8.3) predominate and the tissue fragments show a "shower effect," the lesion is likely a hyperplastic nodule. These tissue fragments do not have well demarcated borders; instead they seem to spill multiple rosettes and tubules into the surrounding area of the smear. If microfollicles (either empty or filled with colloid) are seen, then the lesion is probably a follicular neoplasm. Papillary fragments *per se* are not diagnostic of papillary carcinoma (13,14).

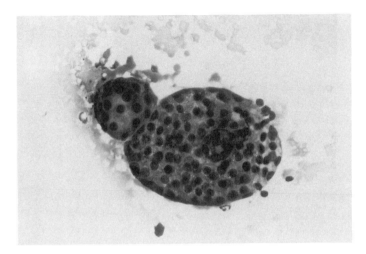

Fig. 8.1. Two spherules. These represent non-neoplastic follicles. Many RBC's lie in the background. Diff-Quik stain, x400.

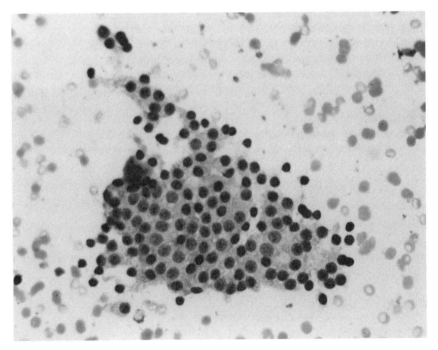

Fig. 8.2. Sheet of follicular epithelial cells with round, regular nuclei approximately equidistant from one another, causing the so called "honeycomb" pattern. Diff-Quik stain, x400.

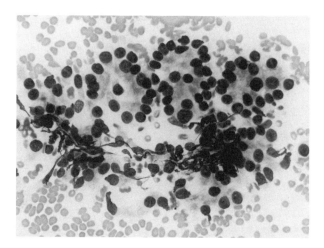

Fig. 8.3. Follicular epithelial cells arranged in rosettes. There are "lympho-epithelial tangles" below them. Diff-Quik stain, x400.

Cellular features

The size of the epithelial cells, particularly the size of the nuclei, is important. Non-neoplastic cells frequently have nuclei no larger than 10-15 µ in diameter (twice the size of an erythrocyte). The types of cells present are relevant, and also whether it is a polymorphous or a monotonous population. The former is consistent with non-neoplastic lesions, whereas a monotonous or monomorphic cellular population is most likely from a neoplasm.

Nomenclature

On reviewing the literature, the author has noted the frequent variations in the diagnostic terms utilized, especially in regard to benign lesions. It is encouraging to note that efforts towards uniform terminology are being made (15).

Non-neoplastic lesions

These are the most frequently aspirated lesions. We should strive to use uniform terminology.

Adenomatoid nodule (s)

This may represent a dominant nodule in a multinodular goiter or may be a single nodule. Its composition varies. In some there is a large amount of colloid, and we refer to these as adenomatoid nodule(s) with abundant colloid. Others use the term colloid nodule (4) or colloid-rich nodule. Frequently these nodules undergo cystic changes. In other instances the cellular component predominates over the colloid, and we use the term cellular adenomatoid nodule (16). Some authors call them parenchymatous nodules (17,18). Our diagnostic criteria are summarized in Table 8-1) (Figs. 8.1-8.3). In our opinion, patients believed to have cellular adenomatoid nodules should undergo suppressive therapy for six to nine months; then another aspiration should be performed. If the lesion does not decrease in size, does not undergo cystic change, the colloid remains scanty, and the cellularity does not decrease, then it should be excised.

Table 8-1. Differences between adenomatoid nodule and cellular
adenomatoid nodule

Cytologic Features	Adenomatoid Nodule	Cellular Adenomatoid Nodule
Cellularity of smears	Usually scant	Marked
Arrangement of follicular cells	Predominantly in sheets and spherules	Predominantly in rosettes and tubules
Tissue fragments	Well defined outlines, contain spherules	"Shower effect," many cords, some empty follicles
Nuclear size	Up to twice the size of an erythrocyte	Variable, usually larger than twice the size of an erythrocyte
Colloid	Moderate to abundant, in the background	Scant
Cystic change	Frequent	Sometimes seen

Multinodular goiter

This is a clinical diagnosis and not a cytologic diagnosis. The findings on the smears are as described under adenomatoid nodule. If we have seen and aspirated the patient, our report will read as follows: "adenomatoid nodules most consistent with multinodular goiter." If we are interpreting smears submitted by other physicians, the cytopathology report will read "adenomatoid nodule(s)."

Graves' disease

Although some reports describe diagnostic cytologic criteria for Graves' disease (19-21), we believe this is a clinical and chemical diagnosis. The so-called cytoplasmic flares are ubiquitous (Fig. 8.4). If you search for them, you will find them in both neoplastic and non-neoplastic entities.

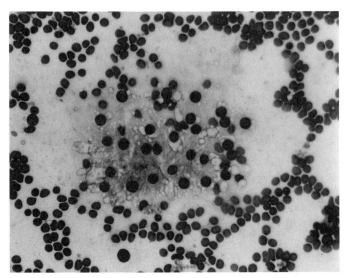

Fig. 8.4.   Sheet of follicular epithelial cells with peripheral cytoplasmic vacuoles (or "flares").
Numerous RBC's are visible. Diff-Quik stain, x400.

Thyroglossal duct cyst

FNA contributes to an accurate preoperative diagnosis of thyroglossal cysts,
allowing a Sistrunk procedure to be performed in these patients rather than an
inappropriate local resection. Smears have scant cellularity. Inflammatory cells are
more numerous than epithelial cells. Histiocytes (mono- or multinucleated, foamy
or hemosiderin-laden), and polymorphonuclear leukocytes predominate (22).
Squamous cells are present more frequently than ciliated columnar epithelial cells;
groups of thyroid follicular epithelial cells are rare.

Inflammatory processes

Most inflammatory processes are infrequent.   Hence, the cytologic literature on
acute suppurative thyroiditis and thyroiditis secondary to fungal infections is rather
sparse (23,24).   In the last few years several cases of *Pneumocystis carinii*
thyroiditis diagnosed on aspirates have been reported (25-28).   Although our
university hospital has a large AIDS population, we have not seen a case yet.

Subacute thyroiditis

We have seen very few cases of subacute (granulomatous, viral, or de Quervain's)
thyroiditis. Because these cases resolve either spontaneously or after symptomatic
medication and have a characteristic clinical picture, no tissue diagnosis is required.
The few patients that we have aspirated have experienced marked pain. Sheets of
small follicular cells with paravacuolar cytoplasmic granules are present.
Macrophages, lymphocytes, polymorphonuclear leukocytes, epithelioid histiocytes,

and multinucleated histiocytes are readily seen (23). Variable amounts of colloid are present and are usually in close proximity to or phagocytosed by macrophages.

Lymphocytic thyroiditis

It is also known as Hashimoto's thyroiditis, autoimmune thyroiditis, chronic nonspecific thyroiditis, and struma lymphomatosa. Most patients present with a multinodular gland, rubbery on palpation. Occasionally there are single or dominant nodules mimicking a neoplasm. The classic cytologic pattern (Fig. 8.5)

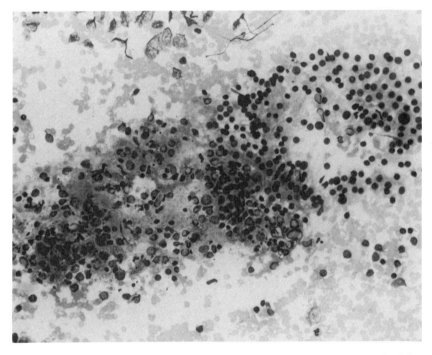

Fig. 8.5. Chronic lymphocytic (Hashimoto's) thyroiditis. Sheet of follicular cells lie to the right, and many lymphoid cells are present on the left. Diff-Quik stain, x200.

consists of numerous lymphocytes (some may be atypical), "lymphoid tangles" (crushed cells), macrophages containing "tingible-bodies" in their cytoplasm, plasma cells, multinucleated histiocytes, and epithelial cells (23,24). The latter may be arranged in sheets with a honeycomb appearance and have "paravacuolar" cytoplasmic granules, or they may have oxyphilic cytoplasm (Askanazy/Hürthle cells). Clearing of the nuclear chromatin of the lymphocytes is a frequently observed artifact (Fig. 8.6). Fragments of fibrocollageous tissue and skeletal muscle are found often (29). The proportion of cellular elements will vary according to the stage of the disease. In early phases the lymphoid cells predominate. It is important to remember that Hashimoto's thyroiditis is the leading source of false positive diagnosis of cancer. Smears have been misdiagnosed as papillary carcinoma, oxyphilic neoplasms, and malignant lymphoma (24,30).

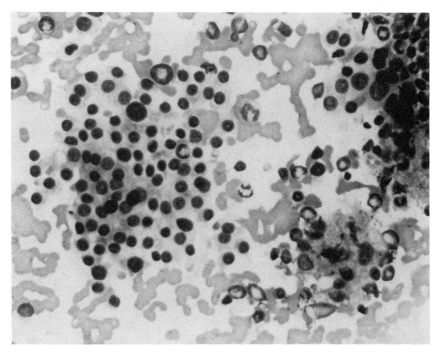

Fig. 8.6. Chronic lymphocytic (Hashimoto's) thyroiditis. There are numerous follicular cells, especially to the left. Lymphoid cells are present throughout, many with "clearing" of the chromatin. Compare with the intranuclear cytoplasmic inclusions seen in Fig. 8.8. Diff-Quik stain, x400.

Neoplastic lesions

The classification we follow is that of the WHO (31) with some of the modifications by the AFIP (13). Thyroidal tumors may be either primary or secondary (metastatic from other organs). The latter are rare. The **primary** tumors of the thyroid fall into two categories: Epithelial and Non-epithelial. The primary epithelial tumors may be of (1) follicular cell differentiation, (2) "C" cell differentiation, and (3) combined follicular cell and "C" cell differentiation.

Primary epithelial tumors

A. Follicular cell differentiation
   I.   Benign
        1.   Follicular adenoma (conventional)
        2.   Follicular adenoma of oxyphilic cell type

   II. Indeterminate
        1.   Atypical follicular adenoma
        2.   Hyalinizing trabecular neoplasm

   III. Malignant
        1.   Better differentiated
             a.   Follicular carcinoma
             b.   Papillary carcinoma
                  • Classic
                  • Microcarcinoma
                  • Follicular variant
                  • Encapsulated
                  • Cystic
                  • Diffuse sclerosing
                  • Oxyphilic cell type
                  • Solid/trabecular
                  • Tall cell
                  • Columnar cell

        2.   Poorly differentiated carcinoma
             a.   Insular
             b.   Others

        3.   Undifferentiated or anaplastic carcinoma
        4.   Squamous cell carcinoma
        5.   Mucoepidermoid carcinoma

B. "C" cell differentiation
   Medullary carcinoma

C. Combined follicular cell and "C" cell differentiation (rare)

Primary non-epithelial tumors

Benign
        Leiomyoma
        Schwannoma

Malignant
>   Lymphoma
>   Sarcoma

Miscellaneous neoplasms

Secondary or metastatic tumors

Follicular neoplasms

Cytologically we cannot differentiate between a follicular adenoma and a follicular carcinoma. We believe, as do others (13,32), that this requires multiple sections through the periphery of the surgically resected tumor to determine the presence (or absence) of capsular and/or vascular invasion. Hence, on FNA smears we only make the diagnosis of "follicular neoplasm," and this category encompasses both the benign and malignant follicular tumors. Some authors have reported that differentiation between adenoma and carcinoma can be made on smears (24).

Follicular adenoma (conventional)/follicular carcinoma

Follicular adenoma is a benign, usually encapsulated tumor with an essentially uniform internal structure different from the surrounding thyroid parenchyma. Often the adjacent follicles are compressed. In contrast the usual adenomatoid nodule (which is considered non-neoplastic) has a varied internal architecture, often contains much colloid, frequently lacks a capsule, and is prone to retrogressive changes. Obviously, there is considerable overlap between adenomas and adenomatoid nodules.

These neoplasms bleed easily on aspiration and many samples are diluted by blood and appear hypocellular. However, a more experienced aspirator may obtain hypercellular smears ("tumor cellularity"). The most characteristic cytologic pattern consists of enlarged follicular cells arranged in rosettes, tubules, and microfollicles containing dark blue inspissated colloid (Diff-Quik stained smears) (Fig. 8.7). These neoplastic follicles have enlarged cells with delicate cytoplasm of pale pink or bluish tint. The rounded nuclei have chromatin of variable density which gives them a mottled appearance. The nuclear borders are slightly irregular. The nucleoli are usually visible. There is no colloid in the background, but red blood cells are numerous.

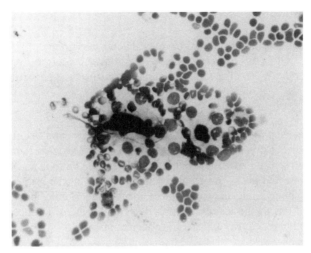

Fig. 8.7. Follicular neoplasm (follicular adenoma in histologic sections). Two neoplastic follicles have dense inspissated colloid in their lumen. Many RBC's are present. Compare with the non-neoplastic follicles in Fig. 8.1 at the same magnification. Diff-Quik stain, x400.

Follicular adenoma/carcinoma of oxyphilic cell type

Oxyphilic cells also are called oncocytes, Askanazy cells, Hürthle cells and mitochondrion-rich cells. We reiterate that cytologically we cannot differentiate between an oxyphilic cell follicular adenoma and carcinoma. See the comment under follicular neoplasms.

The smears are usually markedly cellular. Oxyphilic cells, usually similar to one another, are arranged in tissue fragments, clusters, and singly. The cellular borders are well demarcated. The cytoplasm is abundant, dense, and stains grayish-pink or grayish-blue with Diff-Quik. The nuclei are enlarged, usually round, and have well defined borders; the nucleoli are conspicuous. Binucleation is frequent. Neoplastic follicles, are easily detected; empty follicles are more numerous than those with inspissated colloid (10,33).

Hyalinizing trabecular neoplasm

Although most reported cases have been benign (adenoma), a few have shown local invasion and/or lymph node metastasis (34). The smears are hypercellular with single cells and clusters of cells that may have spindled shapes and a tendency to palisading. Intranuclear cytoplasmic inclusions are frequently present. Also, amorphous hyalin material somewhat reminiscent of amyloid may be observed (35). This has lead to an erroneous cytologic diagnosis of medullary carcinoma or papillary carcinoma. (35-37).

Papillary carcinoma

This is the most common thyroidal cancer. The histologic patterns are remarkably varied. We will only describe those that have cytologic features that are sufficiently distinctive to allow the pathologist to suspect the particular type.

Classic type

The tumors consist of mixtures of neoplastic follicles and papillae formed by distinctive cells, often with considerable dense fibrosis present. They are characteristically very firm on palpation. On aspiration there is a gritty sensation as the needle is inserted (as if one would be inserting the needle into an apple). If the smears are hypocellular, the subsequent aspirations should be taken from the peripheral portions of the lesion. This is detected by the difference in consistency of the thyroidal parenchyma and the fibrotic neoplasm.

The richly cellular smears show neoplastic cells arranged in clusters and sheets with crowded and overlapping nuclei, papillary fragments (with or without vascular cores), and single cells. These cells are enlarged, their cytoplasm is often dense with well demarcated borders. The nuclei are frequently three times the size of the erythrocytes, but considerable variation in size and shape is evident. The chromatin is dense, the nuclear outline is sharp, and nucleoli are inconspicuous. Intranuclear cytoplasmic inclusions are seen frequently (Fig. 8.8). Nuclear grooves are more readily seen in Papanicolaou stained smears (24). Multinucleated histiocytes are common. Psammoma bodies occur in 30% to 40% of these cancers. Colloid is usually scant, but in our experience the characteristic dense, pink colloid (ropy colloid, bubble-gum colloid) is more important than the amount present.

Follicular variant

The smears are very cellular. Rosettes and tubules may be the dominant pattern, but tissue fragments with empty follicles are often evident. Most neoplastic cells are enlarged, but their cytoplasm is not as dense as in the classic type. The nuclei are hyperchromatic, have smooth contours, and vary in size and shape. Some have a triangular shape reminiscent of arrowheads. Dense, pink staining colloid appears as balls and strands in the background, and as clusters of small granules in the lumen of occasional follicles. Multinucleated histiocytes, psammoma bodies, and intranuclear cytoplasmic inclusions are less common than in the classic papillary carcinoma (38).

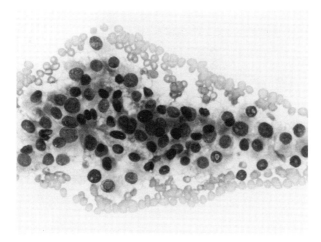

Fig. 8.8 Papillary carcinoma. Group of neoplastic follicular cells with enlarged nuclei. Note the variation in nuclear size, shape, and density of chromatin. Intranuclear inclusions are apparent. Diff-Quik stain, x400.

Cystic papillary carcinoma

These tumors may present as masses of different sizes and consistency. Some are soft while others are hard (fluid under tension). On aspiration the amount, color, and consistency of the fluid vary from 1 ml. to over 20 ml., from light yellow to dark brown, and from watery to syrupy. If the fluid reaccumulates within a few minutes after aspiration, this is suspicious for papillary carcinoma.

These lesions have created concern about the efficacy of fine needle aspiration because they are a source of false negative diagnosis. We believe that this is the result of applying the cytologic diagnostic criteria of classic papillary carcinoma to these cystic cancers. Instead, different cytologic criteria, described below, have to be applied.

Usually the smears show many macrophages (both foamy and hemosiderin-laden and also multinucleated histiocytes) in a background of thin colloid with scattered cellular debris. Squamous metaplastic cells may be present. These features are similar to those seen in smears from an adenomatoid nodule with cystic degeneration. Smears from cystic papillary carcinoma (see Table 8.2) show subtle differences: sheets and small groups of well preserved epithelial cells out of place in this degenerative milieu, single degenerated neoplastic cells with clear cytoplasm and enlarged nuclei (resembling atypical macrophages), and tight clusters of atypical epithelial cells often having pale cytoplasm at the periphery with smooth scalloped borders (10). Numerous psammoma bodies are found often. Balls of pink colloid may be present.

Table 8-2. Differences between adenomatoid nodule with cystic degeneration and cystic papillary carcinoma

Cytologic features	Adenomatoid nodule with cystic degeneration	Cystic papillary carcinoma
Sheets of follicular cells	Nuclei are small and hyperchromatic ("raisins")	Nuclei are twice or three times the size of RBC's ("grapes")
Single cells	Macrophages (foamy and hemosiderin-laden)	Macrophages. Cells with clear cytoplasm and large nuclei mimicking "atypical" macrophages
Clusters of cells	Follicular cells, some with oxyphilic cytoplasm	Atypical epithelial cells with pale cytoplasm. Scalloped borders of clusters
Colloid	Abundant, bluish, thin	Pink balls
Psammoma bodies	Extremely rare	Frequent, numerous

Oxyphilic cell variant

The initial impression is that of an oxyphilic cell (Hürthle cell) follicular neoplasm. More detailed examination reveals the absence of conspicuous nucleoli and of neoplastic follicles (39), frequent presence of papillae (40), and the presence of multinucleated histiocytes (usually extremely rare in follicular neoplasms), psammoma bodies, and intranuclear cytoplasmic inclusions

Tall cell variant

This uncommon variant has been reported as having relatively large cells with abundant eosinophilic cytoplasm, frequent intranuclear cytoplasmic inclusions, and rare psammoma bodies. Some authors have reported the presence of papillary structures (41), but others have not found them consistently (42,43) or not found them at all (44).

Columnar cell variant

The report of a case (45) with Papanicolaou stained smears describes papillary fragments with columnar cells at their periphery, and also fragments with gland-like spaces. The nuclei were hyperchromatic and ovoid or elongated, the nucleoli were indistinct, and the cytoplasm was pale. No colloid was identified.

Undifferentiated or anaplastic carcinoma

In some cases there is marked fibrosis, so multiple aspirates are required to obtain cellular material. Also, extensive necrosis and hemorrhage may be present, and therefore some smears may be hypocellular. However, the few cells observed may be bizarre. In other cases the smears are hypercellular and composed of spindled cells and/or pleomorphic cells. Multinucleated cells may be frequent; they are either histiocytic (osteoclast-like) or pleomorphic neoplastic cells (9,10,24).

The so called small cell carcinoma is extremely rare, and most reported cases are malignant lymphomas.

Medullary carcinoma

We consider this a cytologic diagnosis of exclusion, because the smears are extremely variable, not resembling any of the more common thyroidal neoplasms. Smears are markedly cellular (Fig. 8.9). Loosely cohesive clusters of rounded, polygonal, or spindled cells are observed in a hemorrhagic background with many single neoplastic cells. In some cases the neoplastic cells have round nuclei, eccentrically located, which produces a plasmacytoid appearance (46,47). In other cases the spindled cells predominate. Frequently, large neoplastic cells with enlarged single or multiple nuclei are present. Intranuclear cytoplasmic inclusions are observed in some cases (48). Nucleoli are rarely visible. The cytoplasm has variable tinctorial characteristics, from dense and bluish-pink in the plasmacytoid cells to attenuated and pale blue in the bizarre neoplastic cells. The presence of calcitonin cytoplasmic granules that stain bright pink with hematological stains has been overemphasized in the literature (49,50). In our experience we find them in about one-third of the cases, and only after a tedious search.

The features we find most helpful in making this diagnosis are tumor cellularity, lack of cellular cohesiveness, plasmacytoid appearance of many cells (in some cases), scattered very large tumor cells with bizarre single or multiple nuclei, and the general absence of visible nucleoli.

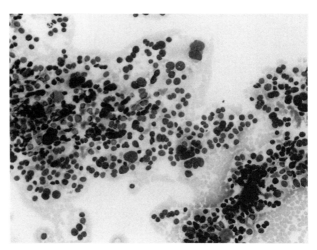

Fig. 8.9. Medullary carcinoma. Hypercellular smear with marked variation in size and shape of the neoplastic nuclei. Diff-Quik stain, x200.

Non-epithelial neoplasms

This category includes the malignant lymphomas and the benign and malignant soft tissue tumors (which rarely occur in the thyroid) (51,52).

Malignant lymphoma

Most thyroid glands involved by a primary lymphoma are the site of autoimmune (lymphocytic) thyroiditis. Therefore, FNA may obtain the benign lymphoplasmacytic infiltrates and altered follicular epithelial cells characterizing the thyroiditis. These findings do not explain the clinical picture that led to the suspicion of lymphoma, so multiple aspirates from the enlarged gland often are needed.

Lymphocytic thyroiditis has a varied population of small and large lymphocytes (including activated lymphocytes or "basket cells"), plasma cells, and "tingible-body" macrophages. Also, sheets of follicular epithelial cells, some with oxyphilic cytoplasm, are found with relative ease in many cases. The smears from the lymphoma show a monotonous lymphoid population, fairly numerous mitotic figures and a notable absence of follicular epithelial cells (24,30).

Secondary or metastatic tumors

Although the thyroid is well vascularized, metastatic tumors are uncommon. Usually such a lesion presents as a single nodule, although we have seen examples appearing as a multinodular goiter. The most frequent primary neoplasms that spread to the thyroid are carcinomas of the lung, kidney, and breast, and malignant melanoma (24). Malignant lymphoma and leukemia may secondarily involve the thyroid.

Miscellaneous tumors

Lipomas of the anterior neck can be mistaken for thyroid neoplasms, both on physical examination and on radionuclide scan. FNA allows a definite diagnosis, thereby avoiding unnecessary suppressive therapy or surgery (53).

Other cervical lesions that may be mistaken for masses in the thyroid include parathyroid tumors or cysts and soft tissue lesions such as nodular fasciitis.

References:

1. Ashcraft MW, Van Herle AJ. Management of thyroid nodules. II: Scanning techniques, thyroid suppressive therapy, and fine needle aspiration. Head Neck 1981;3:297-322.
2. Miller JM, Kini SR, Hamburger JI, Meissner WA. Needle Biopsy of The Thyroid. Current Concepts. 1st ed. New York: Praeger, 1983.
3. Khafagi F, Wright G, Castles H, Perry-Keene D, Mortimer R. Screening for thyroid malignancy: the role of fine-needle biopsy. Med J Aust 1988;149:302-7.
4. Gharib H, Goellner JR, Johnson DA. Fine-needle aspiration cytology of the thyroid. A 12-year experience with 11,000 biopsies. Clin Lab Med 1993;13:699-709.
5. Sabel MS, Staren ED, Gianakakis LM, Dwarakanathan S, Prinz RA. Effectiveness of the thyroid scan in evaluation of the solitary thyroid nodule. Am Surg 1997;63:660-4.
6. Hayes AA, Hay ID, Gorman CA. Solitary thyroid nodule: fine needle aspiration, the first investigation. Nucl Med Commun 1989;10:768-71.
7. Kaplan MM. Progress in thyroid cancer. Endocrinol Metab Clin North Am 1990;19:469-78.
8. Oertel YC. Fine-needle aspiration of the thyroid. In: Moore WT, Eastman RC, eds. Diagnostic Endocrinology. 2nd ed. St. Louis: Mosby-Year Book, Inc, 1996:211-28.
9. Oertel YC. Fine-needle aspiration and the diagnosis of thyroid cancer. Endocrinol Metab Clin North Am 1996;25:69-91.
10. Oertel YC. Fine-needle aspiration in the evaluation of thyroid neoplasms. Endocr Pathol 1997;8:215-24.
11. Hamburger JI. Extensive personal experience. Diagnosis of thyroid nodules by fine needle biopsy: Use and abuse. J Clin Endocrinol Metab 1994;79:335-9.
12. Oertel YC. A pathologist's comments on diagnosis of thyroid nodules by fine needle aspiration. J Clin Endocrinol Metab 1995;80:1467-8.
13. Rosai J, Carcangiu ML, DeLellis RA. Tumors of The Thyroid Gland. Washington, D.C.: A.F.I.P., 1992 (Rosai J, Sobin LH, eds. Atlas of Tumor Pathology. 3rd Series; Fascicle 5).
14. Faser CR, Marley EF, Oertel YC. Papillary tissue fragments as a diagnostic pitfall in fine- needle aspirations of thyroid nodules. Diagn Cytopathol 1997;16:454-9.
15. Suen KC, The Papanicolaou Society of Cytopathology task force on standards of practice. Guidelines of the Papanicolaou Society of Cytopathology for the examination of fine-needle aspiration specimens from thyroid nodules. Mod Pathol 1996;9:710-5.
16. Busseniers AE, Oertel YC. "Cellular adenomatoid nodules" of the thyroid: Review of 219 fine-needle aspirates. Diagn Cytopathol 1993;9:581-9.
17. Welsh RA, Correa P. The comparative pathology of goiter in a nonendemic and an endemic area. Arch Pathol Lab Med 1960;69:694-700.
18. Harach HR, Soto MS, Zusman SB, Saravia Day E. Parenchymatous thyroid nodules: a histocytological study of 31 cases from a goitrous area. J Clin Pathol 1992;45:25-9.

19.   Kyriakos G, Ioannidou M, Tolis G. Evaluation of fine-needle aspiration biopsy findings in treatment of Grave's disease. In: Goerttler K, Feichter GE, Witte S, eds. New Frontiers in Cytology. Berlin: Springer-Verlag, 1988:320-3.

20.   Jayaram G, Singh B, Marwaha RK. Grave's (sic) disease. Appearance in cytologic smears from fine needle aspirates of the thyroid gland. Acta Cytol 1989;33:36-40.

21.   Bhalotra R, Jayaram G. Overlapping morphology in thyroiditis (Hashimoto's and subacute) and Grave's disease. Cytopathology 1990;1:371-2.

22.   Shaffer MM, Oertel YC, Oertel JE. Thyroglossal duct cysts. Diagnostic criteria by fine-needle aspiration. Arch Pathol Lab Med 1996;120:1039-43.

23.   Persson PS. Cytodiagnosis of thyroiditis. A comparative study of cytological, histological, immunological and clinical findings in thyroiditis, particularly in diffuse lymphoid thyroiditis. Acta Med Scand 1968;183(Suppl. 483):1-100.

24.   Kini SR. Thyroid. 2n ed. New York: Igaku-Shoin, 1996 (Kline TS, ed. Guides to Clinical Aspiration Biopsy).

25.   Gallant JE, Enriquez RE, Cohen KL, Hammers LW. Pneumocystis carinii thyroiditis. Am J Med 1988;84:303-6.

26.   Walts AE, Pitchon HE. Pneumocystis carinii in FNA of the thyroid. Diagn Cytopathol 1991;7:615-7.

27.   Battan R, Mariuz P, Raviglione MC, Sabatini MT, Mullen MP, Poretsky L. *Pneumocystis carinii* infection of the thyroid in a hypothyroid patient with AIDS: Diagnosis by fine needle aspiration biopsy. J Clin Endocrinol Metab 1991;72:724-6.

28.   Ragni MV, Dekker A, DeRubertis FR, et al. *Pneumocystis carinii* infection presenting as necrotizing thyroiditis and hypothyroidism. Am J Clin Pathol 1991;95:489-93.

29.   Poropatich C, Marcus D, Oertel YC. Hashimoto's thyroiditis: Fine-needle aspirations of 50 asymptomatic cases. Diagn Cytopathol 1994;11:141-5.

30.   Mazzaferri EL, Oertel YC. Thyroid Lymphoma. In: Mazzaferri EL, Samaan NA, eds. Endocrine Tumors. 1st ed. Boston: Blackwell Scientific Publications, Inc, 1993:348-77.

31.   Hedinger C, Williams ED, Sobin LH. Histological Typing of Thyroid Tumours. World Health Organization International Histological Classification of Tumours. 2nd ed. Berlin: Springer-Verlag, 1988.

32.   Brown CL. Pathology of the cold nodule. Clin Endocrinol Metab 1981;10:235-45.

33.   Gonzalez JL, Wang HH, Ducatman BS. Fine-needle aspiration of Hürthle cell lesions. A cytomorphologic approach to diagnosis. Am J Clin Pathol 1993;100:231-5.

34.   Sambade C, Franssila K, Cameselle-Teijeiro J, Nesland J, Sobrinho-Simoes M. Hyalinizing trabecular adenoma: A misnomer for a peculiar tumor of the thyroid gland. Endocr Pathol 1991;2:83-91.

35.   Bondeson L, Bondeson A-G. Clue helping to distinguish hyalinizing trabecular adenoma from carcinoma of the thyroid in fine-needle aspirates. Diagn Cytopathol 1994;10:25-9.

36.   Goellner JR, Carney JA. Cytologic features of fine-needle aspirates of hyalinizing trabecular adenoma of the thyroid. Am J Clin Pathol 1989;91:115-9.

37.   Strong CJ, Garcia BM. Fine needle aspiration cytologic characteristics of hyalinizing trabecular adenoma of the thyroid. Acta Cytol 1990;34:359-62.

38.   Gallagher J, Oertel YC, Oertel JE. Follicular variant of papillary carcinoma of the thyroid: Fine-needle aspirates with histologic correlation. Diagn Cytopathol 1997;16:207-13.

39.   Chen KTK. Fine-needle aspiration cytology of papillary Hürthle-cell tumors of thyroid: A report of three cases. Diagn Cytopathol 1991;7:53-6.

40.   Kaur A, Jayaram G. Thyroid tumors: Cytomorphology of Hürthle cell tumors, including an uncommon papillary variant. Diagn Cytopathol 1993;9:135-7.

41.   Harach HR, Zusman SB. Cytopathology of the tall cell variant of thyroid papillary carcinoma. Acta Cytol 1992;36:895-9.

42.   Bocklage T, DiTomasso JP, Ramzy I, Ostrowski ML. Tall cell variant of papillary thyroid carcinoma: Cytologic features and differential diagnostic considerations. Diagn Cytopathol 1997;17:25-9.

43.   Gamboa-Domínguez A, Candanedo-González F, Uribe-Uribe NO, Angeles-Angeles A. Tall cell variant of papillary thyroid carcinoma. A cytohistologic correlation. Acta Cytol 1997;41:672-6.

44.   Kaw YT. Fine needle aspiration cytology of the tall cell variant of papillary carcinoma of the thyroid. Acta Cytol 1994;38:282-3.

45.   Hui P-K, Chan JKC, Cheung PSY, Gwi E. Columnar cell carcinoma of the thyroid. Fine needle aspiration findings in a case. Acta Cytol 1990;34:355-8.

46. Kini SR, Miller JM, Hamburger JI, Smith MJ. Cytopathologic features of medullary carcinoma of the thyroid. Arch Pathol Lab Med 1984;108:156-9.

47. Collins BT, Cramer HM, Tabatowski K, Hearn S, Raminhos A, Lampe H. Fine needle aspiration of medullary carcinoma of the thyroid. Cytomorphology, immunocytochemistry and electron microscopy. Acta Cytol 1995;39:920-30.

48. Schäffer R, Müller H-A, Pfeifer U, Ormanns W. Cytological findings in medullary carcinoma of the thyroid. Pathol Res Pract 1984;178:461-6.

49. Mendonça ME, Ramos S, Soares J. Medullary carcinoma of thyroid: a re-evaluation of the cytological criteria of diagnosis. Cytopathology 1991;2:93-102.

50. Bose S, Kapila K, Verma K. Medullary carcinoma of the thyroid: A cytological, immunocytochemical, and ultrastructural study. Diagn Cytopathol 1992;8:28-32.

51. Thompson LDR, Wenig BM, Adair CF, Heffess CS. Peripheral nerve sheath tumors of the thyroid gland: A series of four cases and a review of the literature. Endocr Pathol 1996;7:309-18.

52. Thompson LDR, Wenig BM, Adair CF, Shmookler BM, Heffess CS. Primary smooth muscle tumors of the thyroid gland. Cancer 1997;79:579-87.

53. Butler SL, Oertel YC. Lipomas of anterior neck simulating thyroid nodules: Diagnosis by fine-needle aspiration. Diagn Cytopathol 1992;8:528-31.

9 THE ROLE OF MEDICAL IMAGING IN THE DIAGNOSIS AND FOLLOW-UP OF RECURRENT OR METASTATIC THYROID CANCER

Kyuran A. Choe, M.D.
Harry R. Maxon, M.D.
University of Cincinnati
Cincinnati, Ohio

Location and Prevalence of Metastatic or Recurrent Differentiated Thyroid Cancer

In an extensive review of this subject, 1095/3083 (35.5%) patients with papillary carcinoma and 102/797 (12.8%) patients with follicular carcinoma were found to have lymph node metastases at the time of initial diagnosis of their cancer (1). In children, the prevalence may be as high as 70% (2). Of patients thought to be disease free after their initial treatment, 252/2684 (9.4%) with papillary and 43/641 (6.7%) with follicular carcinoma subsequently developed nodal metastases (1).

Distant metastases outside of the neck were present at the time of initial diagnosis in 161/4227 (3.8%) of patients with papillary and 182/1107 (16.4%) of those with follicular carcinoma and appeared later in 109/2684 (4.1%) of papillary cancer patients and in 83/641 (13.0%) of follicular cancer patients who were considered to have been disease free after initial therapy (1). Up to 20% of children with thyroid cancer present with distant metastases (2). When distant metastases occur, they usually are located in the lungs (~ 46%), bone (~ 30%), lung and bone (~ 10%), mediastinum alone (~ 7%), brain (~ 5%) or liver (~ 2%). Mediastinal metastases often are associated with lung metastases (3).

Recurrent thyroid cancer in the neck occurs in about 6% of papillary and 8% of follicular cancer patients (1).

Based on the likelihood of recurrent or metastatic disease in a given patient, specific diagnostic and follow-up imaging protocols should be determined individually for each patient.

Radioiodine Imaging

Concentration of Radioiodine by Recurrent or Metastatic Thyroid Cancer

In 1971, Pochin noted that only 50-80% of differentiated thyroid carcinomas took up radioiodine (4). A more recent review found that 268/369 (72.6%) of recurrent or metastatic differentiated thyroid cancers concentrated radioiodine and that there was no significant difference in this ability between papillary and follicular cancers (1). The likelihood of recurrent thyroid carcinoma concentrating radioiodine appears to be less than that of the original cancer (5), and metastatic lesions may lose their ability to concentrate radioiodine over time (6). Occasionally, metastases that appear to have lost their ability to concentrate radioiodine may regain it later (7).

Preparation of the Patient for Radioiodine Imaging

In brief, the patient is rendered hypothyroid either by thyroid hormone withdrawal or is prepared by using recombinant human thyrotropin (rhTSH). A low iodine diet is begun one week prior to the initiation of diagnostic radioiodine imaging. A detailed discussion of patient preparation is given in Chapter 12.

Formulation of [131]I

Because of the ease of administration to the patient, encapsulated radioiodine is used commonly for diagnostic studies. Some capsule formulations may result in a 7-8% decrease in absorption of the radioiodine, and care must be exercised to ensure that the patient has absorbed the radioiodine (8,9). We insist that the patient be n.p.o. except for water for 3 hours before and 3 hours after the administration of the radioiodine to ensure adequate time for dissolution and absorption. With this protocol and the use of capsule formulations that do not contain magnesium steroid (9), we rarely, if ever, find absorption problems in people with normal gastrointestinal function.

Selection of Diagnostic Administered Activity of [131]I

In 1951, Rawson and colleagues reported that 4/20 patients who received large "diagnostic" [131]I in amounts up to 25 mCi failed to concentrate subsequent "therapeutic" administrations of ^{131}I to the same degree (10). Park et al found that 2/5 (40%) patients who received diagnostic administrations of 3 mCi of ^{131}I and that 16/18 (89%) who received diagnostic administrations of 10 mCi of ^{131}I showed a subsequent decrease in concentration of their therapeutic ^{131}I administrations by their thyroid remnants and/or metastatic lesions. When such "stunning" did occur, it could persist for weeks to months (11) . Jeevanram et al demonstrated that, as the radiation dose to residual thyroid tissue from diagnostic ^{131}I increased, the subsequent fractional uptake by the same tissue progressively decreased. The mean reduction in the 72 hour uptake by residual thyroid tissue 1 week after the diagnostic administration of 5 mCi of ^{131}I was 54% (12). Muratet and coworkers evaluated the impact of diagnostic ^{131}I on the success of a 100 mCi ^{131}I dosage to ablate postoperative thyroid remnants. Success was defined as a negative 3 mCi ^{131}I scan and an undetectable TSH stimulated serum thyroglobulin level 6-15 months later. Treatment given 9 days after the diagnostic scan was successful in 62/74 (74%) patients who received 1 mCi and in 60/120 (50%) patients who received 3 mCi diagnostic ^{131}I administrations (p < 0.001) (13). McDougall compared 48-72 hour 2 mCi ^{131}I scans with approximately 8 day post 30-200 mCi therapy scans in 147 patients (14). Post therapy scans showed less uptake in one region than was seen on the 2 mCi ^{131}I diagnostic scan in only 2/147 (1.4%) patients. The post treatment scan showed more lesions in 12/147 (8%) patients, but in only 4 of the 12 patients was the stage of disease changed. Three had unexpected lung metastases , and one had unexpected lymph node metastases.

As detailed in Chapter 12, a 2 mCi diagnostic administered activity of ^{131}I may result in about a 20% decrease in the subsequent radiation dose to thyroid remnants and/or metastatic foci. We consider a 2 mCi diagnostic administration of ^{131}I to be the best compromise between imaging sensitivity and the need to avoid adverse effects on treatment.

^{123}I or ^{124}I as Alternatives to ^{131}I

Radioiodine-123 is widely used in routine thyroid imaging. A standard 0.3 mCi capsule will deliver a radiation dose to normal thyroid tissue that is only about 0.2% of that delivered by 2 mCi of ^{131}I and is not associated with an adverse impact on subsequent ^{131}I therapy (11).

Park et al evaluated 128 patients who had radioiodine scans 6 weeks after a total or near total surgical thyroidectomy for differentiated thyroid cancer. The accuracy of their diagnostic scans was found to be 89.5% (77/86) for 24 hour 0.3 mCi ^{123}I and 92.9% (39/42) for 48-72 hour 3-10 mCi (average 7.1 mCi) ^{131}I scans. In contrast, when they evaluated 89 patients who previously had undergone both total/near total surgical thyroidectomy and 100-200 mCi ^{131}I therapy, then the diagnostic accuracy of 24 hour 0.3 mCi ^{123}I scans was only 69.4% (25/36) as compared with 92.5% (49/53) for 48-72 hour 3-10 mCi (average 8.6 mCi) ^{131}I scans. However, because of "stunning" that occurred after the 3-10 mCi diagnostic administrations of ^{131}I, success rates for the second attempt to ablate persistent remnants were similar for both the ^{123}I and the ^{131}I diagnostic scan groups (15). They concluded that 0.3 mCi ^{123}I diagnostic scans were a reasonable alternative to ^{131}I in the first postoperative studies of patients expected to have thyroid remnants.

Berbano et al compared diagnostic images using 10 mCi of ^{123}I with scans obtained 5-7 days after therapy with 75-200 mCi of ^{131}I in 16 patients (16). In 10/16 patients only residual thyroid tissue was noted on both scans. Of the remaining patients, 3/6 had metastases in the same location on both scans, 2/6 had equivocal additional metastases on the ^{123}I study that were not confirmed on the ^{131}I scans, and 1/6 had more metastases seen on the ^{131}I than the ^{123}I scans. They found no advantage to 48 hour post ^{123}I imaging as compared with 24 hour imaging.

In 1993, we reported 13 diagnostic administrations of 20.1 mCi of ^{123}I to 11 patients with thyroid cancer who previously had undergone surgical and ^{131}I treatment (17). We determined that the detectable photon yield from 20 mCi of ^{123}I would equal that of the following activities of ^{131}I, depending on the time of imaging: 2-3 hours, 40 mCi; 15 hours, 27 mCi; 25 hours, 13 mCi; 40 hours, 4 mCi. Imaging at 2 hours post ^{123}I resulted in false negative scans in 5/13 (38%) cases. Imaging at 18-24 hours post 20 mCi of ^{123}I resulted in no false negatives using scans obtained 48-72 hours after ^{131}I therapy as the gold standard. However, 48-72 hour 2 mCi ^{131}I scans were just as accurate and only 10-20% as costly. Reliable quantitative dosimetry could not be obtained with ^{123}I (17).

Bautovich et al evaluated 10 patients who previously had undergone thyroid ablation for thyroid cancer and who were thought to be at high risk for metastatic disease (18). They compared 24 and 48 hour 27 mCi ^{123}I scans with 72 hour 5 mCi ^{131}I scans and found 13 more foci of uptake on the ^{123}I scans than on ^{131}I scans. Overall, the ^{123}I scans were considered to be superior in 8/10 patients (18). Based on the report of Park et al (15), we estimate that 30 mCi of pure ^{123}I would result in about 15% of the radiation dose to residual thyroid tissue from 2 mCi of ^{131}I at 10-20 times the cost. Therefore our routine continues to be to use 2 mCi ^{131}I diagnostic scans whenever quantitative dosimetry is desired or the patient has had prior thyroid ablative therapy.

Radioiodine-124 is not available commercially in the United States at this time. However, it has good imaging characteristics when appropriate high energy positron imaging equipment is available and, with a 4.2 day physical half life, should permit quantitative dosimetry. Its radiation dose to residual thyroid tissue is about 60% of that from the same activity of ^{131}I (15) so administered activities would be limited to only 3 mCi if "stunning" were to be kept at the same level as that from 2 mCi of ^{131}I.

Techniques of ^{131}I Imaging

The Society of Nuclear Medicine has published guidelines for the use of scintigraphy in the diagnosis of residual functioning thyroid tissue and/or thyroid cancer (19). Although they are generic and are not designed to be applied rigidly to every patient, they are succinct and are highly recommended for review by physicians engaged in the care of patients with differentiated thyroid cancer.

As detailed in Chapter ---, we prefer a quantitative dosimetric approach that is designed to optimize ^{131}I therapy for each patient. After determining that the patient has been prepared properly and after obtaining a negative menstrual history and negative pregnancy test on all women of child bearing years, the patient is instructed to empty their bladder and to avoid urinating or defecating until after their 2 hour post administration counts are obtained. An appropriate 2 mCi capsule of ^{131}I then is administered by mouth after it has been assayed in the dose calibrator and recorded. The patient is given 8 ounces of water by mouth to ensure that the capsule has been swallowed. The patient's height and weight are measured and recorded.

The following procedure then is followed for whole body quantification using a dual head whole body scanning unit. The results permit diagnostic imaging as well as calculation of the patient's effective whole body half life of ^{131}I which, in turn, is used to determine whole blood and red bone marrow dosimetry and eligibility for outpatient therapy (see Chapter 12):

- Obtain data at 2, 24, 48, and 72 hours post ^{131}I administration.

- Use collimators appropriate for ^{131}I.

- Peak the camera for ^{131}I using a 15% window.

- With the lower head as close to the table as possible and the upper had as far above the table as possible, obtain background counts using a scan speed of 224 cm/minute.

- Position the patient on the table with the mid coronal plane parallel to the face of the detectors, and the mid sagittal line running through the center of the table. The patient's arms are positioned at their side.

- Image at 224 cm/min to obtain a fast survey scan on the computer. These count data will be used to determine the effective whole body half life. Do at 2, 24, 48, and 72 hours.

- Repeat the scan at 24, 48 and 72 hours using a speed to obtain the highest information density possible (approximately 2-3 million total counts per probe at 24 hours) within 30-40 minutes.

- Measure the distance from the mid-line of the patient to the surface of the table and image a standard positioned at the same distance using a speed of 224 cm/minute.

Lesion quantification is carried out whenever abnormal areas of ^{131}I uptake are noted on whole body images. Their presence initially is confirmed using high count density images with the patient upright and after eating and drinking to remove any artifact from saliva in the mouth or esophagus. Other potential sources of artifact also are checked and removed. Quantification of uptake in and retention by discrete lesions then is performed as follows:

- Using an appropriate collimator, the camera is peaked for ^{131}I using a 10% window.

- Place a support pillow under the patient's shoulders to hyperextend the neck as much as possible.

- On the gamma camera take 300 second images, storing the data on the computer simultaneously in a 64 x 64 word mode.

    a) Anterior views: with the patient supine and their neck hyperextended, place the collimator parallel to the mid-coronal plane at a distance about 3 inches from the anterior neck surface. Record the distance from the surface of the neck to the collimator, the view, and the number of counts collected in 5 minutes.

    b) Posterior views: with a pillow under their chest, have the patient lie prone with the head straight down, facing the table. A small pad under the forehead will aid in the ease of breathing. Repeat a 5 minute image and data collection as above.

    c) Standard: for a small lesion, a standard of approximately 50 uCi is used in about 0.3 ml in a 1 cc syringe; for a larger lesion, approximately 100 uCi in a 1 ml volume in a 3 cc syringe is used. A rubber cap is put on the nipple of the syringe instead of a needle. This standard should be assayed before each set of quantification data is obtained, and the assayed amount recorded on the data sheet along with the time of assay. Acquire a 5 minute image of this on the computer. The distance from the standard to the collimator should be equal to the distance from the collimator to the lesion on the anterior view (about one inch plus the distance from the anterior neck to the collimator face). Put the source under the center of the collimator, record the time, distance, and counts on the data sheet.

    d) Background - record the same data for a 5 minute background acquisition each day.

    e) Transmission images are needed to determine the density of the patient at the level of the lesion. This should be obtained as soon as any areas of abnormal uptake become evident, usually at 48 hours.

        1. The transmission data are accumulated with the patient in the same position as for the anterior view. The source is slipped behind the patient and placed directly behind the lesion noted on the positioning oscilloscope. This positioning is very important! Once again, a 5 minute data collection is acquired on the computer and the relevant facts are recorded on the data sheet.

        2. Measure the distance from the transmission source to the collimator face and record on the data sheet.

        3. The transmission standard must also be imaged (put in the center of the collimator area) and data stored on the computer. The distance

from the collimator face to source should be the same as the distance from the collimator in the transmission picture in #2 above.

4. These transmission data usually need be obtained only once, whereas the remainder of the images and data (anterior, posterior, standard and background) need to be repeated every day.

The radiation dose to the thyroid remnants or to a discrete metastasis then is calculated as follows:

$$\text{Dose (rad)} = 0.63 \times C \times T_{1/2lesion}$$

Where C = the calculated absolute initial concentration of ^{131}I in the lesion in microcuries/gram using back extrapolation from the quantitative data from the patient and the standards to determine the concentration and the mass as determined by methods outlined in Chapter 12. The $T_{1/2lesion}$ is the effective half-life of ^{131}I in the lesion in hours as determined by the quantification procedure. In the event that the effective half-life is protracted, curve fit is poor, and the patient is unable to return for additional data points, a maximum default value of 156 hours may be used. Details of the mathematics used in the calculations have been published previously (20, 21).

Imaging Shortly After ^{131}I Therapy

Nemec et al compared the results of diagnostic, 24 hour, 0.2 - 0.5 mCi ^{131}I scans with 1-5 day post 80-120 mCi therapy scans in 97 patients. In 16/97 (16%) patients the post therapy scans showed unexpected foci of residual and/or metastatic thyroid cancer (22). We compared 92 sets of 2 mCi diagnostic scans obtained at 24, 48, and 72 hour and 2-14 day post ^{131}I therapy (209 ± 35 mCi) scans and found additional lesions in 8% of the patients. However, unexpected distant metastases were found only in 4/92 (4.3%) post therapy scans (23). Sherman and colleagues compared 143 pairs of 48-72 hour, 2-5 mCi diagnostic ^{131}I scans and 5-12 day, 30-200 mCi post ^{131}I therapy scans from 43 patients with well differentiated thyroid cancer (24). They found that 17/143 (11.9%) post treatment scans demonstrated ^{131}I uptake in metastatic lesions that were already known from prior studies but that had not been seen on the current diagnostic scan; 14/143 (9.8%) post treatment scans showed new, unexpected locations of metastatic disease; and 7/143 (4.9%) post therapy scans were unable to confirm a focus of uptake seen on the diagnostic scan. Presumably this latter finding represented either "stunning" or artifact on the diagnostic examination. Immediate post therapy imaging appeared to be most useful in patients who previously had undergone ^{131}I therapy. The optimal imaging time after ^{131}I therapy appears to be 4-5 days (25), with additional imaging as needed to allow differentiation between artifacts and true abnormalities.

Need for Protracted Follow-Up

Hoie and colleagues observed that, when distant metastases from papillary thyroid cancer became evident, they did so within the first year after diagnosis in 43% of patients; between years 1 and 5 in 25%; between years 5 and 10 in 23%, and at more than 10 years in 9% (26). When we evaluated the time from diagnosis to death from differentiated thyroid cancer (27), we found that about two thirds of deaths from either papillary or follicular cancer occur within 10 years of diagnosis; 14% of deaths from papillary and 29% of deaths from follicular cancer occur between years 11 and 20 following diagnosis; and 20% of deaths from papillary and 3% of deaths from follicular cancer occur at 21 years or more after diagnosis. Based on these considerations, we continue to follow our patients until they are at least 20 years after their last known evidence of thyroid cancer. The follow-up generally includes annual ^{131}I scans until they are negative, then an ^{131}I scan 2 years later, and then another scan every 5 years thereafter. In the case of patients with low risk lesions that are not considered to warrant radioiodine therapy, obviously ^{131}I scans do not constitute part of the follow-up (see Chapter 12).

Artifacts in Radioiodine Imaging

Radioiodine appears normally in the lacrimal glands, nasal and vaginal mucosa, salivary glands, gastric mucosa, and sweat glands. Cardiac and pulmonary blood pool activity may appear early but usually clears by 24 hours unless a large amount of radioiodinated protein is released from residual thyroid tissue, residual cancer, or metastases. Diffuse hepatic uptake in the absence of liver metastasis may be seen in 12% of 48 hour, 2-10 mCi diagnostic ^{131}I scans and 36% of 3-5 day, 30-200 mCi post ^{131}I therapy scans and is correlated with levels of ^{131}I-labeled thyroglobulin in the patient's serum (28). In about 4% of patients diffuse hepatic uptake may be the earliest scintigraphic finding in occult thyroid remnants or recurrent/metastatic cancer (28). Radioiodine normally is excreted from the kidneys, resulting in visualization of the urinary bladder. On later scans, gut activity becomes more apparent as radioiodine from the lacrimal, nasal, salivary, and gastric secretions become mixed with stool and passes through the intestines.

The most common artifacts are those created by radioactivity in nasal and pharyngeal secretions that either are partially swallowed and lie in the esophagus or are on handkerchiefs or tissues that the patient has used and then put into a shirt or pants pocket. Technologists must look for these artifacts and ask specifically that tissues, handkerchiefs, and so on be removed prior to scanning and that the patient drink water just prior to scanning. Artifacts from drops of contaminated urine or spittle on the skin, clothing, or imaging equipment, occasionally appear and also must be considered before the patient is released.

A variety of nonthyroidal conditions have been reported to concentrate ^{131}I, albeit rarely. These include the following (1, 29-39):

Non-Thyroidal Neoplasms
carcinomas of the salivary gland or stomach

carcinomas of the lung or bronchus

meningiomas

struma ovarii or ovarian teratomas

Inflammatory Conditions
acute or chronic inflammatory lung/bronchial disease

folliculitis, skin burns, psoriatic plaques

infected sebaceous cyst

chronic sinusitis

dacryocystitis

chronic cholecystitis

sialoadenitis

gingivitis

Other Conditions
post traumatic porencephalic cyst

frontal sinus mucocele

saliva or sweat around a false eye, in braided hair, or on the skin or clothing

lymphoepithelial cyst of the parotid or Wharton's duct stone

ectasia of the common carotid with stasis

thymus: normal or hyperplastic

esophagus: normal retained secretions, Zenker's diverticulum, strictures, achalasia, colonic "pull-though" graft, hiatal hernia

displacement of the cardiac blood pool by pectus excavation

pericardial effusion or pleuropericardial cyst

lactating, postpartum, or stimulated breast

dilated intrahepatic ducts

single or multiple renal cysts

There are occasions when patients have been treated with ^{131}I for what was artifactual uptake. Clearly, it is crucial that the scans be interpreted in light of the patient's complete clinical history and with care to exclude artifacts.

Other Nuclear Medicine Agents

Thallium 201 Chloride

Thallium 201 is a potassium analogue that enters cells via the sodium-potassium ATPase pump. It has been used as a cardiac imaging agent and has been shown to be taken up in tumors in a non-specific fashion. Several researchers have investigated the use of ^{201}Tl for the detection of recurrent and metastatic thyroid carcinoma and have compared ^{201}Tl to ^{131}I scans and serum thyroglobulin levels. Interest in ^{201}Tl is due to the incidence of non-iodine avid recurrences and metastases of well-differentiated thyroid cancer (1) and the the ability to study patients using ^{201}Tl without thyroid hormone withdrawal. However, the studies of ^{201}Tl have produced variable results. Evaluation of these reports demonstrates variability in the study populations and administered ^{131}I activities.

Tonami et al (40) evaluated 28 patients with well-differentiated thyroid cancer. Fifteen of these patients had been treated with total thyroidectomy, and 13 had residual thyroid tissue. In the athyrotic group, 8 patients were shown to have recurrent or metastatic disease, of whom 7 had abnormal ^{201}Tl scans in comparison with only 3 patients with abnormal ^{131}I scans. The authors noted that the poor results of ^{131}I scanning may have been due to insufficient periods of thyroid hormone withdrawal. Metastatic lymph nodes were detectable by ^{201}Tl imaging only when larger than 1.5 cm in diameter. None of the metastatic lymph nodes that were smaller than 1.0 cm in diameter were detected. Similarly, Ohnishi (41) demonstrated that ^{201}Tl scans of the neck were able to detect 14 of 39 tumor foci greater than 2 cm in diameter, whereas no focus less than 1.5 cm was detected.

Hoefnagel (42) compared ^{201}Tl and ^{131}I scans with serum thyroglobulin or calcitonin/CEA levels. The patient population consisted of 301 patients with either papillary or follicular carcinoma. In addition, there were 6 patients with anaplastic carcinoma, 1 with giant cell carcinoma, and 18 with medullary carcinoma of the thyroid. Calculation of sensitivity and specificity was based on patients in whom both ^{201}Tl and ^{131}I scans and tumor marker assays were performed. These included 50 patients with metastatic thyroid carcinoma, 8 of whom had medullary carcinoma, and 1 with giant cell carcinoma, both of which typically are not iodine avid. Therefore, the reported sensitivities for detection of patients with metastatic disease of ^{201}Tl as 94% and ^{131}I as 48% may be somewhat misleading.

Conversely, Brendel et al (43) compared ^{201}Tl to immediate post-ablative ^{131}I scans. Of 51 sites of tumor, ^{201}Tl was positive in 23, and ^{131}I was positive in 43. However, Pacini et al (44) and Sherman et al (24) demonstrated that post-treatment ^{131}I scans will detect additional metastatic foci in comparison with diagnostic ^{131}I scans. Therefore, the number of positive ^{131}I scans in the study by Brendel may have been lower if only diagnostic activities of ^{131}I had been used.

Studies by Carril (45), Dadparvar (46) , Ramanna (47) and Tonami (40) have included patients both prior to and after ^{131}I ablative therapy. In the patients who had not undergone prior ablative therapy, ^{131}I activity in the thyroid bed frequently was felt to be due to residual thyroid tissue. The appearance of this area on ^{201}Tl scans was variable: (47) 6/21 patients had no ^{201}Tl uptake and 7/21 patients had mild, diffuse uptake in the thyroid bed.

Lorberboym (48) studied 50 patients with well-differentiated thyroid carcinoma using ^{201}Tl and ^{131}I whole body scans (60 pairs of examinations). Within this study, 16 ^{201}Tl examinations demonstrated false positive results, the most common location being in the right lower mediastinum. Burman (49) noted a false positive ^{201}Tl examination caused by a stitch abscess in the neck. Charkes (50) noted false positive ^{201}Tl uptake both in the lungs of patients with coronary artery disease and in foci of metastatic breast cancer. Thallium uptake is non-specific and may be seen in other malignant disease, in reactive lymphadenopathy (51), and in pneumonia (52).

Charkes (50) compared planar and single photon tomographic (SPECT) imaging with [201]Tl. Planar imaging yielded 12 of 20 metastatic foci whereas SPECT demonstrated 17 of 20 foci. Two of the ^{201}Tl negative foci were ^{131}I positive. One palpable cervical lymph node that was not seen with ^{201}Tl imaging was demonstrated to be a cystic nodal metastasis. Pulmonary metastases that were less than 1.5 cm in diameter could not be visualized by ^{201}Tl but were documented by ^{131}I imaging or chest x-ray. Diffuse micronodular pulmonary metastases were seen by SPECT but not by planar imaging with [201]Tl. Brandt-Mainz et al (53) evaluated 162 patients with ^{201}Tl and demonstrated a sensitivity of 88% for cervical and mediastinal nodal metastases that decreased to only 58% for metastases in other locations.

In 1993, van Sorge-van Boxtel et al (54) compared ^{201}Tl and ^{131}I imaging and serum thyroglobulin levels in 86 patients with well-differentiated thyroid carcinoma who had undergone prior surgical thyroidectomy and ^{131}I ablation. The serum thyroglobulin test demonstrated sensitivities of 97% off thyroid hormone replacement and 92% on T4, with a specificity of 100%. [131]I scans yielded sensitivities of 77% following therapeutic administrations and of 57% after 5 mCi diagnostic activities, with a specificity of 98%. [201]Tl provided a sensitivity of 55% and a specificity of 91%. However, foci of persistent or recurrent tumor were visualized in 8/38 patients only on ^{201}Tl scans, and these represented 8 of 11 patients who were ^{131}I scan negative.

Therefore, due to ongoing variability in the outcomes of studies using ^{201}Tl, current recommendations for monitoring patients with well-differentiated thyroid cancer include serum thyroglobulin measurements and ^{131}I whole body scans under adequate TSH stimulation. In patients in whom the suspicion of recurrent or residual cancer is high (e.g., elevated thyroglobulin levels) and whose ^{131}I scans fail to demonstrate tumor foci, evaluation with ^{201}Tl may be beneficial (55).

[99m]Technetium Sestamibi

[99m]Tc-sestamibi was developed as a myocardial perfusion agent, but non-specific uptake in tumors has been described (56). ^{99m}Tc-sestamibi has been used both for differentiated thyroid cancers in general and specifically for non-^{131}I avid medullary and Hurthle cell carcinomas.

Nemec et al (57) evaluated ^{99m}Tc-sestamibi in 200 patients with differentiated (papillary and follicular) thyroid carcinoma. Patients were evaluated for tumor recurrence in the neck and for metastatic spread to the lungs or bones. The diagnoses were confirmed by other imaging methods, including ^{131}I diagnostic and post-therapeutic scans. In 105 patients with local disease, ^{99m}Tc-sestamibi demonstrated an 81% sensitivity with a 71% specificity. In 19 patients with pulmonary metastases, both 95% sensitivity and specificity were noted. For the 17 patients with osseous metastases, a 100% sensitivity and 99% specificity were cited. In a comparison between ^{99m}Tc-sestamibi, ^{201}Tl, and post therapy ^{131}I scans, Miyamoto et al (58) evaluated 27 patients with well-differentiated thyroid carcinoma. They determined that ^{99m}Tc-sestamibi identified 75% of pulmonary metastases, 100% of lymph node metastases, and 94% of osseous metastases. [201]Tl scans were able to identify a similar number of lesions. [131]I post-therapy scans identified 85%, 42%, and 87% of lung, nodal, and osseous lesions respectively.

In contrast, Dadparvar et al (59) compared ^{99m}Tc-sestamibi with ^{201}Tl and ^{131}I scans in 34 patients, 16 of whom were studied prior to ^{131}I ablative therapy and 29 of whom were evaluated after such ablation. The patient population was mixed: 32 patients had papillary or follicular carcinoma, 1 had Hurthle cell, and 1 had medullary carcinoma. Evaluation of the 29 post ablation patients demonstrated a sensitivity for metastatic disease of 36% for both ^{201}Tl and ^{99m}Tc-sestamibi with a high concordance rate (97%) of imaging findings between these two tests. The sensitivity with ^{131}I was higher at 55%. False negative ^{201}Tl and ^{99m}Tc-sestamibi studies were noted if the lesion in the chest or neck were less than 1 cm. The patients who had not received prior ^{131}I ablation included 3 patients who had undergone only a lobectomy. The concordance rate (69%) for ^{201}Tl and ^{99m}Tc-sestamibi was lower in this patient group.

For patients with medullary carcinoma, which is not iodine avid, ^{99m}Tc-sestamibi with SPECT has been compared to radiographic CT scans. Learoyd et al (60) noted that SPECT imaging was useful in defining the location of a lesion, but that it did not provide additional lesion detection as compared with planar imaging with ^{99m}Tc-sestamibi. In a lesion-by-lesion analysis, in the soft tissues of the neck and mediastinum, ^{99m}Tc-sestamibi detected a larger number of lesions (22/25) than did CT (11/25). This may be due to difficulty in differentiating post-operative changes from tumor in the neck and chest by CT. In this patient population, ^{99m}Tc-sestamibi detected only 6/17 (35%) of osseous metastases, unlike the study by Nemec (57). Due to its hepatic uptake and excretion, ^{99m}Tc-sestamibi was unable to identify any of the 47 liver lesions detected by CT.

[99m]Tc-sestamibi also has been evaluated in patients with Hurthle cell carcinoma, a subtype of follicular carcinoma. Yen et al (61) described the results of ^{99m}Tc-sestamibi imaging in 37 patients with previous thyroidectomy for Hurthle cell carcinoma who also had ^{201}Tl and ^{131}I scans. Of 22 patients with elevated serum thyroglobulin levels, 4 had positive 3 mCi diagnostic ^{131}I scans, 15 had positive ^{201}Tl scans, and 18 had positive ^{99m}Tc-sestamibi scans. However, no pathologic

correlation of the findings were presented. It has been postulated that the high frequency of uptake in Hurthle cell carcinoma may be due to the large number of mitochondria present in the more common form of this tumor and to the fact that ^{99m}Tc-sestamibi localizes in mitochondria (61,62).

[99m]Tc-sestamibi can be used as an alternative to [201]Tl. The imaging characteristics of the ^{99m}Tc label are favorable. However, the costs of using this agent are slightly higher. At our institution, the cost of a dosage of ^{201}Tl is about $50 less than ^{99m}Tc-sestamibi.

[99m]Technetium Tetrofosmin

Like ^{99m}Tc-sestamibi, ^{99m}Tc-tetrofosmin is primarily a cardiac perfusion imaging agent. However, it also has been used for tumor imaging, and studies have been performed to evaluate its utility in thyroid cancer. Lind et al (63) evaluated ^{99m}Tc-tetrofosmin in patients with well-differentiated thyroid carcinoma while on TSH suppressive hormone therapy. Of 7 patients with local recurrence, ^{99m}Tc-tetrofosmin was able to identify disease in all patients. Two of these patients also were found to have distant metastases by the ^{99m}Tc-tetrofosmin scan. In 17 patients with known distant metastases, ^{99m}Tc-tetrofosmin identified lesions with 86% sensitivity. In 9 of 17 patients, ^{99m}Tc-tetrofosmin avid metastases were not identified on the diagnostic or therapeutic ^{131}I scan. The authors also noted that abdominal images needed to be performed early in the study due to interference from the normal biliary clearance of this agent. Spanu et al (64) evaluated ^{99m}Tc-tetrofosmin in conjunction with ^{131}I scans and serum thyroglobulin levels in patients who had undergone prior thyroidectomy and ^{131}I ablation. This study evaluated the chest and neck and used SPECT in addition to planar imaging. Sixteen patients had elevated thyroglobulin levels and normal ^{131}I scans. ^{99m}Tc-tetrofosmin detected 32 lesions in this group, 10 of which were identified only on the SPECT images. In patients with abnormal ^{131}I scans, ^{99m}Tc-tetrofosmin identified more lesions, but there were 3 lesions seen on the ^{131}I scans that were not demonstrated on the ^{99m}Tc-tetrofosmin studies. Two patients who had both normal thyroglobulin levels and ^{131}I scans were noted to have abnormal foci on the ^{99m}Tc-tetrofosmin scans. Both of these patients had biopsy proven metastatic disease that corresponded to the abnormal scan foci.

[18]F FDG PET

^{18}F-FDG PET has been compared to ^{131}I scans and ^{99m}Tc-sestamibi. In a recent study published by Feine and coworkers (65) comparing ^{18}F-FDG PET and ^{131}I scans in a population of 41 patients with papillary and follicular carcinoma, including Hurthle cell, variability in ^{18}F-FDG and ^{131}I uptake was noted. This included foci with ^{131}I avidity without ^{18}F-FDG uptake, ^{18}F-FDG uptake without ^{131}I avidity, and lack of uptake by either method. These patterns may vary within a metastatic focus and within a patient. The authors suggested that ^{131}I avidity indicates greater differentiation, while ^{18}F-FDG uptake, indicating a higher metabolic rate, is a sign of more aggressive malignancy. A similar suggestion was

made by Grunwald et al (66,67) who noted similar findings. Fridich et al (68) evaluated ^{18}F-FDG in conjunction with ^{131}I (diagnostic and therapeutic dosages), PET, and ^{99m}Tc-sestamibi. Not unexpectedly, the tomographic evaluation was more sensitive than rectilinear scans with ^{18}F-FDG, and therapeutic administrations of ^{131}I demonstrated more lesions than did diagnostic ^{131}I scans. ^{99m}Tc-sestamibi also demonstrated a few more lesions than the ^{18}F-FDG.

Agents for Medullary Thyroid Carcinoma

Due to the absence of iodine avidity in medullary carcinoma of the thyroid, multiple other agents have been evaluated for the identification and localization of metastatic foci in the setting of abnormal serum calcitonin and/or CEA levels. In addition to ^{201}Tl and ^{99m}Tc-sestamibi, ^{131}I-MIBG, pentavalent ^{99m}Tc(V)-DMSA, ^{111}In octreotide, and labeled CEA antibody have been used. A review of the literature concerning the use of ^{131}I-MIBG in medullary cancer (69) demonstrated a sensitivity of 30% with a false negative rate of 52%. In the evaluation of ^{99m}Tc(V)-DMSA, studies have been small (70,71,72) but cumulative data reviewed by Skowsky yielded a true positive rate of 78% and a false positive rate of 24%. A comparison of ^{99m}Tc(V)-DMSA, ^{99m}Tc-MDP, and ^{131}I-MIBG performed by Clarke (73) in 9 patients with persistently elevated serum calcitonin levels yielded an overall sensitivity of 95% with ^{99m}Tc(V)-DMSA and 12% with ^{131}I-MIBG. ^{99m}Tc(V)-DMSA was able to detect 94% of osseous and 100% of soft tissue metastases. Conversely, ^{131}I-MIBG identified only 10% of the osseous and 13% of soft tissue metastases. Not unexpectedly, ^{99m}Tc-MDP identified 100% of the osseous metastases and none of the soft tissue metastases. Kurturan (74) evaluated ^{99m}Tc(V)-DMSA as a tool in the pre-operative staging of medullary carcinoma and demonstrated that it was unable to identify any of the lymph nodes with disease. All involved nodes were less than 2 mm in size.

Medullary carcinoma has been demonstrated to have somatostatin receptors, which has prompted use of the labeled somatostatin analog ^{111}In-octreotide. Baudin et al (75) evaluated 12 patients with gross evidence of disease by clinical examination or conventional imaging. Amongst these 12 patients, ^{111}In-octreotide identified only 50% of liver and osseous lesions, 33% of chest lesions, and 25% of neck lesions. Only 2 of 7 patients who had positive ^{111}In-octreotide scans (of 12 patients with gross disease) demonstrated concordance with conventional imaging. They also studied 12 patients with no evidence of disease by conventional imaging. One patient with abnormal uptake in the chest had a 1 cm mediastinal metastasis. Multiple other studies (76,77,78,79) have demonstrated that ^{111}In-octreotide is unable to identify liver metastases. False positive studies that have been noted include mediastinal uptake, presumed to be related to previous radiation therapy, and a uterine fibroid (75). Kwekkeboom et al (80) performed a cost analysis of somatostatin receptor scintigraphy and found that, in the evaluation of medullary carcinoma of the thyroid, ^{111}In-octreotide scans added significant cost with only a low yield (2.5%) in further localization of disease and did not increase the identification of patients with metastatic disease.

In addition to serum calcitonin levels, serum CEA concentrations can be utilized to assess patients for recurrent or metastatic disease. Imaging with radiolabeled antibody to CEA has been used to detect metastatic medullary thyroid carcinoma in patients with abnormally elevated serum CEA levels. Anti-CEA has been labeled with ^{123}I, ^{131}I, and [99m]Tc (81). Preliminary evaluation of various forms of antibodies and fragments with different tracers in patients with elevated serum calcitonin and CEA levels was performed using both diagnostic and potentially therapeutic administrations. A total of 26 patients were studied, and each form of radiolabeled antibody was used in only a small number of patients. A lesion-by-lesion analysis yielded a sensitivity of 76-100%. There were no patients included in this study with normal serum CEA and calcitonin levels. Moreover, development of human antimouse antibodies (HAMA) may preclude repetitive use of these agents.

Other Radiologic Imaging Techniques

Local Recurrence and Nodal Disease in the Neck

In well-differentiated thyroid carcinoma, local nodal involvement is present at the time of diagnosis in 35% of patients with papillary carcinoma and in 13% of patients with follicular carcinoma (1). Nodal disease at diagnosis is more common in medullary carcinoma, occuring in 50-75% of patients (82). Recurrent disease in the thyroid bed and local lymph nodes occurs in 5.6% and 9.4% respectively in patients with papillary carcinoma and 7.8% and 6.7% respectively in patients with follicular carcinoma (1). By clinical examination, only 15-28% of recurrences are palpable (83,84). Evaluation of the thyroid bed and cervical lymph nodes may be performed by ultrasound, CT, and MRI (85). Each of these modalities utilizes size criteria for the identification of potentially malignant lymph nodes.

Attempts at differentiation between benign and malignant lymph nodes with sonography have utilized morphologic characteristics (86), color (87) and power doppler and doppler waveforms (88,89,90), in addition to sonographic contrast agents (91). However, it is not possible to reliably differentiate between reactive and malignant lymph nodes or to identify normal sized but malignant lymph nodes. Nodes with a more rounded configuration (86,92) or with increased vascularity (87,88,90) can be seen with malignant involvement, but these are not reliable indicators (89,91). Ultrasound has the ability to provide real-time guidance for biopsy and fine needle aspiration of suspicious lesions (84,92,93). The role of sonography in the follow-up of patients with thyroid cancer also has been studied (83,94,95). Simeone et al (83) reported a sensitivity of 96% and specificity of 23%. However, this assessment excluded 32 patients (of a total of 73 patients) with abnormal sonograms without clinical or pathologic confirmation. Antonelli et al (94) noted that 16 of 63 patients had findings on ultrasound suspicious for recurrence and that 12 of 16 (75%) were documented to have disease by fine needle aspiration.

Both computed tomography (CT) and magnetic resonance imaging (MRI) provide tomographic imaging of the body. Detection of lesions is dependent on multiple factors, including image contrast and resolution. In CT, image contrast is based on differences in density between adjacent tissues which may be augmented by the administration of iodinated intravenous contrast agents. However, in patients awaiting treatment for thyroid carcinoma, this can have important implications since the intravenous contrast is iodine based. In MRI, soft tissue contrast is created by the differing quantities of mobile protons in tissue and the differences in their local chemical environment. MRI contrast agents can augment image contrast and are based on paramagnetic and ferromagnetic nuclei. Image resolution within the plane of imaging is dependent on the image size and acquisition matrix. In general, image resolution is greater in CT, but image contrast can be greater in MRI. Image fusion with nuclear medicine SPECT studies may be performed with either CT or MRI (96,97). In both CT and MRI, identification of nodal metastases is dependent on node size, as in ultrasound. However, these imaging methods are less operator dependent and tend to be more reproducible than ultrasound. The CT and MRI appearances of nodal metastases in thyroid cancer can be variable depending on the presence of calcification, hemorrhage, cystic change, and thyroglobulin content (98). In a comparison with ^{201}Tl, Ohnishi (41) and coworkers demonstrated that MRI is more sensitive than ^{201}Tl in the detection of recurrent disease in the neck, using a lesion by lesion analysis with surgical correlation. MRI was able to differentiate between post-operative changes and recurrent tumor in the thyroid bed. In addition, recent research (99,100) with MRI contrast agents suggest that MRI may be useful for differentiation between normal and metastatic lymph nodes in the future.

Pulmonary Metastases

Intra-thoracic metastases can involve the pulmonary parenchyma, mediastinum, or hila. The presence of distant metastases has been correlated with decreased survival in all types of thyroid cancer (101). Approximately 63-80% (26,102,103,104) of patients with papillary carcinoma and distant metastases have thoracic involvement; whereas 32% of patients with follicular carcinoma and distant metastases have pulmonary involvement (104). About 13% of pulmonary metastases are not evident on diagnostic ^{131}I scans or on chest x-ray (1). However, these patients usually have elevated serum thyroglobulin levels.

Patterns of pulmonary parenchymal metastases on chest x-ray include a normal chest x-ray in 30%, micronodular metastases in 33%, and macronodular metastases in 37% (105). In their patient population with papillary carcinoma, Dineen found micronodular metastases more common (77%) (102). Hoie (26) also described a pattern of "infiltration" with mediastinal and hilar enlargement in 34% of their patient population. This description suggests lymphatic obstruction or invasion with tumor and is indicative of more advanced disease. The pattern of parenchymal metastases has prognostic implication, with macronodular disease having a higher risk of death than micronodular disease when compared to patients with normal chest x-rays (105). CT of the chest is more sensitive than chest tomography or chest x-ray for detection of pulmonary nodules (106), and evaluation of the chest with CT does not require the use of intravenous contrast. Schlumberger (105) found that pulmonary metastases were identified on chest CT in 51% of patients with a normal chest x-ray but positive ^{131}I scans or elevated serum thyroglobulin levels. Piekarski (107) found that 14 of 19 patients with normal chest x-rays and functioning pulmonary metastases documented by ^{131}I scan were shown to have micronodular metastases on chest CT. Current techniques using spiral (helical) CT can increase detection of pulmonary nodules by 42% in comparison to axial CT (108). This is due to a reduction of respiratory artifact and slice misregistration (109).

MRI is not routinely used for the detection of pulmonary nodules. However, a comparison of MRI to CT (110) showed that CT demonstrated more small nodules due to its higher resolution. However, due to better contrast resolution, MRI was able to delineate nodules adjacent to vessels better than CT. As with most pulmonary metastases, the CT density of pulmonary metastases is that of soft tissue. However, calcified metastases have been described in medullary carcinoma (111). Evaluation of the mediastinum for metastatic disease to the lymph nodes is again based on size criteria (112,113,114). Detection of normal sized but metastatic lymph nodes and differentiation between metastatic and reactive enlarged lymph nodes is not possible at this time.

Osseous Metastases

Distant metastatic disease to bone occurs in 15% of patients with follicular carcinoma (115,116) and 1-2% of patients with papillary carcinoma (26,102,115) and is associated with a lower survival (104,117,118). Skeletal metastases most commonly occur in the axial skeleton, with 68% occurring in the vertebral column, pelvis or ribs (115). The typical radiographic appearance of untreated thyroid metastases is lytic (119). However, detection of osseous metastases by plain radiography requires significant bone loss (approximately 50%) (120). In other neoplastic diseases, nuclear medicine bone scans are used for the detection of osseous metastases, providing a survey of the entire skeleton. Early reports of the use of bone scans in well-differentiated thyroid cancer suggested that 59% of lesions detected by ^{131}I scan and plain radiography were not detected on bone scan and that 19% of metastases detected only demonstrated minimally increased uptake (121). A recent study by Tenenbaum et al (122) evaluated patients with known osseous metastases. Of 63 osseous lesions in 15 patients, 47 (75%) were detected by bone scan with ^{99m}Tc-HMDP. The scintigraphic patterns included increased activity in 29 lesions, decreased activity in 7 lesions, and heterogeneous uptake in 7 foci. One false positive lesion was demonstrated to be a vertebral angioma. They also noted that ^{131}I was more accurate in the skull; whereas the ^{99m}Tc-HMDP bone scan was more accurate in the thorax and spine. They also studied a second group of 9 patients with bone pain and negative ^{131}I scans. There were 8 osteolytic lesions noted on radiographs obtained prior to scintigraphy. Bone scans detected 29 additional lesions that were confirmed by radiographs. There was one false negative bone scan of a metastatic focus in the petrous bone diagnosed by CT.

Alam et al (123) recently published a study evaluating bone scans and ^{201}Tl scintigraphy for differentiated thyroid carcinoma. They had 27 patients with 77 bone lesions confirmed by ^{131}I scans, histology, MRI, or CT. On bone scan, 75% of the lesions were detected. By ^{201}Tl, 69% of lesions were detected. Moreover, of the 19 lesions that were not seen on bone scan, 14 demonstrated increased ^{201}Tl uptake. Using both techniques yielded a sensitivity of 94%. Of interest, ^{131}I scans detected 82% of lesions.

Although MRI is reported to be more sensitive than bone scans for the detection of osseous lesions (124,125,126,127), it does not routinely provide whole body assessment. Recently, Kosuda et al (124) compared nuclear medicine bone SPECT and MRI of the vertebral column. Although MRI diagnosed the most lesions (86/88) compared with planar and SPECT bone scans, SPECT was able to detect more lesions that were located outside of the vertebral body. A recent report by Eustace et al (128) evaluated whole body MRI and bone scans. Their preliminary results suggest that whole body MRI is more sensitive than planar bone scan. MRI also is more sensitive than CT for the detection of osseous metastases and provides excellent anatomic delineation of lesions. CT, however, is better at delineation of the bone cortex. If CT evaluation is desired, contrast enhancement is not required for the evaluation of the bone.

Abdominal Metastases

Sites of metastatic disease in the abdomen include liver and, less commonly, abdominal lymph nodes and the adrenal glands. Evaluation of the liver may be performed by ultrasound, CT, or MRI. The most sensitive techniques for identification of hepatic metastases, intra-operative ultrasound and CT arterial portography, are invasive and are not suitable for long-term follow-up of oncologic patients. Early comparison studies between ultrasound and contrast enhanced CT demonstrated similar detection rates for metastatic foci (129,130,131). However, earlier CT scanners were unable to scan rapidly through the liver during optimal hepatic enhancement. In recent comparative studies with abdominal CT, trans-abdominal ultrasound demonstrated sensitivities of 53-66% (132,133), which are lower than those for contrast enhanced CT.

CT examination of the abdomen may be performed without or with intravenous iodinated contrast. However, evaluation of the liver without intravenous contrast detects fewer metastatic lesions when compared to contrast enhanced CT (134,135,136). Contrast enhancement of the liver is complex due to its dual blood supply, and the differential blood supply of normal hepatic parenchyma and tumors has important indications in lesion detection (137,138). Thyroid metastases are hypervascular and therefore may be isodense in the portal venous phase of enhancement. Early reports suggested the use of routine noncontrast CT in conjunction with contrast enhanced CT to improve lesion detection (139) when studying hypervascular lesions. However, with rapid helical scanning, arterial phase imaging can increase the detection of hypervascular lesions. A few studies (134,135,140) have investigated the need for both noncontrast CT and contrast enhanced CT in patients with suspected hypervascular metastases and have concluded that noncontrast CT no longer need be performed when contrast CT is to be utilized. Case reports of CT examinations of hepatic metastases in patients with medullary carcinoma have demonstrated calcification within the metastatic foci (141,142).

MRI has been shown to be an alternative modality with similar sensitivities for lesion detection (143). Increased lesion detection can be achieved using MRI contrast agents. In addition to the extracellular gadolinium chelates (144,145), two new liver contrast agents have become available. Feroximides are iron agents that are taken up by the reticuloendothelial system (145). Manganese DPDP is a manganese based agent that is taken up by hepatocytes (145,146). Early work suggests that these agents will increase lesion detection in comparison with noncontrast MRI (146,147,148,149).

For all imaging modalities (US, CT, MRI) lesion detection is dependent upon lesion size. All of the imaging methods demonstrate lower sensitivity for lesions smaller than 1 cm in diameter (133,150) with improved lesion detection as lesion diameter increases (133).

As in the neck and chest, detection of metastatic lymph nodes in the abdomen is based on size criteria. At this time, non nuclear medicine imaging studies cannot detect normal sized, but pathologic lymph nodes.

CNS Metastases

Metastases to the brain are uncommon. Imaging of the brain may be performed by either CT or MRI. However, optimal CT evaluation requires the administration of iodinated intravenous contrast. In addition, MRI has demonstrated sensitivities greater than single or double dose contrast enhanced head CT for the detection of metastatic foci (151,152). MRI also has the advantage of using contrast agents that do not contain iodine. For evaluation of the spinal column, MRI continues to be the imaging modality of choice.

Summary

In summary, ^{131}I whole body scans remain the primary imaging modality in patients with iodine avid tumor. In patients with elevated tumor markers and negative ^{131}I scans or with non-iodine avid tumors, imaging with ^{201}Tl or ^{99m}Tc-sestamibi may be beneficial. Further imaging is dependent on the most likely sites of tumor recurrence or metastases. Recurrences in the neck are more likely with papillary and medullary carcinoma. Pulmonary metastases are common in all forms of thyroid cancer, but are more commonly seen in papillary carcinoma. Evaluation of the chest can be performed well with chest x-ray and non-contrast CT. Osseous metastases are less commonly seen in papillary carcinoma, but are approximately equal in incidence to pulmonary metastases in follicular carcinoma. If evidence of distant metastatic disease or skeletal symptoms are present, bone scans can be useful. If the bone scan is negative and the patient has localized symptoms, further evaluation may be made with MRI. Less commonly, abdominal metastases occur. If intravenous contrast cannot be administered due to the iodine load, MRI may prove to be an appropriate alternative, particularly with liver specific contrast agents. CNS metastases, although uncommon, are best evaluated by MRI.

References

1. Maxon HR & Smith HS. Radioiodine-131 in the diagnosis and treatment of metastatic well differentiated thyroid cancer. Endo Metab Clin N Am 1990; 19: 685-718.
2. Yeh SDJ & LaQuaglia MP: [131]I therapy for pediatric thyroid cancer. Sem Ped Surg 1997; 6:128-133.
3. Beierwaltes WH, Nishiyama RH, Thompson NW, et al. Survival time and "cure" in papillary and follicular thyroid carcinoma with distant metastases: statistics following University of Michigan therapy. J Nucl Med 1982; 23: 561-568.
4. Pochin EE. Radioiodine therapy of thyroid cancer. Semin Nucl Med 1971; 1: 501-515.
5. Maheshwari YK, Hill CS, Jr., Haynie TP, III, et al. [131]I therapy in differentiated thyroid carcinoma: M.D. Anderson Hospital experience. Cancer 1981; 47: 664-671.
6. Krishna L, Dadparvar S, Brady L, et al. Paradoxical changes in iodine-131 scintigraphic findings in advanced follicular thyroid cancer. J Nucl Med 1993; 34: 1574-1576.
7. Oyen, WJG, Mudde AH, van den Broek WJM, and Lorstens FHM. Metastatic follicular carcinoma of the thyroid: Reappearance of radioiodine uptake. J Nucl Med 1995; 36: 613-615.
8. Green JP, Wilcox JR, Marriott JD, et al. Thyroid uptake of [131]I: further comparisons of capsules and liquid preparations. J Nucl Med 1976; 17: 310-312.
9. Hung JC. Radioiodine dispensing and usage in a centralized hospital nuclear pharmacy. Thyroid 1997; 7: 289-294.
10. Rawson RW, Ball JE, Peacock W. Limitations and indications in the treatment of cancer of the thyroid with radioactive iodine. J Clin Endocrinol 1951; 11: 1128-1142.
11. Park HM, Perkins OW, Edmondson JW, et al. Influence of diagnostic radioiodine on the uptake of ablative dose of iodine-131. Thyroid 1994; 4: 49-54.
12. Jeevanram RK, Shah DH, Sharma SM, Ganatra RD. Influence of initial large dose on subsequent uptake of therapeutic radioiodine in thyroid cancer patients. Nucl Med Biol 1986; 13: 277-279.
13. Muratet JP, Giraud P, Daver A, et al. Do scanning doses of I-131 stun thyroid remnants? A comparison of 37 vs. 111 MBq before first I-131 ablative therapy in patients with differentiated thyroid carcinoma. J Nucl Med 1997; 38: 46P (abstract).
14. McDougall IR: 74 MBq radioiodine ^{131}I does not prevent uptake of therapeutic doses of [131]I (i.e. it does not cause stunning) in differentiated thyroid cancer. Nuc Med Commun 1997; 18: 505-512.
15. Park HM, Park YH, Zhou XH. Detection of thyroid remnant/metastasis without stunning: an ongoing dilemma. Thyroid 1997; 7: 277-280.
16. Berbano R, Naddaf S, Echemendia E, et al: Use of iodine-123 as a diagnostic tracer for neck and whole body scanning in patients with well-differentiated thyroid cancer. Endocr Pract 1998; 4: 11-16.
17. Maxon HR, Thomas SR, Washburn LC, Hinnefeld JD. High activity I-123 for the diagnostic evaluation of patients with thyroid cancer. J Nucl Med 1993; 34: 42P (abstract).
18. Bautovich GJ, Towson JE, Eberl S, et al. Comparison of iodine-123 and iodine-131 as a scanning agent for the detection of metastatic thyroid cancer. J Nucl Med 1997; 38: 150P-151P (abstract).
19. Becker D, Charkes ND, Dworkin H, et al. Procedure guideline for extended scintigraphy for differentiated thyroid cancer: 1.0. J Nucl Med 1996; 37: 1269-1271.
20. Thomas SR, Maxon HR, Kereiakes JG, et al. Quantitative external counting techniques enabling improved diagnostic and therapeutic decisions in patients with well-differentiated thyroid cancer. Radiology 1997; 122: 731-737.
21. Thomas SR, Maxon HR, Kereiakes JG. In vivo quantitation of lesion radioactivity using external counting methods. Med Phys 1976; 3: 253-255.
22. NČmec J, Röhling S, Zamrazil V, et al. Comparison of the distribution of diagnostic and thyroablative ^{131}I in the evaluation of differentiated thyroid cancers. J Nucl Med 1979; 20: 92-97.

23. Maxon HR, Englaro EE, Hertzberg VS, Chen LS. Chest x-ray, bone scans, and immediate post treatment I-131 scans: utility in well differentiated thyroid cancer. J Nucl Med 1992;33(S): 894 (abstract).

24. Sherman SI, Tielens ET, Sostre S, et al. Clinical utility of post treatment radioiodine scans in the management of patients with thyroid carcinoma. J Clin Endocrinol Metab 1994; 78: 629-634.

25. Briele B, Hotze A, Grunwald F, et al. Whole body scan with [131]I: advantage of delayed images for the detection of thyroid cancer metastases. Nuklearmedizin 1990; 29: 264-268.

26. Hoie J, Stenwig AE, Kullmann G, Lindegaard M. Distant metastases in papillary thyroid cancer: a review of 91 patients. Cancer 1988; 61: 1-6.

27. Maxon HR, Thomas SR, Book SA, et al. Induction of thyroid cancer by ionizing radiation. National Council on Radiation Protection and Measurements Report 80, Bethesda, Maryland, 1985, p 61.

28. Chung JK, Lee YJ, Jeong JM, et al. Clinical significance of hepatic visualization on iodine-131 whole body scan in patients with thyroid carcinoma. J Nucl Med 1997; 38: 1191-1195.

29. Bakheet SM, Powe J, Hammami MM. Radioiodine uptake in the chest. J Nucl Med 1997; 38: 984-986.

30. Bakheet SM & Hammami MM. False-positive radioiodine whole body scan in thyroid cancer patients due to unrelated pathology. Clin Nucl Med 1994; 19: 325-329.

31. McDougall, IR. Whole-body scintigraphy with radioiodine-131: A comprehensive list of false-positives with some examples. Clin Nucl Med 1995; 20: 869-875.

32. Kipper MS & Krohn LD. Increased submandibular gland uptake on thyroid scintigraphy due to Wharton's duct stone. Clin Nucl Med 1996; 21: 881-882.

33. Giuffado D, Garofalo MR, Cacciaguerra G, et al. False positive ^{131}I total body scan due to an ectasia of the common carotid. J Endocrinol Invest 1993; 16: 207-211.

34. Matheja P, Lerch H, Schmid KW, et al. Frontal sinus mucocele mimicking a metastasis of papillary thyroid carcinoma. J Nucl Med 1997; 38: 1022-1024.

35. Andreas J, Bruhl K, Eissner D. False positive I-131 whole body imaging after I-131 therapy for a follicular carcinoma. Clin Nucl Med 1997; 22: 123-124.

36. Guiffrida D, Fornito MC, Pellegriti G, et al. False positive ^{131}I total body scan due to bilateral polycystic renal disease. J Endocrinol Invest 1997; 20: 342-344.

37. Brucker-Davis F, Reynolds JC, Skarulis M, et al. False positive iodine-131 whole body scans due to cholecystitis and sebaceous cyst. J Nucl Med 1996; 37: 1690-1693.

38. Kinuya S, Yokoyama K, Michigishi T, Tonami N. I-131 accumulation in folliculitis of the scalp. Clin Nucl Med 1996; 21: 807-808.

39. You DL, Tzen KY, Chen JF, et al. False positive whole body iodine-131 scan due to intrahepatic duct dilatation. J Nucl Med 1997; 38: 1977-1979.

40. Tonami N, Hisada K. [201]Tl scintigraphy in postoperative detection of thyroid cancer: a comparative study with [131]I. Radiology 1980; 136: 461-464.

41. Ohnishi T, Noguchi S, Murakami N, Jinnouchi S, Hoshi H, Futami S, Watanabe K. Detection of recurrent thyroid cancer: MR versus thallium-201 scintigraphy. AJNR 1993; 14: 1051-1057.

42. Hoefnagel CA, Delprat CC, Marcuse HR, de Vijlder JJM. Role of thallium-201 total-body scintigraphy in follow-up of thyroid carcinoma. J Nucl Med 1986; 27: 1854-1857.

43. Brendel AJ, Guyot M, Jeandot R, Lefort G, Manciet G. Thallium-201 imaging in the follow-up of differentiated thyroid carcinoma. J Nucl Med 1988; 29: 1515-1520.

44. Pacini F, Lippi F, Formica N, Elisei R, Anelli S, Ceccarelli C, Pinchera A. Therapeutic doses of iodine-131 reveal undiagnosed metastases in thyroid cancer patients with detectable serum thyroglobulin levels. J Nucl Med 1987; 28: 1888-1891.

45. Carril JM, Quirce R, Serrano J, Banzo I, Jiminez-Bonilla J, Tabuenca O, Barquin RG. Total-body scintigraphy with thallium-201 and iodine-131 in the follow-up of differentiated thyroid cancer. J Nucl Med 1997; 38: 686-692.

46. Dadparvar S, Krishna L, Brady LW, Slizofski WJ, Brown SJ, Chevres A, Micaily B. The role of iodine-131 and thallium-201 imaging and serum thyroglobulin in the management of differentiated thyroid carcinoma. Cancer 1993; 71: 3767-3773.

47. Ramanna L, Waxman A, Braunstein G. Thallium-201 scintigraphy in differentiated thyroid cancer: Comparison with radioiodine scintigraphy and serum thyroglobulin determinations. J Nucl Med 1991; 32: 441-446.

48. Lorberboym M, Murthy S, Mechanick J, Bergman D, Morris JC, Kim CK. Thallium-201 and iodine-131 scintigraphy in differentiated thyroid carcinoma. J Nucl Med 1996; 37: 1487-1491.

49. Burman KD, Anderson JH, Wartofsky L, Mong DP, Jelenik JJ. Management of patients with thyroid carcinoma: application of thallium-201 scintigraphy and magnetic resonance imaging. J Nucl Med 1990; 31: 1958-1964.

50. Charkes ND, Vitti RA, Brooks K. Thallium-201 SPECT increases detectability of thyroid cancer metastases. J Nucl Med 1990; 31: 147-153.

51. Dunkley SM, Roach PJ. Thallium-201 uptake in reactive lymphadenopathy. Clin Nucl Med 1997; 22: 125-126.

52. Toney MO, Williams S. Focal Thallium-201 uptake in pneumonia. Clin Nucl Med 1997; 22: 183-184.

53. Brandt-Mainz K, Mηller SP, Sonnenschein W, Reiners C, Sciuk J, Bocklsch A. The influence of the location of thyroid cancer metastases on tumor detectability with thallium-201. J Nucl Med 1997; 38(S): 237P.

54. VanSorge-VanBoxtel RAJ, VanEck-Smit BLF, Goslings GM. Comparison of serum thyroglobulin, ^{131}I and ^{201}Tl scintigraphy in the post-operative follow-up of differentiated thyroid cancer. Nuc Med Commun 1993; 14: 365-372.

55. Mallin WH, Elgazzar AH, Maxon HR. Imaging modalities in the follow-up of non-iodine avid thyroid carcinoma. Am J Otolaryngol 1994; 15: 417-422.

56. Sutter CW, Stadalnik RC. Noncardiac uptake of technetium-99m sestamibi: an updated gamut. Sem Nucl Med 1996; 26: 135-140.

57. Němec J, Nývitová O, Blažek T, Viček P, Racek P, Novák Z, Preiningerová M, Hubáčková M. Positive thyroid cancer scintigraphy using technetium-99m methoxyisobutylisonitrile. Eur J Nucl Med 1996; 23: 69-71.

58. Miyamoto S, Kasagi K, Misaki T, Alam MS, Konishi J. Evaluation of technetium-99m-MIBI scintigraphy in metastatic differentiated thyroid carcinoma. J Nucl Med 1997; 38: 352-356.

59. Dadparvar S, Chevres A, Tulchinsky M, Krishna-Badrinath L, Khan AS, Slizofski W. Clinical utility of technetium-99m methoxyisobutylisonitrile imaging in differentiated thyroid carcinoma: comparison with thallium-201 and iodine-131 Na scintigraphy, and serum thyroglobulin quantitation. Eur J Nucl Med 1995; 22: 1330-1338.

60. Learoyd DL, Roach PJ, Briggs GM, Delbridge LW, Wilmshurst EG, Robinson BG. Technetium-99m-sestamibi scanning in recurrent medullary thyroid carcinoma. J Nucl Med 1997; 38: 227-230.

61. Yen T, Lin H, Lee C, Chang S, Yeh S. The role of technetium-99m sestamibi whole-body scans in diagnosing metastatic Hurthle cell carcinoma of the thyroid gland after total thyroidectomy: a comparison with iodine-131 and thallium-201 whole body scans. Eur J Nucl Med 1994; 21: 980-983.

62. Balon HR, Fink-Bennett D, Stoffer SS. Technetium-99m-sestamibi uptake by recurrent Hurthle cell carcinoma of the thyroid. J Nucl Med 1992; 33: 1393-1395.

63. Lind P, Gallowitsch HJ, Langsteger W, Kresnik E, Mikosch P, Gomez I. Technetium-99m tetrofosmin whole-body scintigraphy in the follow-up of differentiated thyroid carcinoma. J Nucl Med 1997; 38: 348-352.

64. Spanu A, Solinas ME, Bagella C, Nuvoli S, Langer M, Madeddu G. The usefulness of Tc-99m tetrofosmin scan in the follow-up of differentiated thyroid carcinoma. J Nucl Med 1997; 38(S): 236P.

65. Feine U, Lietzenmayer R, Hanke J, Held J, W̄ hrle H, Mηller-Schauenburg W. Fluorine-18-FDG and iodine-131-iodide uptake in thyroid cancer. J Nucl Med 1996; 37: 1468-1472.

66. Grηnwald F, Schomburg A, Bender H, Klemm E, Menzel C, Bultmann T, Palmedo H, Ruhlmann J, Kozak B, Biersack H. Fluorine-18 fluorodeoxyglucose positron emission tomography in the follow-up of differentiated thyroid cancer. Eur J Nucl Med 1996; 23: 312-319.

67. Grunwald F, Menzel C, Bender H, Palmedo H, Willkomm P, Ruhlmann J, Franckson T, Biersack H. Comparison of [18]FDG-PET with [131]iodine and ^{99m}Tc-sestamibi scintigraphy in differentiated thyroid cancer. Thyroid 1997; 7: 327-335.

68. Fridich L, Messa C, Landoni C, Lucignani G, Moncayo R, Kendler D, Riccabona G, Fazio F. Whole-body scintigraphy with ^{99m}Tc-MIBI, ^{18}F-FDG and ^{131}I in patients with metastatic thyroid carcinoma. Nuc Med Commun 1997; 18: 3-9.

69. Skowsky WR, Wilf L. Iodine-131 Metaiodobenzylguanidine scintigraphy of medullary carcinoma of the thyroid. South Med J 1991; 84: 636-641.

70. Clarke SEM, Lazarus C, Mistry R, Maisey MN. The role of technetium-99m pentavalent DMSA in the management of patients with medullary carcinoma of the thyroid. Br J Radiol 1987; 60: 1089-1092.

71. Mojiminiyi OA, Udelsman R, Soper NDW, Shepstone BJ, Dudley NE. Pentavalent Tc-99m DMSA scintigraphy: prospective evaluation of its role in the management of patients with medullary carcinoma of the thyroid. Clin Nucl Med 1991; 16:259-262.

72. Ohta H, Yamamoto K, Endo K, Mori T, Hamanaka D, Shimazu A, Ikekubo K, Makimoto K, Iida Y, Konishi J, Morita R, Hata N, Horiuchi K, Yokoyama A, Torizuka K, Kuma K. A new imaging agent for medullary carcinoma of the thyroid. J Nucl Med 1984; 25:323-325.

73. Clarke SEM, Lazarus CR, Wraight P, Sampson C, Maisey M. Pentavalent [^{99m}Tc]DMSA, [^{131}I]MIBG, and [^{99m}Tc]MDP - An evaluation of three imaging techniques in patients with medullary carcinoma of the thyroid. J Nucl Med 1988; 29:33-38.

74. Kurtaran A, Scheuba C, Angelberger P, Kaserer K, Niederle B, Virgolini I. Clinical value of In-111-DTPA-D-PHE-1-Octreotide (In-111-Oct) and Tc-99m Dimercaptosuccinic acid (Tc-99m-DMSA-V) scans for preoperative staging of primary medullary thyroid carcinoma (MTC). J Nucl Med 1997; 38(S):237P.

75. Baudin E, Lumbroso J, Schlumberger M, Leclere J, Giammarile F, Gardet P, Roche A, Travagli JP, Parmentier C. Comparison of octreotide scintigraphy and conventional imaging in medullary thyroid carcinoma. J Nucl Med 1996; 37:912-916.

76. Dorr U, Sautter-Bihl M, Bihl H. The contribution of somatostatin receptor scintigraphy to the diagnosis of recurrent medullary carcinoma of the thyroid. Sem in Oncology 1994; 21(Supp 13):42-45.

77. Kwekkeboom DJ, Reubi JC, Lamberts SWJ, Bruining HA, Mulder AH, Oei HY, Krenning EP. In Vivo somatostatin receptor imaging in medullary thyroid carcinoma. J Clin Endocrinol Metab 1993; 76:1413-1417.

78. O'Byrne KJ, O'Hare N, Sweeney E, Freyne PJ, Cullen MJ. Somatostatin and somatostatin analogues in medullary thyroid carcinoma. Nuc Med Commun 1996; 17:810-816.

79. Krausz Y, Ish-Shalom S, Dejong RBJ, Shibley N, Lapidot M, Maaravi Y, Glaser B. Somatostatin-receptor imaging of medullary thyroid carcinoma. Clin Nuc Med 1994; 19:416-421.

80. Kwekkeboom DJ, Lamberts SWJ, Habbema JDF, Krenning EP. Cost-effectiveness analysis of somatostatin receptor scintigraphy. J Nucl Med 1996; 37:886-892.

81. Juweid M, Sharkey R, Behr T, Swayne LC, Rubin AD, Herskovic T, Hanley D, Markowitz A, Dunn R, Siegel J, Kamal T, Goldenberg DM. Improved detection of medullary thyroid cancer with radiolabeled antibodies to carcinoembryonic antigen. J Clin Oncol 1996; 14:1209-1217.

82. Sessions RB, Davidson BJ. Thyroid Cancer. Med Clin NA 1993; 77:517-538.

83. Simeone JF, Daniels GH, Hall DA, McCarthy K, Kopans DB, Butch RJ, Mueller PR, Stark DD, Ferrucci JT, Wang CA. Sonography in the follow-up of 100 patients with thyroid carcinoma. AJR 1987; 148:45-49.

84. Sutton RT, Reading CC, Charboneau JW, James EM, Grant CS, Hay ID. US-guided biopsy of neck masses in postoperative management of patients with thyroid cancer. Radiology 1988; 168:769-772.

85. van den Brekel MWM, Castelijns JA, Snow GB. Imaging of cervical lymphadenopathy. Neuroimag Clin NA 1996; 6:417-434.

86. Sakai F, Kiyono K, Sone S, Kondo Y, Oguchi M, Watanabe T, Sakai Y, Imai Y, Takeda S, Yamamoto K, Ohta H. Ultrasonic evaluation of cervical metastatic lymphadenopathy. J Ultrasound Med 1988; 7:305-310.

87. Na DG, Lim HK, Byun HS, Kim HD, Ko YH, Baek JH. Differential diagnosis of cervical lymphadenopathy: Usefulness of color doppler sonography. AJR 1997; 168:1311-1316.

88. Giovagnorio F, Rusticali A, Araneo AL. Color and pulsed doppler evaluation of benign and malignant adenopathy. Clin Imaging 1997; 21:163-169.

89. Giovagnorio F, Caiazzo R, Avitto A. Evaluation of vascular patterns of cervical lymph nodes with power doppler sonography. J Clin Ultrasound 1997; 25:71-76.

90. Choi MY, Lee JW, Jang KJ. Distinction between benign and malignant causes of cervical, axillary, and inguinal lymphadenopathy: Value of doppler spectral waveform analysis. AJR 1995; 165:981-984.

91. Maurer J, William C, Schroeder R, Hidajad N, Hell B, Bier J, Weber S, Felix R. Evaluation of metastases and reactive lymph nodes in doppler sonography using an ultrasound contrast enhancer. Invest Radiol 1997; 32:441-446.

92. Takashima S, Sone S, Nomura N, Tomiyama N, Kobayashi T, Nakamura H. Nonpalpable lymph nodes of the neck: Assessment with US and US-guided fine-needle aspiration biopsy. J Clin Ultrasound 1997; 25:283-292.

93. Boland GW, Lee MJ, Mueller PR, Mayo-Smith W, Dawson SL, Simeone JF. Efficacy of sonographically guided biopsy of thyroid masses and cervical lymph nodes. AJR 1993; 161:1053-1056.

94. Antonelli A, Miccoli P, Ferdeghini M, Di Coscio G, Alberti B, Iacconi P, Baldi V, Fallahi P, Baschieri L. Role of neck ultrasonography in the follow-up of patients operated on for thyroid cancer. Thyroid 1995; 5:25-28.

95. Frank K, Raue F, Lorenz D, Herfarth C, Ziegler R. Importance of ultrasound examination for the follow-up of medullary thyroid carcinoma: Comparison with other localization methods. Henry Ford Hosp Med J 1987; 35:122-123.

96. Scott AM, Macapinlac H, Zhang J, Daghighian F, Montemayor N, Kalaigian H, Sgouros G, Graham MC, Kolbert K, Yeh SDJ, Lai E, Goldsmith SJ, Larson SM. Image registration of SPECT and CT images using an external fiduciary band and three-dimensional surface fitting in metastatic thyroid cancer. J Nucl Med 1995; 36:100-103.

97. Perault C, Schvartz C, Wampach H Liehn J-C, Delisle M-J et al. Thoracic and abdominal SPECT-CT image fusion without external markers in endocrine carcinoma. J Nucl Med 1997; 38:1234-1242.

98. Som PM, Brandwein M, Lidov M, Lawson W, Biller HF. The varied presentations of papillary thyroid carcinoma cervical nodal disease: CT and MR findings. AJNR 1994; 15:1123-1128.

99. Anzai Y, Blackwell KE, Hirschowitz SL, Rogers JW, Sato Y, Yuh WTC, Runge VM, Morris MR, McLachlan SJ, Lufkin RB. Initial clinical experience with dextran-coated superparamagnetic iron oxide for detection of lymph node metastases in patients with head and neck cancer. Radiology 1994; 192:709-715.

100. Harika L, Weissleder R, Poss K, Papisov M. Macromolecular intravenous contrast agent for MR lymphography: Characterization and efficacy studies. Radiology 1996; 198:365-370.

101. Sherman SI, Brierley J, Sperling M, Maxon HR III. Initial Analysis of Staging and Outcomes from a Prospective Multicenter Study of Treatment of Thyroid Carcinoma. Thyroid 1996; 6(supp 1):39.

102. Dinneen SF, Malimaki MJ, Bergstralh EJ, Goellner JR, Gorman SA, Hay ID. Distant metastases in papillary thyroid carcinoma: 100 cases observed at one institution during 5 decades. J Clin Endocrinol Metab 1995; 80:2041-2045.

103. Mazzaferri EL, Jhiang SM. Long-term impact of initial surgical and medical therapy on papillary and follicular thyroid cancer. Am J Med 1994; 97:418-428.

104. Ruegemer JJ, Hay ID, Bergstralh EJ, Ryan JJ, Offord KP, Gorman CA. Distant metastases in differentiated thyroid carcinoma: A multivariate analysis of prognostic variables. J Clin Endocrinol Metab 1988; 67: 501-508.

105. Schlumberger M, Tubiana M, de Vathaire F, Hill C, Gardet P, Travagli J-P, Fragu P, Lumbroso J, Caillou B, Parmentier C. Long-term results of treatment of 283 patients with lung and bone metastases from differentiated thyroid carcinoma. J Clin Endocrinol Metab 1986; 63:960-967.

106. Heaston DK P utman CE, Rodan BA, Nicholson E, Ravin CE, Korobkin M, Chen JTT, Seigler HF. Solitary pulmonary metastases in high-risk melanoma patients: A prospective comparison of conventional and computed tomography. AJR 1983; 141:169-174.

107. Piekarski DJ, Schlumberger M, Leclere J, Couanet D, Masselot J, Parmentier C. Chest computed tomography (CT) in patients with micronodular lung metastases of differentiated thyroid carcinoma. Int J Radiation Oncology Biol Phys 1985; 11:1023-1027.

108. Remy-Jardin M, Remy J, Giraud F, Marquette C-H. Pulmonary nodules: Detection with thick-section spiral CT versus conventional CT. Radiology 1993; 187:513-520.

109. Collie DA, Wright AR, Williams JR, Hashemi-Malayeri B, Stevenson AJM, Turnbull CM. Comparison of spiral-acquisition computed tomography and conventional computed tomography in the assessment of pulmonary metastatic disease. Br J Radiol 1994; 67:436-444.

110. Mηller NL, Gamsu B, Webb WR. Pulmonary nodules: Detection using magnetic resonance and computed tomography. Radiology 1985; 155:687-690.

111. Jiminez JM, Casey SO, Citron M, Khan A. Calcified pulmonary metastases from medullary carcinoma of the thyroid. Comp Med Imag Graph 1995; 19:325-328.

112. Staples CA, Mηller NL, Miller RR, Evans KG, Nelems B. Mediastinal nodes in bronchogenic carcinoma: Comparison between CT and mediastinoscopy. Radiology 1988; 167:367-372.

113. Libshitz HI, McKenna RJ. Mediastinal lymph node size in lung cancer. AJR 1984; 143:715-718.
114. Feigin DS, Friedman PJ, Liston SE, Haghighi P, Peters RM, Hill JG. Improving specificity of computed tomography in diagnosis of malignant mediastinal lymph nodes. J Comput Tomogr 1985; 9:21-32.
115. Marcocci C, Pacini F, Elisei R, Schipani E, Ceccarelli C, Miccoli P, Arganini M, Pinchera A. Clinical and biologic behavior of bone metastases from differentiated thyroid carcinoma. Surgery 1989; 106:960-966.
116. Brennan MD, Bergstralh EJ, van Heerden J, McConahey WM. Follicular thyroid cancer treated at the Mayo Clinic, 1946 through 1970: Initial manifestations, pathologic findings, therapy, and outcome. Mayo Clin Proc 1991; 66:11-22.
117. Leeper RD. The effect of ^{131}I therapy on survival of patients with metastatic papillary or follicular thyroid carcinoma. J Clin Endocrinol Metab 1973; 36:1143-1152.
118. Rossi R, Cady B, Silverman ML, Wool MS, ReMine S, Hodge MB, Salzman FA. Surgically incurable well-differentiated thyroid carcinoma. Prognostic factors and results of therapy. Arch Surg 1988; 123:569-574.
119. Gold RI, Seeger LL, Bassett LW, Steckel RJ. An integrated approach to the evaluation of metastatic bone disease. Rad Clin NA 1990; 28:471-483.
120. Krasnow AZ, Hellman RS, Timins ME, Collier BD, Anderson T, Isitman AT. Diagnostic bone scanning in oncology. Sem Nucl Med 1997; 27: 107-141.
121. Castillo LA, Yeh SDJ, Leeper RD, Benua RS. Bone scans in bone metastases from functioning thyroid carcinoma. Clin Nuc Med 1980; 5:200-209.
122. Tenenbaum F, Schlumberger M, Bonnin F, Lumbroso J, Aubert B, Benali H, Parmentier C. Usefulness of technetium-99m hydroxymethylene diphosphonate scans in localizing bone metastases of differentiated thyroid carcioma. Eur J Nucl Med 1993; 20:1168-1174.
123. Alam S, Takeuchi R, Kasagi K, Misaki T, Miyamoto S, Iida Y, Hidaka A, Konishi J. Value of combined technetium-99m hydroxy methylene diphosphonate and thallium-201 imaging in detecting bone metastases from thyroid carcinoma. Thyroid 1997; 7:705-712.
124. Kosuda S, Kaji T, Yokoyama T, Katayama M, Iriye T, Uematsu M, Kisano. J Nucl Med 1996; 37:975-978.
125. Delbeke D, Powers TA, Sandler MP. Correlative radionuclide and magnetic resonance imaging in evaluation of the spine. Clin Nuc Med 1989; 14:742-749.
126. Gosfield E, Alavi A, Kneeland B. Comparison of radionuclide bone scans and magnetic resonance imaging in detecting spinal metastases. J Nucl Med 1993; 34:2191-2198.
127. Frank JA, Ling A, Patronas N, Carrasquillo NJ, Horvath K, Hickey AM, Dwyer AJ. Detection of malignant bone tumors: MR imaging vs. scintigraphy. AJR 1990; 155:1043-1048.
128. Eustace S, Tello R, DeCarvalho V, Carey J, Wrolblicka JT, Melhem ER, Yucel EK. A comparison of whole-body Turbo-STIR MR imaging and planar ^{99m}Tc-methylene diphosphonate scintigraphy in the examination of patients with suspected skeletal metastases. AJR 1997; 169:1655-1661.
129. Andersson T, Eriksson B, Hemmingsson, A, Lindgren PG, Oberg K. Angiography, computed tomography, magnetic resonance imaging and ultrasonography in detection of liver metastases from endocrine gastrointestinal tumours. Acta Radiol 1987; 28:535-539.
130. Lundstedt C, Ekberg H, Hederstrom E, Stridbeck H, Torfason B, Tranberg K-G. Radiologic diagnosis of liver metastases in colo-rectal carcinoma. Acta Radiol 1987; 28:431-438.
131. Schreve RH, Terpstra OT, Ausema L, Lameris JS, van Seijen A. Detection of liver metastases. A prospective study comparing liver enzymes, scintigraphy, ultrasonography and computed tomography. Br J Surg 1984; 71:947-949.
132. Wernecke K, Rummeny E, Bongartz G, Vassallo P, Kivelitz D, Wiesmann W, Peters PE, Reers B, Reiser M, Pircher W. Detection of hepatic masses in patients with carcinoma: Comparative sensitivities of sonography, CT and MR imaging. AJR 1991; 157:731-739.
133. Gunven P, Makuuchi M, Takayasu K, Moriyama N, Yamasaki S, Hasegawa H. Preoperative imaging of liver metastases. Comparison of angiography, CT scan and ultrasonography. Ann Surg 1985; 202:573-579.
134. Chomyn JJ, Stamm ER, Thickman D. CT of melanoma liver metastases: Is the examination without contrast media superfluous? J Comput Assist Tomogr 1992; 16:568-571.
135. Frederick MG, Paulson EK, Nelson RC. Helical CT for detecting focal liver lesions in patients with breast carcinoma: Comparison of noncontrast phase, hepatic arterial phase, and portal venous phase. J Comput Assist Tomogr 1997; 21:229-235.

136.   Yassa NA, Agostini JT, Tan MS.   Routine pre-contrast CT for liver lesion detection.   A re-examination. Clin Imag 1997; 21:346-349.

137.   Baron RL. Understanding and optimizing use of contrast material for CT of the liver. AJR 1994; 163:323-331.

138.   Oliver JH, Baron RL.   Helical biphasic contrast-enhanced CT of the liver: Technique, indications, interpretation, and pitfalls. Radiology 1996; 201:1-14.

139.   Bressler EL, Alpern MB, Glazer GM, Francis IR, Ensminger WD.   Hypervascular hepatic metastases: CT evaluation. Radiology 1987; 162:49-51.

140.   Patten RM, Byun J-Y, Freeny PC. CT of hypervascular hepatic tumors: Are unenhanced scans necessary for diagnosis? AJR 1993; 161:979-984.

141.   McDonnell CH, Fishman EK, Zerhouni EA.   CT demonstration of calcified liver metastases in medullary thyroid carcinoma. J Comput Assist Tomogr 1986; 10:976-978.

142.   Bankoff MS, Tuckman GA, Scarborough D.   CT appearance of liver metastases from medullary carcinoma of the thyroid. J Comput Assist Tomogr 1987; 11:1102-1103.

143.   Reinig JW, Dwyer AJ, Miller DJ, White M, Frank JA, Sugarbaker PH, Chang AE, Doppman JL. Liver metastasis detection: Comparative sensitivities of MR imaging and CT scanning. Radiology 1987; 162:43-47.

144.   Curati WL, Halevy A, Gibson RN, Carr DH, Blumgart LH, Steiner RE. Ultrasound, CT and MRI comparison in primary and secondary tumors of the liver. Gastroint Radiol 1988; 13:123-128.

145.   Low RN. Contrast agents for MR imaging of the liver. JMRI 1997; 7:56-67.

146.   Birnbaum BA, Weinreb JC, Fernandez MP, Brown JJ, Rofsky NM, Young SW. Comparison of contrast enhanced CT and Mn-DPDP enhanced MRI for detection of focal hepatic lesions. Initial findings. Clin Imaging 1998; 18:21-27.

147.   Rummeny EJ, Nilsen G, Torres CG, Fagertun H.   Detection and characterization of focal liver lesions before and after administration of Mn-DPDP: Results of an independent image evaluation in 300 patients. Radiology 1995; 197(P):415.

148.   Bernardino MR, Young SW, Lee JKT, Weinreb JC.   Hepatic MR imaging with Mn-DPDP: Safety, image quality, and sensitivity. Radiology 1992; 183:53-58.

149.   Petersein J, Saini S, Weissleder R. Liver II: Iron oxide-based reticuloendothelial contrast agents for MR imaging: Clinical review. MRI Clin NA 1996; 4:53-60.

150.   Heiken JP, Weyman PJ, Lee JKT, Balfe DM, Picus D, Brunt EM, Flye MW. Detection of focal hepatic masses: Prospective evaluation with CT, delayed CT, CT during arterial portography, and MR imaging. Radiology 1989; 171:47-51.

151.   Akeson P, Larsson EM, Kristoffersen DT, Jonsson E, Holtas S. Brain metastases - Comparison of gadodiamide injection-enhanced MR imaging at standard and high dose, contrast-enhanced CT and non-contrast-enhanced MR imaging. Acta Radiol 1995; 36:300-306.

152.   Kuhn MJ, Hammer GM, Swenson LC, Youssef HT, Gleason TJ.   MRI evaluation of "solitary" brain metastases with triple-dose gadoteridol: Comparison with contrast-enhanced CT and conventional-dose gadopentetate dimeglumine MRI studies in the same patients.   Comp Med Imag Graph 1994; 18:391-399.

153.   Davis PC, Hudgins PA, Peterman SB, Hoffman JC. Diagnosis of cerebral metastases: Double-dose delayed CT vs contrast-enhanced MR imaging. AJNR 1991; 12:293-300.

10 SURGICAL MANAGEMENT OF THYROID CANCER

Gary R. Peplinski, MD
University of California at San Francisco
San Francisco, California

Samuel A. Wells, Jr., MD
American College of Surgeons
Chicago, Illinois

Introduction

Operations on the thyroid gland have been performed since 952 A.D.[1] Early procedures were complicated by uncontrollable hemorrhage from the vascular thyroid gland often resulting in the death of the patient. Theodor Kocher, a Swiss surgeon and pioneer in thyroid surgery, performed his first thyroidectomy in 1872. By the end of his career, he had performed over 5,000 thyroidectomies with a progressive decrease in operative mortality from 13 percent to 1 percent.[2] Kocher contributed substantially to the field of thyroid surgery. He emphasized meticulous control of bleeding and the importance of identification and preservation of the parathyroid glands. He also recognized the complications of postoperative hypothyroidism.

Since Kocher's time, our knowledge of thyroid physiology and pathophysiology has increased markedly, and the medical and surgical therapies available for patients with thyroid disorders are much more sophisticated. Currently, the operative mortality for thyroidectomy approaches zero and the feared postoperative complications, damage to the recurrent laryngeal nerve and hypoparathyroidism, are infrequent but directly associated with the extent of resection, the size and local infiltration of the thyroid disease, and the skill of the thyroid surgeon. This chapter concerns the surgical management of patients with thyroid carcinoma.

Evaluation of the patient with a thyroid nodule

Well-differentiated thyroid carcinoma typically presents as a thyroid nodule or mass. Clinically evident thyroid nodules are common (the incidence in the adult population in the United States of America [U.S.A.] is approximately 4 percent), however, thyroid carcinoma is relatively uncommon (30-60 per million population per year)[3.] It is important to differentiate benign from malignant tumors since the treatment for the two diseases is different.

A thorough clinical history and physical examination provide essential information in the decision-making process. The clinical findings frequently associated with a thryoid malignancy are listed in Table 1. Laboratory and radiological tests must be interpreted in light of clinical suspicion.

Table 1: Clinical signs and symptoms suggestive of thyroid malignancy

HISTORY	PHYSICAL EXAM	
Previous neck irradiation	1)	Solitary nodule
New neck mass	2)	Firm mass
Enlarging neck mass	3)	Fixation of mass to local neck structure
Hoarseness	4)	Enlarged cervical nodes
Male gender	5)	Hoarse voice
Extremes of age		
Family history of medullary thyroid cancer		

History

It is most important to determine if the patient with a thyroid nodule has a history of prior head and neck irradiation, specifically exposure to external beam radiation therapy during childhood. The risk of thyroid carcinoma in this setting approaches 30 percent. Some surgeons feel that such a history in a patient with a thyroid nodule is indication for a total thyroidectomy. This is because one assumes that all of the thyroid gland was irradiated. Also, in this setting half of the patients having total thyroidectomy are found to have carcinoma in a portion of the thyroid gland separate from the thyroid nodule.

Thyroid carcinoma may also present in a familial setting, in which case it is almost always associated with medullary thyroid carcinoma (MTC). Multiple Endocrine Neoplasia (MEN) type 2A, MEN 2B, and Familial Medullary Thyroid Carcinoma (FMTC) are characterized by the inheritance of MTC in a an autosomal dominant pattern. Patients with MEN 2A and MEN 2B also have pheochromocytomas. Additionally, patients with MEN 2A have parathyroid hyperplasia, whereas patients with MEN2B have mucosal neuromas, ganglioneuromatosis and a characteristic phenotype. Patients with FMTC have MTC without the extrathyroidal manifestations of either MEN 2A or MEN 2B. Approximately 30 percent of patients with MTC have one of these three cancer family syndromes.[7,8] These are discussed also in Chapter 4. In patients with MEN 2A or MEN 2B, it is essential to exclude the presence of a pheochromocytoma before performing a thyroidectomy for MTC. Differentiated thyroid carcinoma of follicular cell origin has also been associated with familial adenomatous polyposis and Gardner's syndrome.[9,10]

The MTC cells secrete the polypeptide hormone calcitonin (CT) which serves as an excellent tumor marker for MTC especially following the intravenous administration of the provocative agents, calcium and pentagastrin. Currently, measurement of plasma CT levels is most useful in evaluating patients following thyroidectomy, as elevated plasma levels indicate the presence of persistent or recurrent disease.

The most sensitive test for familial MTC presenting as MEN 2A, MEN 2B or FMTC is direct DNA testing for characteristic mutations in the RET protooncogene.[11,12] Prophylactic thyroidectomy is indicated in family members shown to have a characteristic RET mutation. Thyroidectomy appears to be curative.[13,14]

Physical Examination

Approximately 15 percent of solitary thyroid nodules are malignant. The majority of patients with a palpable nodule actually have multiple nodules when examined by ultrasound, thyroidectomy, or autopsy.[15] It is important to exclude the non-thyroid lesions, including thyroglossal duct cysts, branchial cleft cysts, and enlarged lymph nodes, which may mimic thyroid nodules since their surgical management is different.

A patient who presents with hoarseness, a painful thyroid nodule fixed to the trachea, or surrounding soft tissue structures, and enlarged cervical lymph nodes very likely has a malignant lesion. Fifteen percent of adults and 85 percent of children with thyroid carcinoma have clinically palpable cervical lymph nodes.[16] It is important to perform an evaluation of the upper airway to evaluate the vocal cords and the integrity of the airway. When the airway is markedly narrowed due to chronic extrinsic pressure the patient may need to remain intubated for a variable period of time after thyroidectomy. Operatively, total thyroidectomy and en bloc removal of surrounding soft tissues and lymph nodes may be necessary to effect a cure.

Radiographic imaging studies of the neck are rarely indicated unless the thyroid nodule is large or there is a question of metastatic disease in the pulmonary parenchyma or bones.

Ancillary Studies

Sampling of the thyroid tissue is the single most important diagnostic test in patients with a thyroid nodule and a major therapeutic determinant.[17]   The diagnostic test of choice for a potentially malignant thyroid nodule is fine needle aspiration biopsy (FNAB).[19,20,21] This technique is an accurate, safe, and cost effective method for screening patients at risk for thyroid carcinoma.[22] Experience with this technique improves diagnostic results. The aspirated specimen is obtained by making several passes through the center of the mass using a 23-gauge needle. The aspirated cells are immediately applied to microscope slides and fixed. Appropriate specimen handling is important for accurate interpretation by cytopathologists (see Chapter 8).

Fine needle biopsy of solid thyroid nodules is accurate in 70-97 percent of cases.[23,24,25] Typically, 5 percent of specimens are positive for thyroid carcinoma, and thyroidectomy is indicated in almost all of these patients, excepting those who have lymphoma or a giant cell anaplastic carcinoma. Approximately 70 percent of samples show no evidence of cancer. However, the false-negative rate of FNAB is 5 percent. Therefore, clinically suspicious thyroid lesions must be followed closely, despite negative FNAB results. Repeat FNAB and thyroidectomy are indicated if the nodule grows in size or other symptoms of malignancy become evident. Even if repeat FNAB is negative, lesions with high clinical suspicion for malignancy should be resected.

In 17 percent of patients, the sample is inadequate or nondiagnostic and repeat FNAB is indicated since it may yield a diagnostic result in half of the patients. In approximately 10 percent of cases where the aspiration biopsy has been inadequate or inconclusive a malignancy is found at subsequent thyroidectomy.[26,27] Biopsy of nodules smaller than 1 cm in size is difficult and ultrasound guided biopsy may improve the accuracy of sampling.

The appropriate management of patients with suspicious or indeterminate FNAB results is more challenging.[28] Most suspicious readings show follicular cells, and the diagnosis of carcinoma cannot be established by cytoanalysis alone because histologic examination of the entire nodule is necessary to assess for vascular or capsular invasion.[29] There have been comparative evaluations of fine needle aspiration biopsy (FNAB) and core needle biopsy of thyroid nodules. Not only has FNAB had a greater sensitivity and specificity but it is associated with fewer complications than core needle biopsy.

Fine needle aspiration biopsy has increased the yield of cancer found in thyroidectomy specimens resected for suspected malignancy (from about 14 percent to 29 percent), and decreased the number of unnecessary thyroidectomies (from 67 percent to 43 percent).[18] Furthermore, a preoperative diagnosis of cancer aids in counseling the patient and in the planning of a definitive surgical procedure.

When the FNAB is suspicious for malignancy it is most often because of the presence of follicular cells. In this setting, a thyroid lobectomy is indicated and a diagnosis of cancer may not be made at frozen section examination. Study of permanent sections is necessary to determine whether the nodule is benign or malignant.

Adjunctive tests

Measurement of serum thyroid hormone levels, and studies such as radionucleid scanning or radiographic imaging studies, ultrasonography, or computed tomography (CT), are rarely necessary in the preoperative evaluation of a thyroid nodule.

Serum thyroglobulin levels do not differentiate benign from malignant lesions preoperatively.[30] However, they are useful in monitoring patients for recurrence after total thyroidectomy for papillary, follicular, or Hurthle cell carcinoma. Plasma calcitonin (CT) levels will be elevated in patients presenting with MTC and a thyroid mass. In patients with early stage C-cell hyperplasia the basel plasma CT levels may be normal but are elevated following intravenous stimulation with pentagastrin and calcium.

Thyroid radionucleide scanning cannot conclusively discriminate between benign and malignant lesions and, therefore, is no longer a routine test for evaluating a thyroid nodule.[31,21] Thyroid ultrasound examination may be indicated when the presence of a nodule is uncertain on physical examination, when multiple thyroid nodules are present, to differentiate solid and cystic lesions, or to temporally follow the size of a nodule. The majority of cystic thyroid nodules have solid elements identified on ultrasound examination and they have a similar risk of malignancy as do purely solid thyroid lesions.[26,33,34] Ultrasound guided biopsy enhances accurate sampling of a thyroid nodule and may be useful in nodules that are difficult to palpate or are residing in a multinodular gland.

Both neck CT scanning and magnetic resonance imaging (MRI) are equivalent in showing anatomic details. Magnetic resonance imaging may differentiate postoperative fibrosis from recurrent or persistent tumor.[35]

Pathology

Papillary thyroid carcinoma (PTC) constitutes 80 percent of primary thyroid carcinomas. Although some are caused by radiation exposure, the majority are not clearly linked to a specific etiology. Most present as a solitary thyroid nodule. Occult thyroid carcinoma may be found in 9-19 percent of thyroidectomy specimens, and almost all are PTCs smaller than 1 cm in diameter.[36,37] On gross inspection, PTC usually is white in color with a firm consistency and a granular cut surface with calcifications. Microscopically, "Orphan Annie-eyed" nuclei are identified in PTC cells, consisting of large size nuclei with a pale-staining, "ground glass" appearance and deep nuclear grooves. The presence of psammoma bodies are highly suggestive of PTC. A follicular variant comprises 8-13 percent of PTC and approximately 25 percent are indistinguishable from follicular neoplasms on cytology.[38] Papillary thyroid carcinoma is multicentric in up to 45 percent of cases. Extrathyroidal invasion occurs in up to 35 percent of patients and is associated with lymph node metastasises, local recurrence, and distant metastasises.

Follicular thyroid carcinoma (FTC) generally effects older patients (greater than 50 years of age). Follicular thyroid carcinoma is more common in areas of endemic goiter. Malignant follicular neoplasms are frequently indistinguishable from benign follicular adenomas on cytology. Clinically evident lymphadenopathy is rare because FTC metastasizes through the bloodstream.

Giant cell anaplastic thyroid carcinoma typically presents in older individuals as a rapidly enlarging neck mass associated with symptoms of dysphagia and hoarseness. Anaplastic thyroid carcinoma is the most aggressive type of thyroid malignancy because it invades locally and metastasizes to distant sites. Cells do not typically concentrate radioiodine. Microscopic examination shows giant cells with intranuclear cytoplasmic invaginations. The frequent presence of residual elements of more differentiated thyroid carcinomas has led to the postulate that anaplastic thyroid carcinoma may evolve from them. Anaplastic carcinomas are best treated with external beam radiation and chemotherapy.

Thyroidectomy

Thyroidectomy is indicated when a patient's thyroid nodule is found to be malignant either by a cytological or histological technique, or when there is strong clinical suspicion of malignancy. With the exception of lymphoma and giant cell anaplastic carcinoma, all solid thyroid cancers are amenable to surgical resection for potential cure. Preoperative patient counseling is essential to describe the nature of the operative procedure, the potential risks, and the possible alternative treatments. Definitive resection should be completed in one operation, if possible. The patient needs to understand the intraoperative management plan including what operative and pathologic findings will influence the extent of thyroidectomy and lymphadenectomy.

Neck exploration

An anterior neck exploration is carried out with the patient under a general anesthetic. The patient is positioned in reverse Trendelenberg with the hips and knees flexed and the neck extended ("lawnchair" position). This position provides adequate access to the neck area and decreases venous distension. A curvilinear incision is made in a skin crease approximately two fingerbreadths above the sternal notch centered about the midline between the sternocleidomastoid muscles (Figure 1). Superior and inferior skin flaps are created in a plane just below the platysma muscle. With adequate retraction the strap muscle fascia is divided vertically in the midline. The muscles are then separated from the surfaces of each thyroid lobe laterally using blunt dissection and cautery. In large masses it may be necessary to divide the strap muscles superiorly. If the strap muscles are tightly adherent to the thyroid mass and there is suspicion of malignancy it may be necessary to resect a portion of the strap muscles.

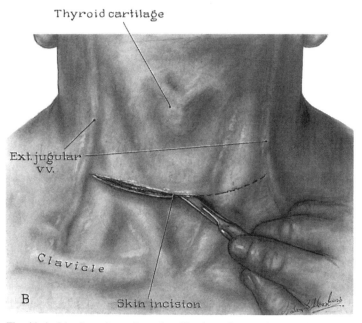

Figure 1. The skin incision is made two finger breadths above the sternal notch. If possible, the incision is placed in a skin crease. (From Wells SA, Jr.: Total thyroidectomy, lymph node dissection for cancer. In: Nyhus LM, Baker RG, Fischer JE, eds. Mastery of Surgery. 3rd ed. Little, Brown and Company, Boston, 1997, p. 498-99; with permission)

A thorough knowledge of normal neck anatomy and the relationship of the thyroid gland to neighboring structures is essential (Figure 2). The normal adult thyroid gland weighs 15 to 20 gm and is composed of two lobes overlying the lower half of the thyroid cartilage laterally and connected by an isthmus which crosses anterior to the trachea below the cricoid cartilage. A pyramidal lobe arises from the isthmus and travels superiorly in 75 percent of patients. The thyroid gland is densely adherent to the trachea and larynx. Posteriorly and laterally, the thyroid lobes overlie, or are adjacent to, the carotid sheath, containing the carotid artery, internal jugular vein, and vagus nerve. Located posteriorly and medially, are the esophagus, recurrent laryngeal nerve, and parathyroid glands. The thyroid gland has a rich blood supply from the superior thyroid artery branching from the external carotid artery and the inferior thyroid artery originating at the subclavian thyrocervical trunk. Additionally there are direct branches from the aorta through the small thyroid ima vessel. Inappropriate vascular control could result in significant blood loss. Venous drainage occurs mainly by way of the superior, middle, and inferior thyroid veins into the jugular and brachiocephalic veins.

At the beginning of the operation the entire thyroid is inspected and palpated. The gross appearance and texture of the gland may suggest the diagnosis of certain thyroid conditions. Important considerations are the location, size, and possible involvement of other neck structures such as the strap muscles, trachea, recurrent laryngeal nerves, or vessels.

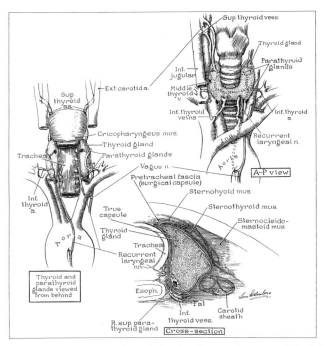

Figure 2. Anterior and posterior views of the neck showing the normal anatomy of the right and left recurrent laryngeal nerves. The location of the superior and inferior parathyroid glands are shown. The cross-sectional view of the left thyroid lobe shows its relation to the carotid sheath, recurrent laryngeal nerve, superior parathyroid gland, esophagus and trachea. (From Wells SA, Jr.: Total thyroidectomy, lymph node dissection for cancer. In: Nyhus LM, Baker RG, Fischer JE, eds. Mastery of Surgery. 3rd ed. Little, Brown and Company, Boston, 1997, p. 498-99; with permission)

Thyroid resection

The ultimate goal of thyroidectomy is to completely resect the cancer with clear margins while preserving vital structures in the neck. The portion of the thyroid harboring the malignancy, as well as locally invaded tissue, is removed *en bloc* with the cancerous mass.

Initially, the thyroid lobe harboring the neoplasm is mobilized using blunt dissection while the strap muscles are retracted laterally. With mobilization, the thyroid lobe is retracted contralaterally and upward into the incision (Figure 3). This is an important maneuver to adequately expose the more posterior thyroid gland, where the superior parathyroid glands and the recurrent laryngeal nerve are found. Great care must be taken to preserve these structures during the course of the procedure.

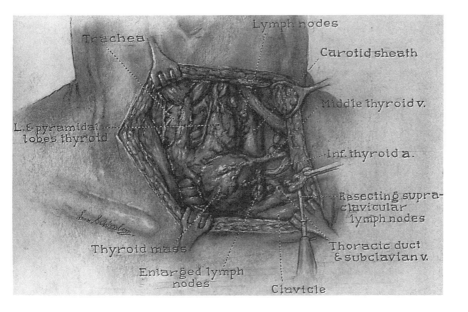

Figure 3. A mass in the inferior portion of the left thyroid pole is shown. Large lymph nodes are evident adjacent to the thyroid mass and in the lateral neck. (From Wells SA, Jr.: Total thyroidectomy, lymph node dissection for cancer. In: Nyhus LM, Baker RG, Fischer JE, eds. Mastery of Surgery. 3rd ed. Little, Brown and Company, Boston, 1997, p. 498-99; with permission)

The more superficially located middle thyroid vein and inferior thyroid artery are found entering the gland laterally at its midportion and are ligated and divided. As structures are divided, the gland is retracted medially, up off the trachea. The "ligament of Berry," near the recurrent laryngeal nerve, especially where it enters the larynx, is carefully divided and the nerve is unroofed (Figure 4). The inferior pole vessels are divided and ligated and the superior thyroid artery and vein are divided close to the gland. It is necessary to place a clamp above the superior thyroid pole, and great care must be taken not to damage the external branch of the superior laryngeal nerve. The thyroid gland is removed from the surface of the trachea using cautery from the lateral to the medial direction, while keeping the recurrent laryngeal nerve and parathyroid glands in view. It is important not to violate the tracheal wall during this part of the dissection.

The thyroid isthmus is removed en bloc with the involved lobe if resection is performed for cancer. In a total thyroidectomy, dissection proceeds to the contralateral thyroid lobe, so that all thyroid tissue is removed as completely as possible. In near total thyroidectomy a small amount of thyroid tissue and capsule (less than 5 gm) is left at the posteromedial aspect of the thyroid gland, where the recurrent laryngeal nerve enters the larynx and the superior parathyroid glands lie in close proximity to the thyroid. The surface of the thyroid specimen is inked by the pathologist and then opened to confirm that the mass in question has been resected in its entirety and that the margins are negative, grossly and microscopically.

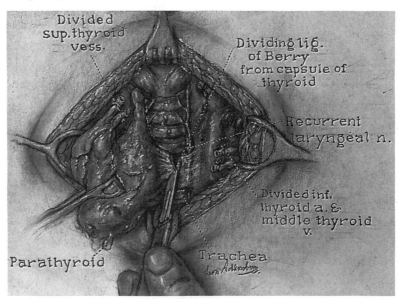

Figure 4. Division of the "ligament of Berry." (For the purposes of illustration this structure is shown thicker than normal.) Notice the position of the recurrent laryngeal nerve. The inferior parathyroid gland will be removed and placed in iced saline for autotransplantation. (From Wells SA, Jr.: Total thyroidectomy, lymph node dissection for cancer. In: Nyhus LM, Baker RG, Fischer JE, eds. Mastery of Surgery. 3rd ed. Little, Brown and Company, Boston, 1997, p. 498-99; with permission)

The neck wound is irrigated and meticulous hemostasis is achieved to avoid postoperative hematoma formation. The uninterrupted course of the recurrent laryngeal nerve is confirmed, and the parathyroid glands are reevaluated. The wound is closed in three layers, approximating the midline strap muscles, the platysma muscle, and then the skin edges. A drain may be placed if the dissection was extensive or if there is concern about ongoing diffuse oozing of blood or lymph.

The recurrent laryngeal nerve

It is very important that the recurrent laryngeal nerve is properly identified. This is accomplished by mobilizing the lateral thyroid lobe medially to provide adequate exposure of the tracheoesophageal groove. The nerve typically courses from lateral to medial deep to the inferior thyroid artery and then travels near the tracheoesophageal groove to enter the larynx in close proximity to the superior thyroid artery (Figure 3). The nerve is commonly identified initially by bluntly dissecting in tissues deep to the inferior thyroid artery. It is important to visualize and follow the entire course of the nerve into the larynx using careful blunt dissection before major structures are divided. Failure to correctly identify the recurrent laryngeal nerve may result in its injury, and lead to one of the most serious complications of thyroidectomy. The nerve may be injured permanently or temporarily by transection, cautery burn, traction, or crush from forceps or clamps.

An important anatomic variant common on the right side than the left is the so called nonrecurrent or direct laryngeal nerve.[39] In this situation the nerve does not travel beneath the right subclavian artery but springs at a right angle from the vagus nerve. The direct laryngeal nerve is most often mistaken for the superior thyroid artery or the middle thyroid vein. If one has difficulty in finding the right recurrent laryngeal nerve, then the direct variant must be considered.

The external branch of the superior laryngeal nerve, which innervates the cricothyroid muscle, courses immediately adjacent to the superior thyroid vessels. Injury to this nerve, which may occur while dividing and ligating the superior thyroid vessels, typically causes decreased voice endurance and loss of high pitch phonation.

Parathyroid gland preservation

Identification of the parathyroid glands and preservation of their fragile blood supply requires knowledge of their normal locations, and an experienced eye. A normal parathyroid gland is about 5 mm in size, with a tan color and a trabeculated surface vascular pattern. Differentiation among parathyroid glands, lymph nodes and fat lobules may be difficult.

The inferior parathyroid glands are most often associated with the thyrothymic ligament, a tongue of tissue, arising from the retrosternal body of the thymus, that attaches to the inferior pole of each thyroid lobe (Figure 5). The inferior glands lie in a somewhat superficial location relative to the tracheoesophageal groove, close to the crossing of the inferior thyroid artery and recurrent laryngeal nerve. The superior parathyroid glands lie near the tracheoesophageal groove at the posteriomedial aspect of the thyroid lobe. The superior glands are often associated with a pad of fatty tissue at the site where the recurrent laryngeal nerve penetrates the larynx. The entire thyroid lobe must be mobilized and retracted upward and medially to gain adequate exposure to identify the superior parathyroid glands.

Each parathyroid gland receives its blood supply from a small vascular pedicle. The parathyroid glands are fragile and should not be directly grasped or handled. Gentle blunt dissection is used to separate the parathyroid glands from the thyroid. Parathyroid autotransplantation during thyroidectomy virtually eliminates permanent postoperative hypoparathyroidism.[40] Parathyroid tissue is minced and reimplanted into sternocleidomastoid muscle pockets (or forearm muscle for patients with MEN 2A) at the conclusion of the procedure.[41] Oral calcium and vitamin D supplementation may be required to treat transient postoperative hypoperathyroidism.

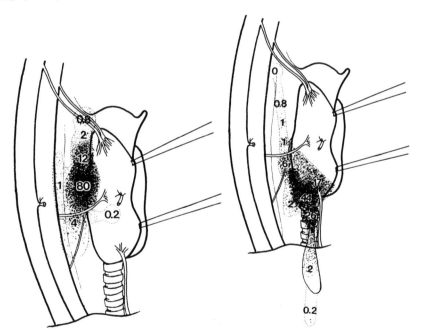

Figure 5. The superior parathyroid glands are located posterior to the thyroid lobe and usually near a fat pad where the recurrent laryngeal nerve enters the larynx. The inferior parathyroid glands are typically situated more superficially in association with the "thyrothymic ligament." The exact location of the parathyroid glands are highly variable. (From Akerström G, Malmaers J, and Bergstrom R: Surgical anatomy of human parathyroid glands. Surgery, 95:17, 1984; with permission)

The parathyroid glands may be situated at ectopic sites ranging from the pharynx to the deep mediastinum. Identification and preservation of at least one parathyroid gland is necessary to prevent postoperative hypoparathyroidism. A time consuming search to find ectopic glands is not necessary during thyroidectomy if at least one parathyroid gland has been definitively identified and preserved. If one is unsure that a tissue in question is parathyroid, a tiny piece need be sent for frozen section examination to confirm the histology of the tissue.

Intraoperative frozen section pathologic analysis

Frozen section pathologic examination is indicated when there has been no preoperative histologic diagnosis of the thyroid nodule, an unsuspected thyroid nodule is found during neck surgery for a non-thyroid condition, or enlarged lymph nodes are found in the operative field.[42]

Routine frozen section examination of a thyroid nodule is not necessary when a preoperative diagnosis is established by adequate FNAB. One prospective study showed that frozen section analysis effected intraoperative decision making in only 2 percent of cases and its routine use was not cost effective.[43]

Suspicious FNAB results are found in follicular neoplasms. Because frozen section evaluation is difficult with follicular lesions, pathologists often defer to permanent section analysis to definitively identify vascular or capsular invasion, the sine qua non to establish the diagnosis of FTC. Therefore, frozen section is rarely useful in this circumstance.

Extent of thyroidectomy

There is substantial controversy about the extent of thyroidectomy for the treatment of well-differentiated thyroid carcinoma. The annual mortality rate from thyroid cancer in the U.S.A. is 6 per million and, regardless of treatment, the majority of patients have a good prognosis.[3] However, some thyroid carcinomas are unpredictably aggressive, invading local structures, metastasizing to distant sites, and causing the death of the patient.[44] Recurrent thyroid carcinomas may be associated with high morbidity and are difficult to manage. Unfortunately, there has never been a prospective, randomized, controlled trial comparing various operative procedures in patients with thyroid carcinoma.

There is general agreement that FTC and MTC require total thyroidectomy for appropriate treatment. Some surgeons recommend lesser procedures for low-risk PTC. Small (less than 1.5 cm), unilateral, PTCs in low-risk patients may be adequately treated only with thyroid lobectomy.[45] Proponents argue that the incidence of recurrent laryngeal nerve injury and postoperative hypoparathyroidism is lower with this approach and that local recurrence rates and survival rates are similar to those observed after total thyroidectomy.[46,47]

For several reasons, we recommend total thyroidectomy whenever a tissue diagnosis of thyroid cancer has been established. Approximately 15 percent of patients with "well-differentiated" thyroid carcinoma do poorly. Lower recurrence rates, including central neck recurrence, have been associated with total thyroidectomy as compared to lesser procedures,[48,49,50] Of patients who develop recurrent thyroid carcinoma in the central neck, 50 percent die from their cancer.[48,51] Papillary thyroid cancer, in particular, is known to be multicentric and may occur in both lobes.[52] Recurrent thyroid carcinoma develops in the contralateral lobe in only five to ten percent of patients who initially undergo unilateral thyroid lobectomy. In addition, uptake of radioactive iodine in remnant thyroid tissue may obscure detection of neck metastases or recurrent tumor. Radioactive iodine treatment of thyroid cancer is more effective in the absence of normal thyroid tissue. In patients who have had complete ablation of all thyroid tissue plasma thyroglobulin levels may be serially measured to screen for recurrent carcinoma.[53] Finally, with experienced surgeons, total thyroidectomy may be accomplished safely with a less than 3 percent complication rate in cases of differentiated cancers contained within the thyroid gland.

When a preoperative histologic or cytologic diagnosis of cancer has not been definitively established the initial surgical procedure is a diagnostic thyroid lobectomy. Immediate frozen section pathologic analysis is performed and if the diagnosis is consistent with benign thyroid disease (approximately 70 percent of cases), no further thyroid resection is indicated. If the mass is a follicular lesion, the pathologist may defer to permanent section analysis to make a definitive diagnosis. In this situation, the surgeon may either complete the total thyroidectomy, if he or she is suspicious that cancer is present, or conclude the procedure and wait for a final pathologic diagnosis. If on subsequent permanent section the histologic diagnosis is follicular carcinoma the patient should undergo completion thyroidectomy as soon as possible. Residual cancer is uncommonly found in the contralateral lobe after unilateral lobectomy for FTC.[54]

Medullary thyroid cancer should be treated with total thyroidectomy. Sporadic MTCs have a low rate of bilaterality. Approximately 40 percent of MTCs are familial, and these tumors are virtually always bilateral and multicentric. When thyroid tissue is left behind, and postoperative plasma CT levels are elevated, it is unknown whether the residual MTC is in the neck or in distant sites.[55]

Lymphadenectomy

Careful inspection and palpation of the exposed neck is performed to evaluate lymph nodes. Involvement with malignancy is suggested by increased size, firmness, or color change to a pale gray. Nodal metastasises occur most frequently in the central compartment, defined as the space between the carotid sheaths, and from the hyoid bone to the sternal notch. This area includes the delphian node, overlying the cricoid cartilage, the nodes in the tracheoesophageal groove, and the nodes in fibrofatty tissue adjacent to the thyroid gland. The second most frequent sites of nodal metastasises are the ipsilateral nodes along the internal jugular chain and the nodes in the supraclavicular fossa. These lymph nodes can be removed as a segment of tissue, while sparing the sternocleidomastoid muscle, internal jugular vein, and spinal accessory nerve (modified neck dissection). This may require extension of the neck incision to the mastoid process for improved exposure. Thyroid carcinoma may also spread to lymph nodes located in the superior mediastinum overlying the thymus and great vessels.

Papillary thyroid carcinoma and MTC first metastasize to regional lymph nodes. Approximately 15 percent of adults with PTC have involved cervical lymph nodes at the time of diagnosis. Modified neck dissection for PTC and MTC is indicated when there is evidence of lymph node involvement and when the primary tumor is greater than 2 cm in diameter and occult lymph node metastases are likely to be present. Central lymph nodes in close proximity to the thyroid gland should be routinely removed with the thyroid specimen. Medullary thyroid carcinoma may remain confined to the cervical lymph nodes for prolonged periods. For MTC, 30 percent of patients with nodal metastases can be cured by extensive lymph node dissection.[56] In contrast, FTC rarely metastasizes to regional lymph nodes, and so modified neck dissection is unnecessary unless enlarged nodes are present. Radioactive iodine is generally not effective in treating node metastases.[57] Radical neck dissection for a thyroid carcinoma is virtually never indicated.

Local invasion of thyroid cancer

Thyroid cancer may involve neck structures in proximity by direct invasion. Preoperative physical examination is important to identify potential spread to neck structures (e.g. hoarse voice, mass fixation to trachea). Many neck structures may be sacrificed and included as part of the *en bloc* resection of the cancer to achieve the optimal surgical goal of complete cancer removal with negative margins. These structures include the recurrent laryngeal nerve unilaterally, the parathyroid glands, small arteries and veins, lymph nodes, and the strap muscles. Because differentiated thyroid cancer is usually a relatively indolent process and other adjuvant therapies are available, resection of other involved neck structures may not be warranted due to inappropriately increased risks, and narrow margins of excision may be acceptable in some circumstances.[58] Resection of recurrent PTC may be required repeatedly over a period of years in order to control local disease.

Recurrent laryngeal nerve involvement. Hoarseness is notoriously associated with recurrent laryngeal nerve involvement by the cancer. This finding may warrant fiberoptic laryngoscopy intraoperatively just prior to endotracheal tube placement in order to document vocal cord function. A nonfunctioning vocal cord is an indication that the ipsilateral recurrent laryngeal nerve is directly involved with cancer, and recovery of function is unlikely. If the nerve is found to be encased in a mass of tumor and the vocal cord is not functioning, the nerve may be resected with the specimen, especially if negative margins have been obtained elsewhere.

With a nonfunctioning vocal cord on one side, extremely meticulous dissection around the contralateral recurrent laryngeal nerve is paramount to preserve its function. If the vocal cord is functioning, the nerve should be preserved by peeling it off the adherent cancer mass. In such cases, postoperative vocal cord function is preserved, and the incidence of local recurrence and overall prognosis does not appear to be effected.[59] Repeat laryngoscopy is indicated during extubation in these circumstances. One must be prepared for immediate reintubation if necessary or, if unsuccessful, emergent tracheostomy.

Involvement of other regional nerves. The vagus and XII cranial nerves may also be sacrificed if involved with large cancerous masses; their function is usually already compromised preoperatively.   Unilateral vagus nerve resection is manifested postoperatively by a hoarseness due to interruption of the recurrent laryngeal nerve.   Twelfth cranial nerve resection results in weakness of the sternocleidomastoid and trapezius muscles. Resection of involved sympathetic ganglia or prevertebral fascia is indicated if the remaining tumor margins are negative. An ipsilateral Horner's syndrome results, which is usually well tolerated. Nerve trunks and cords in the brachial plexus should never be resected.

Tracheal and laryngeal involvement. Intraoperative endoscopy is an important adjunctive procedure to exclude involvement of the tracheal and laryngeal mucosa if the cancer mass appears to be fixed on examination. Mucosal involvement indicates that tracheal or laryngeal resection is necessary to completely excise the cancer. Some surgeons recommend resecting involved portions of the trachea or larynx with reconstruction.[60-62] Others only recommend "shaving" the cancer off the trachea or larynx and leaving tumor behind.

Involvement of major neck vessel. The internal jugular vein can usually be separated from most cancers, although it may also be safely resected on one side with virtually no consequences. Superficial involvement of either the internal or common carotid artery may be managed by resecting the adventitia to obtain a negative margin. With deeper involvement, the internal and common carotid arteries are spared. Since the risks of cerebral ischemia and stroke associated with internal or common carotid resections and reconstructions are not warranted.

Esophageal involvement. The esophagus is uncommonly involved with thyroid cancer and every attempt is made to preserve its continuity during thyroidectomy.

Management of operative complications

Nerve injury

Perhaps the most devastating complication of thyroidectomy is permanent bilateral recurrent laryngeal nerve injury. This is manifested by stridor and poor air movement immediately after extubation. Management consists of immediate reestablishment of an adequate airway. The patient may be simply reintubated, but the surgeon should be ready to perform a tracheostomy if intubation fails. Laryngoscopy during extubation after a complicated procedure may show the functional status of the vocal cords and aid reintubation under direct vision if necessary.

Unilateral recurrent laryngeal nerve injury results in temporary or permanent paralysis of the ipsilateral vocal cord and hoarseness is usually noted immediately postoperatively. Loss of unilateral vocal cord function is generally well tolerated and phonation often returns to normal. The contralateral functioning vocal cord will move past the midline to vibrate against the motionless cord. If the recurrent laryngeal nerve is divided and recognized intraoperatively, then close approximation of the nerve ends may be attempted with fine monofilament suture to enhance regeneration. Aggressive dissection near the nerve, or nerve traction, may cause temporary neuropraxia which generally improves over time.

The immediate concern with unilateral nerve injuries and resultant vocal cord dysfunction is aspiration of saliva and ingested liquids. A speech therapy consultation may be appropriate in order to assess swallowing and aspiration risk. Modified barium swallow exam may show the presence and degree of aspiration with different consistency liquids and foods. Based on these results, ingested foods can then be altered to decrease the risk of aspiration. Injections of different materials directly into the nonfunctioning vocal cord may help appose the nonfunctioning vocal cord with the contralateral normal cord and protect the airway.

Hypoparathyroidism

Hypoparathyroidism usually becomes evident in the first few days following surgery. Common symptoms typically include numbness or tingling in the fingertips and periorally. Chvostek's sign or Tinel's sign may be elicited by examination and should be deliberately checked in all postoperative patients. Measurement of daily serum calcium levels is routine in the immediate postoperative period. A significant decrease in the serum calcium level below normal or the development of typical symptoms are diagnostic of hypoparathyroidism in this postoperative setting and are indications to begin oral calcium and vitamin D supplementation. Rarely, a rapid decrease in the calcium level to low levels accompanied by significant symptoms may warrant intravenous calcium gluconate therapy. Parathyroid function typically recovers if glands remain in place and revascularization ensues.

Other postoperative sequelae

A neck hematoma may occur over the first day postoperatively. Airway compromise is the immediate threat to life, followed by exsaguination from a major artery. Rapid expansion of a neck hematoma postoperatively is best managed by immediate reoperation to identify and control the site of bleeding. Placement of an endotracheal tube to control the airway should be done in the operating suite, if time permits, because bedside endotracheal intubation may induce more severe hemorrhage. The surgeon must be prepared for emergent cricothyrotomy and tracheostomy if an endotracheal tube is unable to be placed.

Neck wound infection is extremely rare in immunocompetent patients given the rich blood supply to the cervical cutaneous tissue. Wounds typically heal with a good cosmetic result if a transverse curvilinear incision within a skin crease is used.

Postoperative management

Patients are typically observed in the hospital overnight after thyroidectomy and a serum calcium level is obtained the following morning after total thyroidectomy. A liquid diet is started the evening of surgery and, if tolerated well, is advanced to regular diet. Patients are discharged from the hospital when there is no evidence of significant neck hematoma, hypoparathyroidism, or aspiration due to vocal cord paralysis. A follow-up visit is scheduled for evaluation of the wound, symptoms of hypoparathyroidism, and phonation.

Patients with PTC are not started on thyroid hormone replacement therapy postoperatively in order to allow TSH levels to increase in anticipation of diagnostic or therapeutic radioactive iodine treatment. Persistent thyroid tissue detected by radioactive iodine scanning may require ablative ^{131}I administration.

Well-differentiated papillary and follicular thyroid cancers. Papillary thyroid carcinoma is a rare cause of death.[49] However, the detection and treatment of recurrences is important in preventing morbidity and mortality. The most common site of recurrence for PTC is in cervical lymph nodes. Cancer recurrence in a node should be resected with consideration of a more extensive ipsilateral lymph node dissection. Radioactive iodine scanning should be performed after resection of recurrent tumor.

The postoperative management of patients with well-differentiated thyroid carcinoma is controversial. Clinical and pathological features may provide an estimate of risk of recurrent disease and mortality and guide therapy. Female patients less than 45 years of age with low grade, intrathyroidal primary tumors less than 1.5 cm in size without metastases and complete gross tumor resection at the initial surgery have an excellent prognosis. For these patients, thyroid hormone replacement to suppress the TSH level to less than 0.1 IU/ml is sufficient therapy after thyroidectomy. Approximately 70 percent of patients with well-differentiated thyroid cancer fall into a low risk group with survival rates of 95 percent as compared to 45 percent in high-risk patients.[63,64]

Poor prognostic features such as age greater than 45 years, male sex, large primary tumor size, high tumor grade, tumor invasion into the thyroid capsule or beyond, and distant metastases are indications for more aggressive treatment. At our institution, thyroid hormone replacement is withheld from these patients postoperatively to allow the TSH level to increase. A total body scan is then performed with ^{131}I. Therapeutic doses of ^{131}I are administered if scan results are positive, and patients are subsequently rescanned. Follow-up consists of frequent physical examinations and measurement of serum thyroglobulin levels to detect recurrent tumor once all normal thyroid tissue is ablated. A rising thyroglobulin level is an indication for radioactive iodine scanning. An elevated thyroglobulin level with a negative scan suggests that the tumor no longer traps iodine. External beam radiation or chemotherapy may be considered in these patients. If tumor growth is indolent and if metastatic tumor is present in only a few sites and is resectable, then surgical resection of the recurrent tumor may be indicated. Patients with intermediate prognosis factors (e.g. tumor size between 1.5 and 4.5 cm, with or without nodal metastasises) are generally treated aggressively at our institution, although this is very controversial.

Anaplastic, poorly differentiated giant and spindle cell thyroid carcinoma. These cancers are rarely cured, and life expectancy averages less than 6 months. Surgery is the only potentially curative option. However, therapy is essentially palliative. Response rates are low even after complete removal of the cancer followed by radioactive iodine, external beam radiation, and multidrug chemotherapy. Given the poor prognosis, resection of recurrent tumor is not indicated in these patients.

Medullary thyroid cancer. The most sensitive method to detect recurrent MTC is the pentagastrin-calcium stimulation test. Increased serum CT levels after stimulation correlate well with volume of persistent or recurrent disease. Physical examination and CT or MRI are used to image and localize recurrent tumor. Response to radioactive iodine and chemotherapy is poor; surgical resection of recurrent disease is indicated, if feasible.[65]

References

1. Halsted WS. The operative story of goiter. Johns Hopkins Hospital Report 1920; 19:71.
2. Becker WP. Pioneers in thyroid surgery. Ann Surg 1977; 185:493-504.
3. Cancer Statistics. CA Cancer J Clin 1998.
4. Samaan NA, Schultz PN, Ordonez NG, et. al. A comparison of thyroid carcinoma in those who have and have not had head and neck irradiation in childhood. J Clin Endocrinol Metab 1987; 64:219-223.
5. Braverstock K, Egloff B, Pinchera A, et. al. Thyroid cancer after Chernobyl. Nature 1992; 359:21-22.
6. Witt TR, Meng RL, Economou SG, et. al. The approach to the irradiated thyroid. Surg Clin North Am 1979;.59:45.
7. Steiner AL, Goodman AD, Powers SR. Study of a kindred with pheochromocytoma, medullary thyroid carcinoma, hyperparathyroidism and Cushing's disease: Multiple endocrine neoplasia, type 2. Medicine 1968; 47:371-409.
8. Farndon JR, Leight GS, Dilley WG, et. al. Familial medullary thyroid carcinoma without associated endocrinopathies: A distinct clinical entity. Br J Surg 1986; 73:278-281.

9.   Plail RO, Bussey HJ, Glazer F, Thomson JP. Adenomatous polyposis: An association with carcinoma of the thyroid. Br J Surg 1987; 74:377-380.

10.   Camiel MR, Mule JE, Alexander LL, Beninghoff DL. Association of thyroid carcinoma with Gardner's syndrome in siblings. N Engl J Med 1968; 278:1056-1058.

11.   Chi DD, Toshima K, Donis-Keller H, Wells SA, Jr. Predictive testing for multiple endocrine neoplasia type 2A (MEN 2A) based on the detection of mutations in the RET protooncogene. Surgery 1994;.116:124-132.

12.   Goodfellow PJ, Wells SA, Jr. RET gene and its implications for cancer. J Natl Cancer Inst 1995;.87:1515-1523.

13.   Lairmore TC, Frisella MM, Wells SA, Jr. Genetic testing and early thyroidectomy for inherited medullary thyroid cancer. Ann Med 1996; 28:401-406.

14.   Wells SA, Jr, Chi DD, Toshima K, Dehner LP, Coffin CM, Dowton SB, Ivanovich JL, DeBenedetti MK, Dilley WG, Moley JF, et. al. Predictive DNA testing and prophylactic thyroidectomy in patients at risk for multiple endocrine neoplasia type 2A. Ann Surg 1994;.220:237-247.

15.   Brander A, Viikinkoski P, Tuuhea J, et. al. Clinical versus ultrasound examination of the thyroid gland in common clinical practice. J Clin Ultrasound 1992;.20:37-42.

16.   Staunton MD, Greening WP. Clinical diagnosis of thyroid cancer. Br Med J 1973;.4:532-535.

17.   Greenspan FS. The role of fine-needle aspiration biopsy in the management of palpable thyroid nodules. Am J Clin Pathol 1997;.108:S26-30.

18.   Hamberger B, Gharib H, Melton LS, et. al. Fine-needle aspiration biopsy of thyroid nodules: Impact on thyroid practice and cost of care. Am J Med 1982;.73:381-384.

19.   Grant CS, Hay ID, Gough IR, et. al. Long-term follow-up of patients with benign thyroid fine-needle aspiration cytologic diagnoses. Surgery 1989;.106:980-986.

20.   Hamburger JI. Consistency of sequential needle biopsy findings for thyroid nodules. Management implications. Arch Intern Med 1987;.147:97-99.

21.   Piromalli D, Martelli G, Del Prato I, et. al. The role of fine needle aspiration in the diagnosis of thyroid nodules: Analysis of 795 consecutive cases. J Surg Oncol 1992;.50:247-250.

22.   Bouvet M, Feldman JI, Gill GN, et. al. Surgical management of the thyroid nodule: Patient selection based on the results of fine-needle aspiration cytology. Laryngoscope 1992; 102:1353-1356.

23.   Liu Q, Castelli M, Gattuso P, Prinz RA. Simultaneous fine-needle aspiration and core-needle biopsy of thyroid nodules. Am Surgeon 1995; 61:628-632.

24.   Ballagh RH, Cramer H, Lampe HB. Accuracy of fine needle aspiration in the preoperative diagnosis of thyroid neoplasia. J Otolaryngol 1994; 23:360-365.

25.   Caruso D, Mazzaferri EL. Fine needle aspiration in the management of thyroid nodules. Endocrinologist 1991; 1:194-202.

26.   Mazzaferri EL. Management of a solitary thyroid nodule. N Engl J Med 1993; 328:553-559.

27.   McHenry CR, Walfish PG, Rosen IB. Non-diagnostic fine needle aspiration biopsy: A dilemma in management of nodular thyroid disease. Am Surg 1993; 59:415-419.

28.   Cersosimo E, Gharib H, Suman VJ, et. al. "Suspicious" thyroid cytologic findings: Outcome in patients without immediate surgical treatment. Mayo Clin Proc 1993; 68:343-348.

29.   Miller JM, Kini SR, Hamburger JI. The diagnosis of malignant follicular neoplasm of the thyroid by needle biopsy. Cancer 1985; 55:2812-2817.

30.   Christensen SB, Bondeson L, Ericsson UB, et. al. Prediction of malignancy in the solitary thyroid nodule by physical examination, thyroid scan, fine-needle biopsy, and serum thyroglobulin. Acta Chir Scand 1984; 150:433-439.

31.   Sabel MS, Staren ED, Gianakakis LM, Dwarakanathan S, Prinz RA: Effectiveness of the thyroid scan in evaluation of the solitary thyroid nodule. Am Surgeon 1997; 63:660-663.

32.   Ashcraft MW, Van Herle AJ. Management of thyroid nodules. II: Scanning techniques, thyroid suppressive therapy, and fine needle aspiration. Head Neck Surg 1981; 3:297-322.

33.   Solbiati L, Volterrani L, Rizzato G, et. al. The thyroid gland with low uptake lesions: Evaluation by ultrasound. Radiology 1985; 155:187-191.

34.   Watters DA, Ahuja AT, Evans RM, et. al. Role of ultrasound in the management of thyroid nodules. Am J Surg 1992; 164:654-657.

35.   Auffermann W, Clark OH, Thurnbar S, et. al. Recurrent thyroid carcinoma: Characteristics on MR images. Radiology 1988; 168:753-757.

36. Sambade MC, Goncalves VS, Dias M, et. al. High relative frequency of thyroid papillary carcinoma in Northern Portugal. Cancer 1983; 51:1754.
37. Yamashita H, Nakayama I, Noguchi S, et. al. Minute carcinoma of the thyroid and its development to advanced carcinoma. Acta Pathol Jpn 1985; 35:377.
38. Harach HR, Zusman SB. Cytologic findings in the follicular variant of papillary carcinoma of the thyroid. Acta Cytol 1992; 36:142.
39. Wijetilaka SE. Non-recurrent laryngeal nerve. Br J Surg 1978; 65:179.
40. Olson JA Jr, DeBenedetti MK, Baumann DS, Wells SA, Jr. Parathyroid autotransplantation during thyroidectomy. Results of long- term follow-up. Ann Surg 1996; 223:472-478.
41. Wells SA Jr, Gunnels JC, Shelburne JD, et. al. Transplantation of the parathyroid glands in man: Clinical indications and results. Surgery 1975; 78:34-44.
42. Hamburger JI, Hambyrger SW. Declining role of frozen section in surgical planning for thyroid nodules. Surgery 1985; 98:307-312.
43. McHenry CR, Raeburn C, Strickland T, Marty JJ. The utility of routine frozen section examination for intraoperative diagnosis of thyroid cancer. Am J Surg 1996; 172:658-661.
44. Beenken S, Guillamondegui O, Shallenberger R, et. al. Prognostic factors in patients dying of well-differentiated thyroid cancer. Arch Otolaryngol Head Neck Surg 1989; 115:326-330.
45. Shah JP, Loree TR, Dharker D, et. al. Lobectomy versus total thyroidectomy for differentiated carcinoma of the thyroid: A matched-pair analysis. Am J Surg 1993; 166:331-335.
46. Brooks JR, Starnes HF, Brooks DC, et. al. Surgical therapy for thyroid carcinoma. A review of 1249 solitary thyroid nodules. Surgery 1988; 104:940-946.
47. Grant CS, Hay ID, Gough IR, et. al. Local recurrence in papillary thyroid carcinoma: Is extent of surgical resection important? Surgery 1988; 104:954-962.
48. Mazzaferri EL, Young RL. Papillary thyroid carcinoma: A 10-year follow-up report of the impact of therapy in 576 patients. Am J Med 1981; 70:511-518.
49. Mazzaferri EL, Jhiang SM. Long-term impact of initial surgical and medical therapy on papillary nd follicular thyroid cancer. Am J Med 1994; 97:418-428.
50. Tollefsen HR, Shah JP, Huvos AG. Papillary carcinoma of the thyroid: Recurrence in the thyroid gland after initial surgical treatment. Am J Surg 1972; 124:468-472.
51. Silverberg SG, Hutter RVP, Foote FW. Fatal carcinoma of the thyroid: Histology, metastasises, and causes of death. Cancer 1970; 25:792.
52. Russel WO, Ibanez ML, Clark RL, et. al. Thyroid carcinoma: Classification, intraglandular dissemination, and clinicopathologic study based upon whole organ section of 80 glands. Cancer 1963; 16:1425.
53. Clark OH, Levin K, Zeng QH, et. al. Thyroid cancer: The case for total thyroidectomy. Eur J Cancer 1988;24:305-313.
54. De Jong SA, Demeter JG, Lawrence AM, et. al. Necessity and safety of completion thyroidectomy for differentiated thyroid carcinoma. Surgery 1992; 112:734-739.
55. Grauer A, Raue F, Gagel RF. Changing concepts in the management of hereditary and sporadic medullary thyroid carcinoma. Endocrinol Metab Clin North Am 1990; 19:613-635.
56. Tisell LE, Hansson G, Jansson S, Salander H. Reoperation in the treatment of asymptomatic metastasizing medullary thyroid carcinoma. Surgery 1986; 99:60-66.
57. Wilson S, Block G. Carcinoma of the thyroid metastatic to lymph nodes of the neck. Arch Surg 1971;102:285-291.
58. Breaux EP, Guillamondegui OM. Treatment of locally invasive carcinoma of the thyroid: How radical? Am J Surg 1980; 140:514-517.
59. Ann Surg 1997;226:85-91.
60. Grillo HC, Zannini P. Resectional management of airway invasion by thyroid carcinoma. Ann Thorac Surg 1986; 42:287-298.
61. Ishihara T, Kobayashi K, Kikuchi K, et. al. Surgical treatment of advanced thyroid carcinoma invading the trachea. J Thorac Cardiovasc Surg 1991; 102:717-720.
62. Friedman M: Surgical management of thyroid carcinoma with laryngotracheal invasion. Otolaryngol Clin North Am 1990; 23:495-507.

63.   DeGroot LJ, Kaplan EL, Straus FH. Does the method of management of papillary thyroid carcinoma make a difference in outcome? World J Surg 1994; 18:123-130.

64.   Samaan NA, Schultz PN, Hickey RC, et. al. The results of various modalities of treatment of well differentiated thyroid carcinomas: A retrospective review of 1599 patients. J Clin Endocrinol Metab 1992; 75:714-720.

65.   Heshmati HM, Gharib H, van Heerden JA, Sizemore GW. Advances and controversies in the diagnosis and management of medullary thyroid carcinoma. Am J Med 1997;103:60-69.

11 THYROID CANCER: IMPACT OF THERAPEUTIC MODALITIES ON PROGNOSIS

Ernest Mazzaferri, M.D., M.A.C.P.
Ohio State University
Columbus, OH

Introduction

The prognosis of thyroid carcinoma is determined by an interaction of three variables: tumor stage, the patient=s age at the time of diagnosis, and the efficacy of therapy. Tumor stage is largely due to the inherent biologic potential of a neoplasm to invade tissues and metastasize to distant sites, and to a lesser extent to the timeliness of diagnosis. Treatment is the only prognostic variable that currently can be modified.

Papillary and follicular thyroid carcinoma, together termed differentiated thyroid carcinoma, displays a wide spectrum of clinical behavior, ranging from slow growing tumors that never seriously threaten survival, to rapidly growing neoplasms that kill within a few years. This chapter will review the prognostic features that alter the behavior of these tumors and will summarize the long-term effects of therapy on prognosis.

Prognosis of differentiated thyroid carcinoma

Current estimates of prognosis

Prognosis may be expressed in terms of cancer-specific mortality and tumor recurrence. Both are important outcomes that gauge the impact of therapy. Although recurrence rates of differentiated thyroid carcinoma are high, mortality rates are relatively low, sometimes giving the clinician a false sense of security about the outcome. Despite the fact that most recurrences can be eradicated, it is a devastating experience for the patient and is sometimes the first signal of a poor outcome.

Mortality. It is estimated that 17,200 new cases of thyroid carcinoma will occur in the U.S. during 1998 (2). Most (90%) are differentiated thyroid carcinomas that occur about three times more often in women than men (3). Only about 1,200 deaths from thyroid cancer are expected in the U.S. during 1998, and most will occur in patients over age 40 who have tumors that are poorly differentiated or well-advanced at the time of diagnosis (Figure 1)(2,4). Over the past several decades, the average 10-year cancer-specific mortality rate for follicular cancer was more than twice that for papillary cancer (27% versus 11%, Table 1).

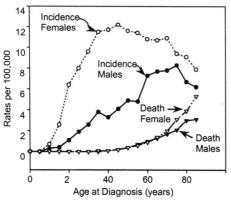

Figure 1. Annual incidence of thyroid cancer (all types) in the United States according to age at the time of diagnosis and patient gender. Adapted from the data in SEER Cancer Statistic Review, 1973-1992

Recurrence. The distinction between recurrent and persistent cancer is often ambiguous. Most ostensibly new recurrences probably are persistent microscopic carcinomas that were not initially eradicated, as opposed to *de novo* cancer developing in a thyroid remnant. An elevated serum Tg may be the only manifestation of microscopic disease, an observation that is less likely to be made when subtotal thyroidectomy is performed. Carcinoma recurs in up to 40% of patients, depending upon its stage and the patient=s age at the time of diagnosis, and the extent of initial therapy. About 80% are in regional

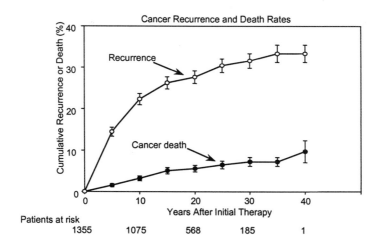

Figure 2. Differentiated thyroid carcinoma recurrence and death rates. Adapted from **Mazzaferri, E. L. and S. M. Jhiang.** 1994 Long-term impact of initial surgical and medical therapy on papillary and follicular thyroid cancer. Am J Med 97:418-428

lymph nodes or soft tissues of the neck and usually can be surgically removed or ablated with ^{131}I, but the others are in distant sites where they often can not be eradicated. The recurrence rate over three decades was 30% in our patients, but varied according to the initial therapy (Figure 2) (1). Local recurrences may be the first sign of a lethal outcome (5-8). In our patients 74% of the recurrences were in cervical lymph nodes, 20% were in thyroid remnants and 6% were in trachea or muscle; 7% of this group died of cancer (1). Distant recurrence sites, usually lungs, were involved in 21% of our patients; half of this group died of cancer. Over half the deaths in our series resulted from recurrent cancer, while the others were due to persistent gross tumor. Mortality rates are lower when recurrences are detected by ^{131}I scans than by clinical signs (8).

Table 1. 10-year survival rates of patients with differentiated thyroid carcinoma*

Author	Year	Country	Patient No.	Age Mean years	10-year survival (%) Papillary	10-year survival (%) Follicular
Byar et al. (9)	1979	Europe	464	---	60	80
Wanebo et al. (10)	1981	USA	157	45	80	77
Forquetet et al. (11)	1983	France	189	55	80	65
Tubiana et al. (12)	1985	France	546	< 45	88	23[a]
Kerr et al. (13)	1986	Scotland	303	47	73	62
Joensuu et al. (14)	1986	Finland	200	52	87[b]	66[b]
Hay et al. (15)	1987	USA	860	45	85	---
Schelfhout et al.(16)	1988	Netherlands	202	49	94	67
Thorensen et al. (17)	1989	Norway	1055	~55	95[b]	88[b]
DeGroot et al. (18)	1990	USA	269	36	94	---
Samaan et al. (19)	1991	USA	1599	40	92	82
Akslen et al. (20)	1991	Norway	2479	55	90	80[c]
Brennan et al. (21)	1993	USA	100	53	---	87
Mazzaferri et al. (1)	1994	USA	1355	36	92	87
Gilliland et al. (22)	1997	USA	14517	39/48[d]	98	92
Tsang et al. (23)	1998	Canada	382	42/55[d]	93	69
Total	---	---	24,677	47[e]	89[e]	73[e]

* Adapted from Mazzaferri (3).

[a] Follicular well differentiated and follicular less well differentiated

[b] Relative survival (observed/expected)

[c] Estimated from life-tables

[d] Median ages for papillary/follicular thyroid carcinoma patients

[e] Weighted average (approximate)

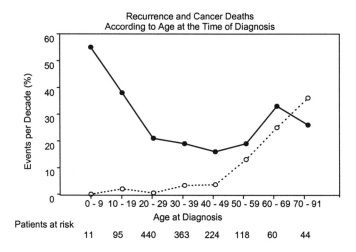

Figure 3. Differentiated thyroid carcinoma recurrence and cancer death rates according to age at the time of diagnosis. Open circles = cancer specific mortalitiy. Closed circles = recurrence. Adapted from **Mazzaferri, E. L. and S. M. Jhiang.** 1994 Long-term impact of initial surgical and medical therapy on papillary and follicular thyroid cancer. Am J Med 97:418-428

Patient Features Influencing Prognosis

Age. Thyroid carcinoma is more likely to be fatal after age 40 and the risk increases with each subsequent decade of life, rising dramatically after age 60 years (Figure 3). However, the pattern of tumor recurrence is much different. Recurrence rates are highest (~ 40%) at the extremes of life, before age 20 years and after age 60 years (Fig. 2) (1,24-27).

Sex. Women have a better prognosis than men, but the difference is usually small (1,12,28). In our study, the risk of death from cancer was about half as great in women as men (1). Men with thyroid carcinoma thus should be regarded with special concern, especially those over age 50.

Tumor Features Influencing Prognosis

Tumor Histology

Papillary carcinoma. The prognosis is more serious for some histologic variants of papillary carcinoma. For example, tall-cell papillary carcinomas, which are large tumors that often occur in older patients and can be identified by fine-needle biopsy, have 10-year mortality rates as high as 25% (29-33). They may have over-expression of the p53 gene but not all have a uniformly poor outcome (34,35). The less common columnar variant of papillary carcinoma is a rapidly growing tumor with a 90%

mortality rate (29,36). About 2% of papillary carcinomas are diffuse sclerosing variants that infiltrate the entire gland and may cause a diffuse goiter without a palpable nodule, which may be mistaken for goitrous autoimmune thyroiditis (29,37). Most metastasize to lymph nodes but up to 25% develop distant metastases and have an unfavorable outcome (29). Nonetheless, the prognosis in younger patients is typically good (29,38). Follicular-variant papillary carcinomas, recognized by their follicular architecture and typical papillary cytology, behave more like papillary carcinomas, although some are more aggressive (3,29,39).

Follicular carcinoma. Widely invasive follicular carcinoma, which is recognized by its aggressive extension into surrounding tissues, has a poor prognosis. Up to 80% of patients with invasive follicular carcinomas develop metastases and about 20% die of their disease (40). Most, however, are minimally invasive encapsulated follicular carcinomas that closely resemble follicular adenomas. The distinction between the two can be made only by study of the permanent histologic sections and not by fine-needle aspiration biopsy or frozen section study, which poses a management predicament at the time of surgery (39,41) The main diagnostic criteria for carcinoma are cells penetrating the tumor capsule and invading blood vessels. The latter has a worse prognosis than capsular penetration alone (42) Few patients with minimally- invasive follicular carcinomas, the main type found in recent years, have distant metastases or die of their disease (1,21,40,43).

The less favorable prognosis of follicular carcinoma is more likely related to the patient's older age and advanced tumor stage at the time of diagnosis than histology alone (1,44). Survival rates with papillary and follicular carcinomas are similar among patients of comparable age and disease stage (12,44-46). Both have an excellent prognosis if they are confined to the thyroid, are small tumors (<1.0 cm) or are minimally invasive (1,5). Both have unfavorable outcomes if they are widely invasive or metastatic to distant sites (45,47).

The 30-year cancer-specific mortality rate, which was 8% in 1,355 patients in our series, (1) was twice as high in the 21% with follicular carcinoma than in the 79% with papillary carcinoma. Those with follicular carcinoma, however, were older and had larger tumors and more advanced disease, including more frequent distant metastases, at the time of diagnosis than patients with papillary carcinoma. Patients with tumors of similar stage had similar 30-year recurrence and cancer-specific mortality rates, regardless of the papillary or follicular histology (1).

Hürthle cell carcinoma. Although the WHO classification considers them as variants of follicular carcinoma, when oncocytic (Hürthle) cells constitute most or all of a tumor, it is usually referred to as Hürthle-cell carcinoma (48). There is some controversy about their diagnosis and management, because fewer than about 500 cases have been reported (48,49). Most nonetheless consider them to be aggressive and unpredictable tumors with a 30-year mortality rate as high as 25%, (50-52) although some find them no more aggressive than similarly-staged follicular carcinomas without Hürthle cells (48,53). In two large series, however, pulmonary metastases occurred in 25% and 35% of patients with Hürthle cell carcinoma, which is about twice the frequency of distant metastases from follicular carcinoma (47,54).

Hürthle-cell variant papillary carcinoma, which is even less common, has higher than usual recurrence and mortality rates in some, (55) but not all studies (56-58).

Tumor Size. The size of a primary tumor has important prognostic implications. High-resolution ultrasonography is capable of detecting many small, impalpable thyroid nodules, most of which are benign. Often referred to as incidentalomas, their prevalence ranges from 30% to 60% in both autopsy and clinical studies (59,60). The risk for malignancy in asymptomatic nodules found by palpation in non-irradiated glands is about 4% and is even lower in tiny (<1cm) nodules found by ultrasonography, most of which can be followed by palpation alone (41).

Papillary carcinomas smaller than 1 cm, termed microcarcinomas, are often found unexpectedly during surgery for benign thyroid conditions (60). They pose no threat to survival and no further surgery is required unless the tumor is multicentric or metastatic, which rarely happens (3,59). In one study, only one cancer death occurred among 454 patients with microcarcinomas (61). Rarely, a multifocal papillary carcinoma smaller than 1 cm may become invasive and metastatic; nonetheless, tumors smaller than 1.5 cm seldom recur and almost never cause death (62). In our series, 30-year recurrence rates in patients with papillary and follicular carcinomas smaller than 1.5 cm were one-third those of patients with larger tumors (1). Small tumors rarely metastasized to distant sites and had a cancer-specific mortality rate of 0.4%, compared with 7% for tumors 1.5 cm or larger. (P<0.001) (1).

There is a linear relationship between tumor size and both recurrence and cancer-specific mortality (Figure 4) (1). For both papillary and follicular carcinomas, the greatest number of adverse events, including distant metastases and cancer deaths, occur with tumors larger than about 4 to 5 cm in diameter (1,28,61).

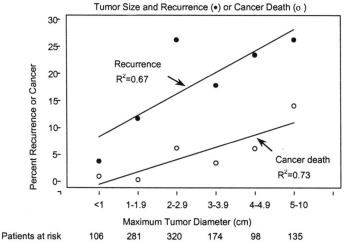

Figure 4. Differentiated thyroid carcinoma recurrence and death rates according to tumor size (maximum diameter in cm) for papillary and follicular thyroid carcinoma. Adapted from **Mazzaferri, E. L. and S. M. Jhiang.** 1994 Long-term impact of initial surgical and medical therapy on papillary and follicular thyroid cancer. Am J Med 97:418-428

Multicentric Primary Tumors. Multiple microscopic intraglandular metastases occur in about 20% of patients with papillary carcinoma when the thyroid is examined routinely and they occur in up to 80% when it is examined in great detail (7,24,63,64). Their clinical importance is debated; however, their presence (which is not usually apparent until the final histologic sections have been studied) has a bearing upon the decision to surgically excise the thyroid remnant or ablate it with [131]I. After unilateral subtotal lobectomy, residual carcinoma is found in up to 30% of the patients who undergo completion thyroidectomy, especially with papillary carcinoma (43,65-67).

Those who routinely perform hemithyroidectomy argue that multiple microscopic tumors are of little clinical consequence (28,68). Others find recurrence rates ranging from 5% to 20% in thyroid remnants and report that pulmonary metastases occur much more often after subtotal than total thyroidectomy (1,69). In one study, patients with multiple intrathyroidal tumors had almost twice the incidence of nodal metastases and three times the rate of pulmonary and other distant metastases than those with single tumors; they also had three times the likelihood of persistent disease than those with single tumors (7). Among our patients with multiple tumors, the 30-year cancer-specific mortality rates were two times those observed in patients with a single primary tumor (1).

Local Tumor Invasion. Microscopic or gross tumor invasion of the surrounding tissues occurs in 5% to 10% of papillary and follicular carcinomas (1,43). Tumor most commonly invades neck muscles and vessels, recurrent laryngeal nerves, larynx, pharynx, and esophagus, although it may extend into the spinal cord and brachial plexus (1,43). The recurrence rates are two times higher with invasive tumors than with noninvasive tumors; moreover, depending upon the extent of invasion, up to one-third die of cancer within the first decade (7,70,71). The primary tumor was locally invasive in 115 of our patients (8% of the papillary and 12% of the follicular carcinomas); their 10-year recurrence rates were 1.5-times higher and their cancer-specific death rates were five times those of patients without local invasion (1).

Lymph Node Metastases. In one review, nodal metastases were reported in 36% of 8,029 adults with papillary carcinoma and in 17% of 1,540 patients with follicular carcinoma (3). They are more common in children, occurring in up to 80% with papillary carcinoma (72,73). An enlarged cervical lymph node, which may be the first sign of thyroid carcinoma, usually is only one of multiple nodal metastases found at surgery (74).

The prognostic impact of cervical lymph node metastases is controversial (7,28,64,75,76). Nonetheless, nodal metastases — especially bilateral cervical or mediastinal lymph node metastases — have been found to be an important risk factor for tumor recurrence and cancer-specific mortality in a number of studies (18,20,71,77-81). For example, in one study, 15% of patients with cervical metastases died of thyroid cancer, whereas none without them died of disease

(P<0.02) (79). In another study, 80% of patients with distantly metastatic papillary carcinoma had mediastinal node metastases at the time cancer was diagnosed (82). When tumor extends through the lymph node capsule into surrounding tissues, one study reported a nine-fold increase in the likelihood of distant metastases (83). We found that patients with papillary or follicular carcinoma who had cervical or mediastinal lymph node metastases had significantly higher 30-year cancer-specific mortality rates than those with no metastases (10% and 6% P<0.01). Mediastinal or bilateral cervical lymph node metastases are associated with an especially unfavorable outcome (Figure 5). The most aggressive tumors are locally invasive with bilateral neck or mediastinal metastases, in patients over age 45 years (1,80).

Distant Metastases. Almost 10% of patients with papillary carcinoma and up to 25% of those with follicular carcinoma develop distant metastases; half are present at the time of diagnosis while the others may appear years later (84). Distant metastases occur even more often (35%) with Hürthle cell carcinoma and in patients older than 40 years (47,54). The most common sites of distant metastases among 1,231 patients reported in 13 studies were lung (49%), bone (25%), both lung and bone (15%), and central nervous system or other soft tissues (10%) (3).

The prognosis with distant metastases is influenced mainly by the patient's age and the tumor=s metastatic site, ability to concentrate ^{131}I, and appearance on chest

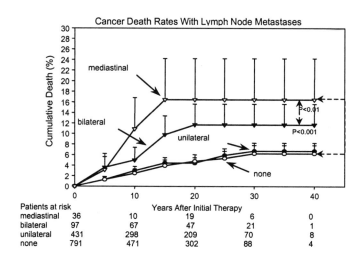

Figure 5. Differentiated thyroid carcinoma death rates according to the presence of nodal metastases found at the time of initial surgery. Adapted from **Mazzaferri, E. L. and S. M. Jhiang.** 1994 Long-term impact of initial surgical and medical therapy on papillary and follicular thyroid cancer. Am J Med 97:418-428

x-ray (47,54,85,86). Some patients survive for decades, especially younger patients with small lung metastases; however, about half die within five years regardless of the tumor=s histology (3). Survival is longest with small pulmonary metastases that concentrate ^{131}I, whereas multiple bone and central nervous system metastases have the most serious prognosis. In one study, when distant metastases were confined to the lung, over half the patients were alive and free of disease at 10 years, while on the contrary no patient with skeletal metastases survived this long (87). In a large study from France, survival rates with distant metastases were 53% at 5 years, 38% at 10 years and 30% at 15 years (88); survival rates were much higher in young patients with pulmonary metastases (86).

Survival is longest with diffuse pulmonary metastases seen only on ^{131}I imaging and not by x-ray (88,89). Some are seen only on a post-treatment ^{131}I whole-body scan done after a large dose of ^{131}I, which has the best prognosis and is compatible with long survival and in some cases an apparent cure (90,91). Prognosis is much worse when the lung metastases do not concentrate ^{131}I or appear as large nodules on chest x-ray; it is intermediate when the tumors are small nodular densities that concentrate ^{131}I (54,82,88,89). A few adults with distant metastases have survived 30 years or longer with very little therapy (92,93).

Staging Systems and Prognosis

There are several staging classifications for thyroid carcinoma, but the TNM classification is perhaps the most widely recommended. (94,95) Eight clinical staging schemes are summarized in Table 2 and the TNM classification is shown in Table 3 (1,9,18,28,61,75,96,97). Cancer mortality can be accurately predicted by these staging systems. When applied to the papillary carcinoma data from the Mayo Clinic, four of the schemes that use age (EORTC, TNM, AMES, AGES) were effective in separating low-risk and high-risk patients in whom, respectively, cancer-specific mortality was 1% and 40% at 20 years (61). Twenty-year survival rates were 99%, 89%, 56%, and 24%, for patients with progressively higher MACIS scores (75). Another study that compared ten different staging systems showed no statistically significant superiority of any system over the TNM classification in predicting cancer-specific mortality (94).

However, young patients typically have extensive disease at the time of diagnosis and generally experience a high recurrence rate but are classified TNM I unless they have distant metastases (98,99). This may be why most clinicians do not alter treatment very much on the basis of a patient=s age (100-102).

When age is not used to define stage, most tumors are classified as stage I. Not surprisingly, a large number of TNM I patients have recurrences and a high number die of disease that by definition should be completely indolent when assigned such a low stage. For example, two large studies (94,95) classified 46% and 75% of patients with differentiated thyroid carcinomas as TNM I. In the larger of the two series, the cancer recurrence and mortality rates were, respectively, 15.4% and 1.7% (TNM I n=516), 22% and 15.8% (TNM II n=57), 46.4% and 30% (TNM III n=104), and 66.7% and 60.9% (TNM IV n=23) (95). The cancer-specific death rates are well separated among the four groups; however, the actual number of patients who experienced tumor recurrence was higher in the TNM I group than TNM II and III groups combined, and nine patients died of cancer in each of the lowest two TNM groups. The authors felt that the small number of patients in TNM stages other than stage I precluded an evaluation of its usefulness as a guide for therapy and supported the practice of total thyroidectomy followed by ^{131}I therapy (when there was radionuclide uptake) of papillary thyroid cancers more advanced than $T_1N_0M_0$ or for multicentric tumors, and for the majority of patients with follicular thyroid carcinoma (95).

Table 2. Staging systems and rating schemes for defining risk category among patients with Papillary (PTC) and Follicular (FTC) thyroid cancer

Variable at the Time of Diagnosis	Staging system and Rating Schemes*							
	TNM [a]	EORTC	AMES	AGES	MACIS	MSK	Chicago	Ohio State
Age	<45	Yes [b]	< 41 M <51 F	Yes [b]	Yes [b]	<45	<45	No
Sex (better prognosis)	No	Yes	Yes	No	No	No	No	No
Tumor Histology	All	All	PTC FTC	PTC	PTC	PTC FTC	PTC FTC	PTC FTC
Grade	No	No	No	Yes	No	No	No	No
Tumor Size diameter (cm)	≤ 1 1-4 > 4	No	< 5 ≥ 5	Yes b	Yes b	≤ 1 1-4 > 4	≤ 1 1-4 > 4	≤ 1.5 1.5-4 ≥ 4.5
Extra-thyroid Invasion	Yes	Yes	Yes	Yes	Yes	Yes	Yes	Yes
Residual Disease	No	Yes	No	No	Yes	No	No	No
Multifocal	No	No	No	No	No	No	No	Yes
Lymph nodes	Yes	No	No	No	No	No	Yes	Yes
Metastases	Yes	Yes	Yes	Yes	Yes	Yes	Yes	Yes

*TNM (96), EORTC (9), AMES (28), AGES (61), MACIS (75) MSK (97) CHICAGO (18) OSU (1)

[a] T = Primary Tumor, T_1 <1 cm; T_2 = > 1cm to 4 cm; T_3 = > 4 cm; T_4 = extension beyond thyroid capsule; N = Regional Lymph Nodes; N_1 = regional lymph node metastases (cervical and upper mediastinal nodes); M = distant metastases present.

[b] continuous

Table 3. TNM Classification (American Joint Committee on Cancer) (96)

TNM	Papillary or Follicular Carcinoma	
	< 45	> 45
I	M0	T1
II	M1	T2-3
III		T4 or N1
IV		M1

According to the TNM classification, 82% of our patients were TNM I. The classification clearly predicted cancer-specific mortality, but recurrence rates were high in all stages (I to IV respectively, 20%, 15%, 35%, 30%). Moreover, 19 cancer deaths (1.8%) occurred with TNM I tumors, the same proportion that was noted in the study cited above (95).

Classified according to The Ohio State system, most patients are stage II (82%), but the recurrence rate was much lower in stage I than stage II (6% and 22%) and no cancer deaths occurred among the 170 patients considered to have stage I tumors (1). We believe this staging system can be used to guide therapy.

The Ohio State classification of 1355 patients with differentiated thyroid carcinoma is shown in Tables 2 and 4 (1). After a median follow-up of almost 16 years, tumor recurrence and cancer-specific mortality rates were progressively and significantly greater with each tumor stage (Table 4). Based on regression modeling on 1322 patients excluding those who presented with distant metastases, the likelihood of death from thyroid carcinoma was increased if age $\geq$40 years, tumor size $\geq$1.5 cm, local tumor invasion or regional lymph node metastases were present, or therapy had been delayed $\geq$12 months. Cancer mortality was reduced in women, by surgery more extensive than lobectomy, and ^{131}I plus T_4 therapy; and unaffected by tumor histologic type.

Regardless of the staging system utilized, its strict application in support of conservative treatment for low-risk patients may lead to inadequate initial therapy. A study from France pointed out that the excess mortality caused by differentiated thyroid carcinoma in children is significant, with a standardized mortality ratio of 6.4, which is a ratio higher than in older patients (98). Rigid application of scoring systems that rely heavily upon the patient's age may result in less than optimal treatment of young patients. Aggressive disease may exist even when patients appear to be at low-risk at the time of diagnosis (1,26,103,104).

Table 4. The Ohio State University Staging of Differentiated Thyroid Carcinoma*

Variables	Stage I	Stage II	Stage III	Stage IV
Tumor size (cm)	<1.5	1.5-4.4 (or)	≥ 4.5	Any size
Cervical metastases	No	Yes [a]	Yes/No	Yes/No
Multiple thyroid tumors (>3) any size	No	Yes [a]	Yes/No	Yes/No
Local tumor invasion	No	No	Yes	Yes/No
Distant metastases	No	No	No	Yes
Outcome				
Age (mean year)	38	34	38	48
P values	---	0.001 [b]	<0.05 [b]	0.01 [b]
No. of recurrences (%)	10 (8)	210 (31)	59 (36)	10 (62)
P values	---	0.001[b]	0.001[b]	NS[b]
No of deaths from cancer	0	34 (6)	19 (14)	17 (65)
P values[l]	---	0.01 [c]	0.001 [c]	0.001 [c]

[a] Includes tumors <1.5 cm with cervical metastases and palpable tumors of uncertain size confined to the thyroid gland; any tumor that fulfills one of the three criteria for size, cervical metastases or multiple intrathyroidal tumors is considered stage 2.
[b] Wilcoxon rank-sum test comparing stage with preceding lower stage (left).
[c] 30-year recurrence or cancer-specific death rate, logrank test comparing stage with preceding lower stage (left).
NS, not significant.
*Data from Mazzaferri and Jhiang (1).

Therapy

Delay in Therapy

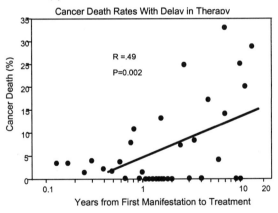

Figure 6. Differentiated thyroid carcinoma death rates according to delay in therapy defined as the time a neck mass was first recognized to the time of initial surgery. Adapted from **Mazzaferri, E. L. and S. M. Jhiang.** 1994 Long-term impact of initial surgical and medical therapy on papillary and follicular thyroid cancer. Am J Med 97:418-428

Although early diagnosis and treatment may have a beneficial effect on outcome of patients with carcinoma, there is a paucity of such evidence for thyroid carcinoma. We found that the median time from the first detection of thyroid cancer - nearly always a neck mass - to initial therapy was 4 months in our patients, but ranged from less than one month to 20 years. Delay in diagnosis correlated with cancer mortality (Figure 6). The median delay was 18 months in those who died of cancer and 4 months in those still living (P<0.001). The 30-year cancer mortality was 6% when patients underwent therapy within a year of diagnosis and 13% when it was delayed (P<0.001). (1)

Extent of Surgery

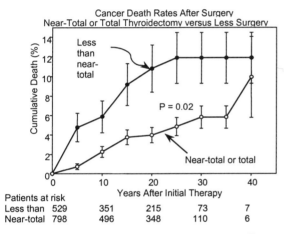

Patients at risk

Less than	529	351	215	73	7
Near-total	798	496	348	110	6

Figure 7. Differentiated thyroid carcinoma death rates according to the extent of thyroidectomy. Adapted from **Mazzaferri, E. L. and S. M. Jhiang**. 1994 Long-term impact of initial surgical and medical therapy on papillary and follicular thyroid cancer. Am J Med 97:418-428

Most now believe that near-total or total thyroidectomy is the surgical treatment of choice for thyroid carcinoma (100,102,105 -107). The extent of surgery closely relates to outcome and influences subsequent decisions concerning medical therapy. Recurrence rates are high with large thyroid gland remnants. For example, in a Mayo Clinic study(24) of patients with papillary thyroid carcinoma, recurrence rates during the first two years after surgery were about four-fold greater after unilateral lobectomy than after total or near-total thyroidectomy (26% vs 6%, P=0.01). Patients with papillary carcinoma whose AGES score was 4 or more had a 25 year cancer mortality rate almost twice as high after lobectomy than after bilateral thyroid resection (65% and 35%, respectively, P=0.06) (15). In another study (18) of patients with papillary carcinoma larger than 1 cm, near-total thyroidectomy decreased the risk of recurrence and death as compared with lobectomy or bilateral subtotal thyroidectomy.

In our study, recurrence and cancer death rates from tumors larger than 1.5 cm were both about 50% lower after near-total or total thyroidectomy as compared with less surgery (Figure 7) (1). We found the 30-year cumulative recurrence rate among 436 patients who had undergone subtotal thyroidectomy was significantly higher than that in 698 patients who had undergone total or near-total thyroidectomy (40% and 26% P<0.002); cancer-specific mortality rates were also higher in the subtotal thyroidectomy group (9% and 6% P=0.02) (1). Surgery more extensive than lobectomy was an independent variable that reduced the likelihood of cancer mortality rate by 60%.

Medical Therapy with Thyroid Hormone (Levothyroxine or T_4)

Effects of Thyrotropin (TSH) Suppression on Tumor Growth. Most papillary and follicular tumors contain functional TSH receptors, although they are more abundant in the latter (108,109). The idea that TSH stimulates the growth of thyroid carcinoma forms the basis for using T_4 to treat differentiated thyroid carcinoma (110,111). However, whether treatment with T_4 alone following surgery improves survival more than treatment with ^{131}I and T_4 is controversial (6,112,113). There have been no prospective trials to test this hypothesis. Yet there is evidence that TSH stimulates tumor growth. For example, differentiated thyroid carcinoma may be more aggressive in patients with Graves' disease, presumably as a result of stimulating TSH receptor antibodies (108,114). In addition, rapid tumor growth sometimes follows T_4 withdrawal during preparation for ^{131}I therapy. There also is evidence that T_4, given as an adjuvant to surgical and ^{131}I therapy, is effective: tumor recurrence rates are higher if T_4 is not given after surgery (115). After 30 years' follow-up, we found that there were 25% fewer recurrences in patients treated with T_4 as compared with no adjunctive therapy (Figure 8, P<0.01), and there were fewer cancer deaths in the T_4 group (6% and 12%, respectively, P<0.001) (1).

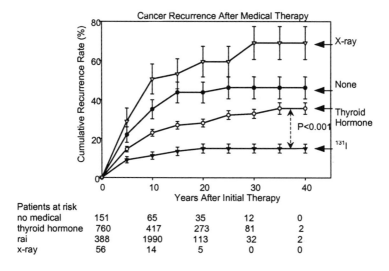

Patients at risk				
no medical	151	65	35	12	0
thyroid hormone	760	417	273	81	2
rai	388	1990	113	32	2
x-ray	56	14	5	0	0

Figure 8. Differentiated thyroid carcinoma recurrence after various forms of postoperative adjunctive medical therapy. The group treated with ^{131}I also was treated with thyroid hormone. Adapted from **Mazzaferri, E. L. and S. M. Jhiang.** 1994 Long-term impact of initial surgical and medical therapy on papillary and follicular thyroid cancer. Am J Med 97:418-428

Patients with thyroid carcinoma are usually given T_4 in sufficient doses to suppress the serum TSH to below normal. One adverse consequence is osteoporosis, which may occur even in children (116). A review on thyroid carcinoma and a meta-analysis of this issue both concluded that TSH suppression contributes to osteoporosis mainly in postmenopausal women (110,117). Alendronate (10 mg/day) therapy may prevent bone loss in elderly patients treated with thyroid hormone (118).

Cardiovascular abnormalities, well recognized to occur among patients with overt thyrotoxicosis, also occur with suppressive doses of T_4 (119). There is an increased risk of atrial fibrillation (120), a higher 24-hour heart rate, more atrial premature contractions per day, and not only increased cardiac contractility but also ventricular hypertrophy that occur with prolonged treatment with T4 given at sufficient doses to lower the third generation TSH to undetectable levels (119).

T4 Dose. Patients who have undergone total thyroid ablation for thyroid carcinoma require more T_4 than those with spontaneous primary hypothyroidism. In one study, the dose of T_4 needed to reduce serum TSH concentrations to normal was 2.11 µg/Kg/day in patients with thyroid carcinoma and 1.62 µg/Kg/day those with non-cancer related hypothyroidism (121). In another study of 180 patients who had undergone total thyroidectomy and remnant ^{131}I ablation, the average dose of T_4 that resulted in an undetectable basal serum TSH concentration and no increase in serum TSH after thyrotropin-releasing hormone (TRH) was 2.7±0.4 µg/kg/day (122). Younger patients need larger doses than older patients do and TSH suppression is more likely when the therapy has been prolonged (122). These data suggest that some T_4 is secreted from residual thyroid tissue in patients with spontaneously occurring hypothyroidism.

As a practical matter, the most appropriate dose of T4 for most patients with thyroid carcinoma is that which reduces the serum concentration to just below the lower limit of the normal range for the assay being used. Some clinicians prefer more TSH suppression, for example, serum TSH concentrations between 0.05 to 0.1 µU/ml in low risk patients and less than 0.01 µU/mL in high risk patients (110) and a few advocate the latter target for all patients (123). There is no published evidence that maintaining serum TSH concentrations less than 0.01 µU/mL has benefits, and it does have some risks.

Radioactive Iodine (^{131}I) Therapy

[131]I has been used for over 40 years to treat differentiated thyroid carcinoma. Given both to ablate remaining normal thyroid tissue and to treat the carcinoma, ^{131}I therapy has gained wide use because these tumors tend to be infiltrative, locally invasive and associated with occult thyroidal and regional lymph node metastases. In addition, recurrence rates are high when patients are treated with surgery and T_4 alone (Figure 8). [131]I is thus a widely accepted therapy for patients with residual or

metastatic thyroid carcinoma but its use to ablate the thyroid remnant remains more controversial. Although effective in both regards, the explicit indications for its use continue to provoke debate (61,106).

Ablation of Residual Normal Thyroid Tissue. Thyroid ^{131}I remnant ablation, the practice of destroying presumably normal thyroid tissue that remains after the initial thyroidectomy, is still under debate (1,61). The controversy centers around the optimal dose of ^{131}I that is required to ablate the thyroid remnant, the efficacy and safety of this practice, and the selection of patients for this treatment. For example, of 233 respondents to a survey of the clinical members of the American Thyroid Association, 86% preferred total or near-total thyroidectomy for a 39-year-old female with a single 2 cm papillary thyroid carcinoma fully contained within the thyroid gland, but only 61% recommended ^{131}I remnant ablation. (102) At an international symposium held in 1987 in The Netherlands, 160 participants who were surgeons, endocrinologists, pathologists, and nuclear medicine specialists, recommended total thyroidectomy followed by postoperative ^{131}I thyroid remnant ablation for most patients with differentiated thyroid carcinoma, regardless of their age (100). A third study (107) based upon the opinions of 157 thyroid experts from around the world found that ablation of the thyroid remnant with ^{131}I was advised by 81% for patients with papillary carcinoma and by 97% for patients with follicular carcinoma.

No prospective trial addresses the issue of remnant ablation, and none is likely to be done, given the low incidence of the disease and its prolonged course. A power analysis for the feasibility of such a clinical trial estimated that each arm of the trial would require nearly 4,000 patients to detect a 10% reduction in mortality after 25 years. (124) It was estimated that it would take 10 years to enroll patients into the study and that the results would be available after 35 years. Their decision analytic model found that thyroid remnant ablation modestly improved life expectancy by 2 to 15 months, depending on the patient's age and sex. Although this is only a modest increase in life expectancy, the absolute gain is comparable to that of other accepted medical interventions such as annual screening mammography for women over age 40 years that increases life expectancy by about 20 days. The model also predicted that the benefit of ablation measured in terms of lowering recurrence and death rates from thyroid carcinoma outweighs the potential risk of leukemia from [131]I.

Although some question remains about routine thyroid remnant ablation with ^{131}I, (125,126) it is widely used and has appeal for several reasons (100,106,107). First, it destroys occult microscopic carcinoma within the thyroid remnant because the malignant cells receive radiation from ^{131}I taken up by adjacent normal thyroid cells. Second, it enables detection of recurrent or persistent disease, particularly in the neck, by imaging. Radioiodine scanning can visualize few metastases when appreciable amounts of normal thyroid tissue remain after surgery. Third, it greatly facilitates the value of serum Tg measurements during follow-up. For these reasons, ^{131}I is commonly used to ablate thyroid gland remnants, even in those without known residual disease who have a very good prognosis. Physicians who do not favor this therapeutic maneuver argue that most patients with papillary or follicular thyroid carcinoma do not require such aggressive therapy because the cancer-specific mortality from the disease is so low. They believe that thyroid remnant ablation should be reserved for patients with tumors that have a more serious prognosis (61). This argument assumes that the risk of ^{131}I therapy is great enough to out-weigh both that of recurrent disease and of death from thyroid carcinoma. This assertion is not true (23,95,105,106,124). These arguments mainly center around treatment of younger patients.

Many report lower recurrence rates after ^{131}I ablation of the thyroid remnant, but not all find this to be the case. For example, at the Mayo Clinic, the recurrence rates were slightly but not significantly higher in 220 patients treated with surgery and ^{131}I ablation than in 726 patients treated with surgery and T$_4$ alone (13.3% and 9.6%). The 10-year cancer-specific mortality rates showed the same trend (3% and 2%).

These results contrast with those reported by others who find a more favorable effect of ^{131}I ablation, even in children (18,106,110,127). We studied 138 patients with no obvious residual disease who were given ^{131}I postoperatively to ablate presumably normal thyroid gland remnants. Their 30-year recurrence rates were less than one-third those not given [131]I (Figure 9) and no patient treated this way has died of thyroid carcinoma (128).

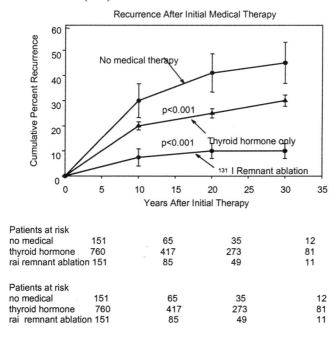

Patients at risk				
no medical	151	65	35	12
thyroid hormone	760	417	273	81
rai remnant ablation	151	85	49	11

Patients at risk				
no medical	151	65	35	12
thyroid hormone	760	417	273	81
rai remnant ablation	151	85	49	11

Figure 9. Differentiated thyroid carcinoma recurrence after thyroid remnant ablation compared with no medical therapy and thyroid hormone alone postoperatively. Adapted from **Mazzaferri, E. L.** 1997 Thyroid remnant ^{131}I ablation for papillary and follicular thyroid carcioma. Thyroid 7:265-271

Low Dose ^{131}I for Thyroid Remnant Ablation. The standard ^{131}I dose for remnant ablation was between 75 and 150 mCi for many years, but now many use about 30 mCi, a dose that will ablate most thyroid remnants if the amount of thyroid tissue remaining after surgery is small (<2 g). This has appeal because hospitalization is not required, the cost is lower and the total-body radiation dose is small. The average whole-body radiation exposure after ^{131}I has been estimated to be 6.1 rem for 30 mCi, 8.5 rem for a 50 mCi, and 12.2 rem for a 60 mCi (129).

Some have found that larger ^{131}I doses are necessary to ablate normal thyroid tissue and to treat residual microscopic carcinoma. For example, one study (125) reported that 100 to 149 mCi is the optimal dose to ablate the thyroid remnant because a single dose of this amount ablated uptake in 87% of patients (125). However, in another study, smaller doses (<30 mCi) ablated thyroid remnant ^{131}I uptake in 77% of patients but was more successful after near-total thyroidectomy than less extensive surgery (90% and 22% respectively) (130). Most (94%) had successful ablation when the surgeon left less than 2 grams of thyroid tissue as compared with a 68% success rate when the remnant was larger (130).

Most studies now indicate that thyroid uptake thus can be ablated in about 80% of patients, providing there is a relatively small thyroid remnant and ablation is defined by diagnostic scans with a 2 to 3 mCi dose of [131]I (129,131,132). Lower success rates are found when large scanning doses are used, regardless of the ablation dose of [131]I (133-135). In a randomized prospective study, the first dose ablated thyroid bed uptake in 81% of patients given 30 mCi and in 84% treated with 100 mCi (136). Regardless of the dose given, however, over 40% had elevated serum Tg concentrations at the time of complete scintigraphic ablation. This may not be a true measure of the long-term effects of ablation because serum Tg concentrations decline slowly after ^{131}I ablation (137).

Tumor recurrence rates are lowered by low-dose ^{131}I remnant ablation. Despite the suggestion that this is not an effective therapeutic strategy on the basis of a nearly 9% recurrence rate in 69 patients given 30 mCi doses of [131]I (132), this rate is about one-third that reported from the same institution in a larger group of patients with papillary carcinoma (24). A study of 831 patients with differentiated thyroid carcinoma found that pulmonary metastases occurred in 11% after partial thyroidectomy, while the rate was reduced by more than half (5%) when subtotal thyroidectomy was supplemented with ^{131}I and dropped to 1.3% after total thyroidectomy and [131]I (69),

In a study from 13 Canadian hospitals of 321 patients treated with ^{131}I given mainly to ablate residual normal thyroid tissue, local disease was controlled significantly more often in those with microscopic residual papillary or follicular carcinoma when treated with either postoperative external radiotherapy or ^{131}I therapy, or both together, than those treated with thyroid hormone alone (P<0.001) (6). Survival at 20 years was less favorable after treatment with surgery alone (about 40%) than after treatment with either ^{131}I or external radiation (about 90%, P<0.01). Radioiodine treatment of patients without obvious residual disease did not increase survival significantly. A subsequent study from Canada (23) showed that age >60, tumor size >4 cm, multifocal tumor, postoperative residual tumor, lymph node involvement, surgery less than near-total thyroidectomy and the lack of use of ^{131}I were significant with regard to local and regional failure.

Our study (128) supports the predictions made by Wong and associates. (124) After 30 years= follow-up we found that thyroid remnant ablation had a favorable effect on tumor recurrence and cancer mortality. The cumulative 30-year recurrence rate was about three-fold lower with thyroid remnant ablation than with thyroid hormone alone or when no adjunctive medical therapy was given postoperatively (P<0.001). Remnant ablation, however, did not lower the recurrence rate of tumors smaller than 1.5 cm that were confined to the thyroid gland (Table 6). In patients with larger primary tumors (with or without lymph node metastases but without local invasion) the 30-year recurrence rate was about three-fold higher when thyroid hormone alone or no medical therapy was given postoperatively compared with thyroid remnant ablation (P=0.001). Distant metastases, which did not occur after thyroid remnant ablation, did so after the other two forms of therapy (Table 6).

The improved recurrence rate after thyroid remnant ablation in our study was associated with a lower cancer-specific mortality rate, (figure 9) (P<0.001). (128) This salutary effect was observed only in those aged 40 years or older and in those with primary tumors 1.5 cm or larger, regardless of the patient=s age or the tumor=s papillary or follicular histology. The 30-year cancer-specific mortality rates among patients with primary tumors 1.5 cm or larger that were confined to the thyroid or only metastatic to regional lymph nodes were lower with thyroid remnant ablation than after treatment with thyroid hormone alone (P<0.05) or no medical therapy (P<0.001). The variables that independently affected cancer and cancer-specific death rates are shown in Table 7.

Table 6. Cancer Recurrence According to Initial Therapy

Variable	No Medical Therapy (%)	Thyroid Hormone Alone (%)	^{131}I Ablation (%)	ANOVA
All Recurrences	35	22	7	0.001
Distant Recurrences	8	3	0	0.002
Age <40 years	34	24	9	0.001
Age ≥40 years	35	19	4	0.003
Papillary Carcinoma	35	23	8	0.001
Follicular Carcinoma	33	17	7	0.03
Tumor size <1.5 cm	21	9	9	NS
Tumor size ≥ 1.5 cm	41	26	4	0.001
Cervical lymph nodes Present	31 46	17 31	7 8	0.001 0.01
Local Invasion Present	33 56	21 39	8 0	0.001 0.03
^{131}I 29- 50 mCi (%) ^{131}I 51-200 mCi	--- 	--- 	3 5	NS**

* ANOVA comparing three modes of post-surgical therapy for variable in each row.
** ANOVA comparing recurrence rates for two ^{131}I dose ranges shown.
Reproduced from Mazzaferri E.L., Thyroid 7:265-271; 1997, with permission of the publisher.

Table 7. Cox Proportional Hazard Model. 1048 Patients With Primary Tumor Larger Than 1.5 cm and Not Invading Through The Thyroid Capsule in Neck Tissues and Not Metastatic to Distant Sites at the Time of Diagnosis

Variable	Hazard Ratio	95% Confidence Interval	P Value
Recurrence			
Cervical Lymph Node Metastases [a]	0.8	0.7 - 0.9	0.001
Tumor stage [b]	1.8	1.5 - 2.3	0.001
Thyroid Remnant Treatment [c]	0.87	0.8 - 0.9	0.001
Cancer Deaths			
Age [d]	13.3	[6.4 - 27.7]	0.001
Carcinoma Recurrence	16.6	[7.5 - 36.8]	0.001
Time to Treatment	3.5	[1.8 - 7.0]	0.001
Thyroid Remnant Treatment	0.5	[0.4 - 0.7]	0.001
Tumor Stage [b]	2.3	[1.0 - 5.3]	0.001

[a] Cervical lymph nodes not present versus present
[b] Tumor stage II and III only; stage III patients with local tumor invasion are not included in this analysis.
[c] Remnant treatment is 1) none, 2) thyroid hormone alone 3) ^{131}I thyroid ablation and thyroid hormone.
[d] Patient age at the time of diagnosis divided into patients under age 40 years and 40 years and older
[e] One year or less versus over one year

Efficacy of ^{131}I Therapy for Macroscopic Residual or Recurrent Disease. The effectiveness of ^{131}I therapy is directly related to a tumor=s capacity to concentrate iodine. Even after meticulous preparation and large ^{131}I doses, many thyroid carcinomas do not concentrate ^{131}I in amounts sufficient to produce a therapeutic response. This is an age- and tumor-dependent phenomenon that occurs mostly among patients older than 40 years and in those with Hürthle cell tumors. In a study of 101 patients with distant metastases, ^{131}I was concentrated by 60% of papillary, 64% of follicular and only 36% of Hürthle cell carcinomas (54). In a study from Czechoslovakia (138), only half of 123 patients with pulmonary metastases had tumors that concentrated ^{131}I. Uptake was achieved more frequently in younger subjects (80%), in papillary cancers and in patients with fine pulmonary metastases on chest films. In a French study (88) two-thirds of 283 patients with lung or bone metastases had tumors that concentrated ^{131}I.

Although most studies report a favorable effect of ^{131}I upon outcome, some have failed to demonstrate this (110). One study reported improved survival with ^{131}I therapy only among patients over age 50 years (76). Another reported more recurrences after [131]I (14% and 1%) and more deaths after [131]I (5% and none) after seven years' follow-up of patients treated with ^{131}I compared with those treated with T_4 alone (139).

Others have reported more favorable results. In 1,599 patients with differentiated thyroid carcinoma treated at the M.D. Anderson Cancer Center between 1948 and 1989, ^{131}I therapy was the single most powerful prognostic indicator for increased disease-free survival (19). Low-risk patients sustained significantly fewer recurrences

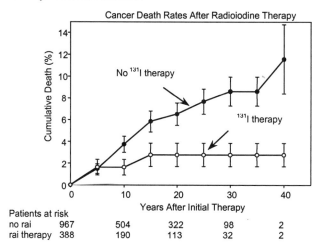

Patients at risk				
no rai	967	504	322	98	2
rai therapy	388	190	113	32	2

Figure 10. Differentiated thyroid carcinoma death rates after radioactive iodine compared with no preoperative radioiodine. Patients treated with ^{131}I had more advanced disease stage at the time of diagnosis. Adapted from Adapted from **Mazzaferri, E. L. and S. M. Jhiang.** 1994 Long-term impact of initial surgical and medical therapy on papillary and follicular thyroid cancer. Am J Med 97:418-428

and deaths after ^{131}I therapy than T_4 alone (P<0.001), while ^{131}I conferred only a slight advantage for high-risk patients.

We found that 30-year recurrence rates were 15% after ^{131}I plus T_4 therapy, 30% with T_4 alone, 40% with no medical therapy, and 63% after external radiation plus T_4, (P<0.001 between and among the four groups, Fig. 8). Although patients treated with ^{131}I had more advanced disease than those treated with T_4 alone, they had lower 30-year recurrence rates (16% versus 38%, P<0.001) and cancer mortality rates (3% versus 9%, P=0.03, Figure 10) than those not so treated.

Choice of Therapy. On the basis of our studies and those by other investigators, we believe that optimal initial therapy for most patients with differentiated thyroid carcinoma is near-total thyroidectomy followed by [131]I. (1,128,140,141) We do not treat patients with ^{131}I when there is no uptake in the thyroid bed and the serum Tg measured by immunometric assay is undetectable postoperatively, but this happens infrequently. We administer 30 mCi of ^{131}I when there is no evidence of carcinoma outside the thyroid and the serum Tg is measurable after surgery; larger doses are given when metastases are present or suspected on the basis of serum Tg concentrations above 10 ng/mL during thyroid hormone withdrawal.

Prognosis and The Impact of Therapy for Children and Young Adults.

Fewer than 10% of differentiated thyroid carcinomas occur in patients younger than 20 years (142). Treatment of children and adolescents is more controversial than it is in adults because not even large retrospective studies with a well-defined treatment protocol exist. Treatment has been so inconsistent that it is almost impossible to determine its influence on outcome (73).

Children and adolescents typically present with more advanced clinical disease, but their prognosis is excellent, although not as good as children without cancer. Survival rates at 15 to 20 years in series published since 1981 are over 90% (143). Some report few or no cancer deaths after three decades of follow-up of patients first treated under age 20 (144,145). Even children with distant metastases survive for long periods. Only one cancer death occurred among 66 children in one study after an average follow-up of about 15 years, although most (84%) had lymph node metastases and many (12%) had pulmonary metastases (146). Another study reported almost the same findings among 54 children treated aggressively and followed for several decades, although most (88%) had lymph node metastases and some (19%) had distant metastases (147). In a study of 72 children younger than age 16 years, 42% developed distant metastases, mostly to lung, but 70% had a complete remission (86).

An analysis of the course of differentiated thyroid carcinoma in 98 children from France followed up to 40 years reached four main conclusions. First, the extent of the disease at the time of initial treatment is advanced in most children. Second, the occurrence of neck (29%) and distant metastases (37%) as relapses are frequent. Third, the excess mortality caused by cancer is significant, with a standardized mortality ratio of 6.4, a ratio higher than in older patients. Fourth, younger age at initial treatment is of great prognostic importance since all six patients who died from thyroid carcinoma were younger than 10 when first treated. (98)

Another study from Italy (148) of 85 children younger than 18 years at the time of diagnosis reported that all patients were alive after a median period of 137 months. The authors concluded that ^{131}I is highly effective in treating lung metastases, but noted that undetectable serum Tg levels were seldom achieved. They felt that total thyroidectomy with ^{131}I therapy is an effective and safe treatment for the majority of patients with differentiated thyroid carcinoma diagnosed during childhood or adolescence.

In a comprehensive study of 140 children and adolescents younger than 19 years, 73% underwent total thyroidectomy and almost half were treated with [131]I (19). Forty percent had recurrences and 19% developed distant metastases, mostly (96%) to the lung. The results suggested that total thyroidectomy was the therapy of choice and that ^{131}I therapy was beneficial. Another study from the same institution reported that nearly 10% of 209 patients under age 25 years had pulmonary metastases at the time of diagnosis (89). Although most the lung metastases concentrated ^{131}I, almost half were not seen on x-ray, indicating that pulmonary metastases may be overlooked unless near-total thyroidectomy is followed by total body ^{131}I scanning in all children with regional lymph node metastases. These observations underscore the need for meticulous treatment of children with this disease and provide evidence that this is not always an indolent disease in the young.

Surgery is the treatment of choice, but there is no consensus concerning the optimal procedure (99). Some perform total or near-total thyroidectomy and cervical lymph node dissection if metastases are present, whereas others perform subtotal thyroidectomy (72,73). Surgical complications occur more frequently in children than in adults, even at large centers (99). Because the risk of cancer death is so low in children, the risk of complications thus constitutes the major reservation about performing more extensive surgery. There are strong arguments for a more aggressive approach in children: the high incidence of primary tumor multicentricity and metastases in children, the high recurrence rate and the fact that life expectancy exceeds 60 years.

Conclusion

Mortality from thyroid carcinoma has diminished in the past several decades. Data published by the National Cancer Institute indicates that there has been a gradual and significant improvement in 5-year survival rates for thyroid carcinoma of all types. Estimated to be around 83% in 1960-63, survival rates have increased from 91.8% in 1974-76 to 94.2% in 1981-86. (4) While several factors may be responsible for this improvement, it is likely that early diagnosis and effective management, particularly of differentiated thyroid carcinoma, accounts for much of it.

REFERENCES:

1. Mazzaferri EL, Jhiang SM. Long-term impact of initial surgical and medical therapy on papillary and follicular thyroid cancer. Am J Med 1994; 97:418-428.
2. Parker SL, Johnston Davis K, Wingo PA, Ries LAG, Heath CW, Jr. Cancer statistics, 998. CA 1998; 48:6-30.
3. Mazzaferri EL Thyroid carcinoma: Papillary and follicular. In: Mazzaferri EL, Samaan N, eds. Endocrine Tumors. Cambridge: Blackwell Scientific Publications Inc., 1993; 278-333.

4. Kosary CL, Ries LAG, Miller BA, Hankey BF, Harras A, Edwards BK. 1995 SEER Cancer Statistic Review, 1973-1992: Tables and Graphs. Bethesda, MD: National Cancer Institute. NIH Pub. No. 96-2789.

5. Crile GJ. Factors influencing the survival of patients with follicular carcinoma of the thyroid gland. Surg Gynecol Obstet 1985; 160:409-413.

6. Simpson WJ, Panzarella T, Carruthers JS, Gospodarowicz MK, Sutcliffe SB. Papillary and follicular thyroid cancer: impact of treatment in 1578 patients. Int J Radiat Oncol Biol Phys 1988; 14:1063-1075.

7. Carcangiu ML, Zampi G, Pupi A, Castagnoli A, Rosai J. Papillary carcinoma of the thyroid. A clinicopathologic study of 241 cases treated at the University of Florence, Italy. Cancer 1985; 55:805-828.

8. Coburn M, Teates D, Wanebo HJ. Recurrent thyroid cancer: Role of surgery *versus* radioactive iodine (I^{131}). Ann Surg 1994; 219:587-595.

9. Byar DP, Green SB, Dor P, et al. A prognostic index for thyroid carcinoma. A study of the E.O.R.T.C. Thyroid Cancer Cooperative Group. Eur J Cancer 1979; 15:1033-1041.

10. Wanebo HJ, Andrews W, Kaiser DL. Thyroid Cancer: Some basic considerations. Am J Surg 1981; 142:474-479.

11. Fourquet A, Asselain B, Joly J. Cancer de la thyroide: Analyse multidimensionnelle des facteurs pronostiques. Ann Endocrinol (Paris) 1983; 44:121-126.

12. Tubiana M, Schlumberger M, Rougier P, et al. Long-term results and prognostic factors in patients with differentiated thyroid carcinoma. Cancer 1985; 55:794-804.

13. Kerr DJ, Burt AD, Boyle P, MacFarlane GJ, Storer AM, Brewin TB. Prognostic factors in thyroid tumors. Br J Cancer 1986; 54:475-482.

14. Joensuu H, Klemi PJ, Paul R, Tuominen J. Survival and prognostic factors in thyroid carcinoma. Acta Radiologica Oncol 1986; 25:243-248.

15. Hay ID, Grant CS, Taylor WF, McConahey WM. Ipsilateral lobectomy versus bilateral lobar resection in papillary thyroid carcinoma: a retrospective analysis of surgical outcome using a novel prognostic scoring system. Surgery 1987; 102:1088-1095.

16. Schelfhout LJ, Creutzberg CL, Hamming JF, Fleuren GJ, Smeenk D, Hermans J. Multivariate analysis of survival in differentiated thyroid cancer: the prognostic significance of the age factor. Eur J Cancer 1988; 24:331-37.

17. Thoresen SO, Akslen LA, Glattre E, Haldorsen T, Lund EV, Schoultz M. Survival and prognostic factors in differentiated thyroid cancer--a multivariate analysis of 1,055 cases. Br J Cancer 1989; 59:231-235.

18. DeGroot LJ, Kaplan EL, McCormick M, Straus FH. Natural history, treatment, and course of papillary thyroid carcinoma. J Clin Endocrinol Metab 1990; 71:414-424.

19. Samaan NA, Schultz PN, Hickey RC, Haynie TP, Johnston DA, Ordonez NG. Well-differentiated thyroid carcinoma and the results of various modalities of treatment. A retrospective review of 1599 patients. J Clin Endocrinol Metab 1992 ; 75:714-720.

20. Akslen LA, Haldorsen T, Thoresen SO, Glattre E. Survival and causes of death in thyroid cancer: a population-based study of 2479 cases from Norway. Cancer Res 1991; 51:1234-1241.

21. Brennan MD, Bergstralh EJ, van Heerden JA, McConahey WM. Follicular thyroid cancer treated at the Mayo Clinic, 1946 through 1970: initial manifestations, pathologic findings, therapy, and outcome. Mayo Clin Proc 1991; 66:11-22.

22. Gilliland FD, Hunt WC, Morris DM, Key CR. Prognostic factors for thyroid carcinoma - A population- based study of 15,698 cases from the surveillance, epidemiology and end results (SEER) program 1973-1991. Cancer 1997; 79:564-573.

23. Tsang RW, Brierley JD, Simpson WJ, Panzarella T, Gospodarowicz MK, Sutcliffe SB. The effects of surgery, radioiodine, and external radiation therapy on the clinical outcome of patients with differentiated thyroid carcinoma. Cancer 1998; 82:375-388.

24. McConahey WM, Hay ID, Woolner LB, van Heerden JA, Taylor WF. Papillary thyroid cancer treated at the Mayo Clinic, 1946 through 1970: Initial manifestations, pathologic findings, therapy and outcome. Mayo Clin Proc 1986; 61:978-996.

25. Viswanathan K, Gierlowski TC, Schneider AB. Childhood thyroid cancer: Characteristics and long-term outcome in children irradiated for benign conditions of the head and neck. Am J Dis Child 1994; 148:260-265.

26. Thoresen S, Akslen LA, Glattre E, Haldorsen T. Thyroid cancer in children in Norway 1953-1987. Eur J Cancer [A] 1993; 29A:365-366.

27. Frankenthaler RA, Sellin RV, Cangir A, Goepfert H. Lymph node metastasis from papillary-follicular thyroid carcinoma in young patients. Am J Surg 1990; 160:341-343.

28. Cady B, Rossi R. An expanded view of risk-group definition in differentiated thyroid carcinoma. Surgery 1988; 104:947-953.

29. LiVolsi VA. Unusual variants of papillary thyroid carcinoma. In: Mazzaferri EL, Kreisberg RA, Bar RS, eds. Advances in Endocrinology and Metabolism. 6th ed. St. Louis: Mosby-Year Book, Inc., 1995; 39-54.

30. Johnson TL, Lloyd RV, Thompson NW, Beierwaltes WH, Sisson JC. Prognostic implications of the tall cell variant of papillary thyroid carcinoma. Am J Surg Pathol 1988; 12:22-27.

31. Harach HR, Zusman SB. 1992 Cytopathology of the tall cell variant of thyroid papillary carcinoma. Acta Cytol (Baltimore) 1992; 36:895-899.

32. Leung C-S, Hartwick RWJ, Bédard YC. Correlation of cytologic and histologic features in variants of papillary carcinoma of the thyroid. Acta Cytol 1993; 37:645-650.

33. Gimm O, Krause U, Wessel H, Finke R, Dralle H. Ectopic intrathyroidal thymus diagnosed as a solid thyroid lesion: Case report and review of the literature. J Pediatr Surg 1997; 32:1241-1243.

34. Rüter A, Dreifus J, Jones M, Nishiyama R, Lennquist S. Overexpression of p53 in tall cell variants of papillary thyroid carcinoma. Surgery 1996; 120:1046-1050.

35. Rüter A, Nishiyama R, Lennquist S. Tall-cell variant of papillary thyroid cancer: Disregarded entity. World J Surg 1997; 21:15-21.

36. Sobrinho-Simoes.M.A., Nesland JM, Johannessen JV. Columnar-cell carcinoma. Another variant of poorly differentiated carcinoma of the thyroid. Am J Clin Pathol 1988; 89:264-267.

37. Fujimoto Y, Obara T, Ito Y, Kodama T, Aiba M, Yamaguchi K. Diffuse sclerosing variant of papillary carcinoma of the thyroid. Clinical importance, surgical treatment, and follow-up study. Cancer 1990; 66:2306-2312.

38. Mizukami Y, Nonomura A, Michigishi T, et al. Diffuse sclerosing variant of papillary carcinoma of the thyroid. Report of three cases. Acta Pathol Jpn 1990; 40:676-682.

39. Tielens ET, Sherman SI, Hruban RH, Ladenson PW. Follicular variant of papillary thyroid carcinoma: A clinicopathologic study. Cancer 1994; 73:424-431.

40. Lang W, Choritz H, Hundeshagen H. Risk factors in follicular thyroid carcinomas:a retrospective follow-up study covering a 14-year period with emphasis on morphologic findings. Am J Surg Pathol 1986; 10:246-255.

41. Mazzaferri EL. Management of a solitary thyroid nodule. N Engl J Med 1993; 328:553-559.

42. van Heerden JA, Hay ID, Goellner JR, et al. Follicular thyroid carcinoma with capsular invasion alone: A nonthreatening malignancy. Surgery 1992; 112:1130-1138.

43. Emerick GT, Duh Q-Y, Siperstein AE, Burrow GN, Clark OH. Diagnosis, treatment, and outcome of follicular thyroid carcinoma. Cancer 1993; 72:3287-3295.

44. Donohue JH, Goldfien SD, Miller TR, Abele JS, Clark OH. Do the prognoses of papillary and follicular thyroid carcinomas differ? Am J Surg 1984; 148:168-173.

45. Beierwaltes WH, Nishiyama RH, Thompson NW, Copp JE, Kubo A. Survival time and "cure" in papillary and follicular thyroid carcinoma with distant metastases: statistics following University of Michigan therapy. J Nucl Med 1982; 23:561-568.

46. Balan KK, Raouf AH, Critchley M. Outcome of 249 patients attending a nuclear medicine department with well differentiated thyroid cancer; A 23 year review. Br J Radiol 1994; 67:283-291.

47. Ruegemer JJ, Hay ID, Bergstralh EJ, Ryan JJ, Offord KP, Gorman CA. Distant metastases in differentiated thyroid carcinoma: a multivariate analysis of prognostic variables. J Clin Endocrinol Metab 1988; 67:501-58.

48. Watson RG, Brennan MD, van Heerden JA, McConahey WM, Taylor WF. Invasive Hurthle cell carcinoma of the thyroid: Natural history and management. Mayo Clin Proc 1984; 59:851-855.

49. Rosen IB, Luk S, Katz I. Hurthle cell tumor behavior: dilemma and resolution. Surgery 1985; 98:777-783.

50. Thompson NW, Dunn EL, Batsakis JG, Nishiyama RH. Hurthle cell lesions of the thyroid gland. Surg Gynecol Obstet 1973; 139:555-560.

51. McDonald MP, Sanders LE, Silverman ML, Chan HS, Buyske J. Hurthle cell carcinoma of the thyroid gland: Prognostic factors and results of surgical treatment. Surgery 1996; 120:1000-1004.

52. Papotti M, Torchio B, Grassi L, Favero A, Bussolati G. Poorly differentiated oxyphilic (Hurthle cell) carcinomas of the thyroid. Am J Surg Pathol 1996; 20:686-694.

53. Arganini M, Behar R, Wu TC, et al. Hurthle cell tumors: a twenty-five-year experience. Surgery 1986; 100:1108-1115.

54. Samaan NA, Schultz PN, Haynie TP, Ordonez NG. Pulmonary metastasis of differentiated thyroid carcinoma: treatment results in 101 patients. J Clin Endocrinol Metab 1985; 60:376-380.
55. Herrera MF, Hay ID, Wu PS, et al. Hurthle cell (oxyphyilic) papillary thyroid carcinoma: a variant with more aggressive biologic behavior. World J Surg 1994; 16:669-674.
56. Beckner ME, Heffess CS, Oertel JE. Oxyphilic papillary thyroid carcinomas. Am J Clin Pathol 1995; 103:280-287.
57. Berho M, Suster S. The oncocytic variant of papillary carcinoma of the thyroid: A clinicopathologic study of 15 cases. Hum Pathol 1997; 28:47-53.
58. Apel RL, Asa SL, LiVolsi VA. Papillary Hürthle cell carcinoma with lymphocytic stroma: "Warthin-like tumor" of the thyroid. Am J Surg Pathol 1995; 19:810-814.
59. Ezzat S, Sarti DA, Cain DR, Braunstein GD. Thyroid incidentalomas: Prevalence by palpation and ultrasonography. Arch Intern Med 1994; 154:1838-1840.
60. Tan GH, Gharib H. Thyroid incidentalomas: Management approaches to nonpalpable nodules discovered incidentally on thyroid imaging. Ann Intern Med 1997; 126:226-231.
61. Hay ID. Papillary thyroid carcinoma. Endocrinol Metabol Clin North Am 1990; 19:545-576.
62. Allo MD, Christianson W, Doivunen D. Not all "occult" papillary carcinomas are "minimal". Surgery 1988; 104:971-976.
63. LiVolsi VA. Papillary lesions of the thyroid. In: LiVolsi VA, ed. Surgical Pathology of the Thyroid. Philadelphia: W.B.Saunders Company, 1990; 136-172.
64. Mazzaferri EL. Papillary thyroid carcinoma: factors influencing prognosis and current therapy. Semin Oncol 1987; 14:315-332.
65. DeGroot LJ, Kaplan EL. Second operations for "completion" of thyroidectomy in treatment of differentiated thyroid cancer. Surgery 1991; 110:936-940.
66. Rao RS, Fakih AR, Mehta AR, Agarwal R, Raghavan A, Shrikhande SS. Completion thyroidectomy for thyroid carcinoma. Head Neck Surg 1987; 9:284-286.
67. Auguste LJ, Attie JN. Completion thyroidectomy for initially misdiagnosed thyroid cancer. Otolaryngol Clin North Am 1990; 23:429-439.
68. Crile GJ, Antunez AR, Esselstyn CBJ, Hawk WA, Skillern PG. The advantages of subtotal thyroidectomy and suppression of TSH in the primary treatment of papillary carcinoma of the thyroid. Cancer 1985; 55:2691-2697.
69. Massin JP, Savoie JC, Garnier H, Guiraudon G, Leger FA, Bacourt F. Pulmonary metastases in differentiated thyroid carcinoma. Study of 58 cases with implications for the primary tumor treatment. Cancer 1984; 53:982-992.
70. Cody HSI, Shah JP. Locally invasive, well-differentiated thyroid cancer. 22 years' experience at Memorial Sloan-Kettering Cancer Center. Am J Surg 1981; 142:480-483.
71. Salvesen H, Njolstad PR, Akslen LA, Albrektsen G, Soreide O, Varhaug JE. Papillary thyroid carcinoma: A multivariate analysis of prognostic factors including an evaluation of the p-TNM staging system. Eur J Surg 1992; 158:583-589.
72. Hung W. Well-differentiated thyroid carcinomas in children and adolescents: a review. Endocrinologist 1994; 4:117-126.
73. De Keyser LFM, Van Herle AJ. Differentiated thyroid cancer in children. Head Neck Cancer 1985; 8:100-114.
74. Attie JN, Setzin M, Klein I. Thyroid carcinoma presenting as an enlarged cervical lymph node. Am J Surg 1993; 166:428-430.
75. Hay ID, Bergstralh EJ, Goellner JR, Ebersold JR, Grant CS. Predicting outcome in papillary thyroid carcinoma: Development of a reliable prognostic scoring system in a cohort of 1779 patients surgically treated at one institution during 1940 through 1989. Surgery 1993; 114:1050-1058.
76. Cunningham MP, Duda RB, Recant W, Chmiel JS, Sylvester JA, Fremgen A. Survival discriminants for differentiated thyroid cancer. Am J Surg 1990; 160:344-347.
77. Scheumann GFW, Gimm O, Wegener G, Hundeshagen H, Dralle H. Prognostic significance and surgical management of locoregional lymph node metastases in papillary thyroid cancer. World J Surg 1994; 18:559-568.
78. Rösler H, Birrer A, Lüscher D, Kinser J. Long-term course in differentiated thyroid carcinoma. Schweiz Med Wochenschr 1992; 122:1843-1857.
79. Sellers M, Beenken S, Blankenship A, et al. Prognostic significance of cervical lymph node metastases in differentiated thyroid cancer. Am J Surg 1992; 164:578-581.
80. Coburn MC, Wanebo HJ. Prognostic factors and management considerations in patients with cervical metastases of thyroid cancer. Am J Surg 1992; 164:671-676.

81. McHenry CR, Rosen IB, Walfish PG. Prospective management of nodal metastases in differentiated thyroid cancer. Am J Surg 1991; 162:353-357.
82. Hoie J, Stenwig AE, Kullmann G, Lindegaard M. Distant metastases in papillary thyroid cancer. A review of 91 patients. Cancer 1988; 61:1-6.
83. Yamashita H, Noguchi S, Murakami N, Kawamoto H, Watanabe S. Extracapsular invasion of lymph node metastasis is an indicator of distant metastasis and poor prognosis in patients with thyroid papillary carcinoma. Cancer 1997; 80:2268-2272.
84. Solan MJ. Multiple primary carcinomas as sequelae of treatment of pulmonary tuberculosis with repeated induced pneumothoraces. Case report and review of the literature. Am J Clin Oncol 1991; 14:49-51.
85. Casara D, Rubello D, Saladini G, et al. Different features of pulmonary metastases in differentiated thyroid cancer: Natural history and multivariate statistical analysis of prognostic variables. J Nucl Med 1993; 34:1626-1631.
86. Schlumberger M, De Vathaire F, Travagli JP, et al. Differentiated thyroid carcinoma in childhood: long term follow-up of 72 patients. J Clin Endocrinol Metab 1987; 65:1088-1094.
87. Brown AP, Greening WP, McCready VR, Shaw HJ, Harmer CL. Radioiodine treatment of metastatic thyroid carcinoma: the Royal Marsden Hospital experience. Br J Radiol 1984; 57:323-327.
88. Schlumberger M, Tubiana M, De Vathaire F, et al. Long-term results of treatment of 283 patients with lung and bone metastases from differentiated thyroid carcinoma. J Clin Endocrinol Metab 1986; 63:960-967.
89. Vassilopoulou-Sellin R, Klein MJ, Smith TH, et al. Pulmonary metastases in children and young adults with differentiated thyroid cancer. Cancer 1993; 71:1348-1352.
90. Mazzaferri EL. Treating high thyroglobulin with radioiodine. A magic bullet or a shot in the dark?. J Clin Endocrinol Metab 1995; 80:1485-1487.
91. Schlumberger M, Mancusi F, Baudin E, Pacini F. 131-I Therapy for elevated thyroglobulin levels. Thyroid 1997; 7:273-276.
92. Hurley DL, Sizemore GW, McConahey WM. Prolonged remission of metastatic follicular thyroid carcinoma. Mayo Clin Proc 1993; 68:1205-1209.
93. Maruyama M, Sugenoya A, Kobayashi S, Masuda H, Shimizu T, Iida F. A case of papillary carcinoma of the thyroid with more than 30 years long-term asymptomatic pulmonary metastases. Clin Endocrinol 1993; 38:331-336.
94. Brierley JD, Panzarella T, Tsang RW, Gospodarowicz MK, O'Sullivan B. A comparison of different staging systems predictability of patient outcome - Thyroid carcinoma as an example. Cancer 1997; 79:2414-2423.
95. Loh KC, Greenspan FS, Gee L, Miller TR, Yeo PPB. Pathological tumor-node-metastasis (pTNM) staging for papillary and follicular thyroid carcinomas: A retrospective analysis of 700 patients. J Clin Endocrinol Metab 1997; 82:3553-3562.
96. American Joint Committee on Cancer. Head and Neck Tumors. Thyroid Gland. In: Beahrs OH, Henson DE, Hutter RVP, Myers MH, eds. Manual for Staging of Cancer. 4th ed. Philadelphia: J.B.Lippincott, 1992; 53-54.
97. Shaha AR, Loree TR, Shah JP. Prognostic factors and risk group analysis in follicular carcinoma of the thyroid. Surgery 1995; 118:1131-1138.
98. Travagli JP, Schlumberger M, De Vathaire F, Francese C, Parmentier C. Differentiated thyroid carcinoma in childhood. J Endocrinol Invest 1995; 18:161-164.
99. Zimmerman D, Hay I, Bergstralh E. 1992 Papillary thyroid carcinoma in children. In: Robbins J, ed. Treatment of thryoid cancer in childhood: Proceedings of a workshop held September 10-11, 1992, at the NIH in Bethesda MD. DOE/EH-0406, Springfield, VA: U.S. Dept of Commerce, 3-10.
100. Van De Velde CJH, Hamming JF, Goslings BM, et al. Report of the consensus development conference on the management of differentiated thyroid cancer in the Netherlands. Eur J Cancer Clin Oncol 1988; 24:287-292.
101. Ottino A, Pianzola HM, Castelletto RH. Occult papillary thyroid carcinoma at autopsy in La Plata, Argentina. Cancer 1989; 64:547-551.
102. Solomon BL, Wartofsky L, Burman KD. Current trends in the management of well differentiated papillary thyroid carcinoma. J Clin Endocrinol Metab 1996; 81:333-339.
103. Rosen IB, Bowden J, Luk SC, Simpson JA. Aggressive thyroid cancer in low-risk age population. Surgery 1987; 102:1075-1080.

104. Jocham A, Joppich I, Hecker W, Knorr D, Schwarz HP. Thyroid carcinoma in childhood: Management and follow up of 11 cases. Eur J Pediatr 1994; 153:17-22.
105. Utiger RD. Follow-up of patients with thyroid carcinoma. N Engl J Med 1997; 337:928-930.
106. Schlumberger MJ. Papillary and follicular thyroid carcinoma. N Engl J Med 1998; 338:297-306.
107. Baldet L, Manderscheid JC, Glinoer D, Jaffiol C, Coste Seignovert B, Percheron C. The management of differentiated thyroid cancer in Europe in 1988 Results of an international survey. Acta Endocrinol (Copenh) 1989; 120:547-558.
108. Filetti S, Belfiore A, Amir SM, et al. The role of thyroid-stimulating antibodies of Graves' disease in differentiated thyroid cancer. N Engl J Med 1988; 318:753-79.
109. Carayon P, Guibout M, Lissitzky S. Thyrotropin receptor-adenylate cyclase system in plasma membranes from normal and diseased human thyroid glands.   J Endocrinol Invest 1978; 1:321-328.
110. Dulgeroff AJ, Hershman JM. Medical therapy for differentiated thyroid carcinoma. Endocrinol Rev 1994; 15:500-515.
111. Dulgeroff AJ, Geffner ME, Koyal SN, Wong M, Hershman JM. Bromocriptine and triac therapy for hyperthyroidism dur to pituitary resistance to thyroid hormone.   J Clin Endocrinol Metab 1992; 75:1071-1075.
112. Rossi RL, Cady B, Silverman ML, et al. Surgically incurable well-differentiated thyroid carcinoma. Prognostic factors and results of therapy. Arch Surg 1988; 123:569-574.
113. Cady B, Cohn K, Rossi RL, et al. The effect of thyroid hormone administration upon survival in patients with differentiated thyroid carcinoma. Surgery 1983; 94:978-983.
114. Mazzaferri EL. Thyroid cancer and Graves' disease. J Clin Endocrinol Metab 1990; 70:826-829.
115. Clark OH. TSH suppression in the management of thyroid nodules and thyroid cancer. World J Surg 1981; 5:39-47.
116. Radetti G, Castellan C, Tatò L, Platter K, Gentili L, Adami S. Bone mineral density in children and adolescent females treated with high doses of L-thyroxine. Horm Res 1993; 39:127-131.
117. Faber J, Galloe AM. Changes in bone mass during prolonged subclinical hyperthyroidism due to L-thyroxine treatment: A meta-analysis. Acta Endocrinol (Copenh) 1994; 130:350-356.
118. Panebianco P, Rosso D, Destro G, et al. Use of disphosphonates in the treatment of osteoporosis in thyroidectomized patients on levothyroxin replacement therapy. Arch Gerontol Geriatr 1997; 25:219-225.
119. Biondi B, Fazio S, Carella C, et al. Cardiac effects of long term thyrotropin-suppressive therapy with levothyroxine. J Clin Endocrinol Metab 1993; 77:334-338.
120. Sawin CT, Geller A, Wolf PA, et al. Low serum thyrotropin concentrations as a risk factor for atrial fibrillation in older persons. N Engl J Med 1994; 331:1249-1252.
121. Burmeister LA, Goumaz MO, Mariash CN, Oppenheimer JH. Levothyroxine dose requirements for thyrotropin suppression in the treatment of differentiated thyroid cancer. J Clin Endocrinol Metab 1992; 75:344-350.
122. Bartalena L, Martino E, Pacchiarotti A, et al. Factors affecting suppression of endogenous thyrotropin secretion by thyroxine treatment: retrospective analysis in athyreotic and goitrous patients. J Clin Endocrinol Metab 1987; 64:849-855.
123. Wartofsky L. Use of sensitive TSH assay to determine optimal thyroid hormone therapy and avoid osteoporosis. Annu Rev Med 1991; 42:341-345.
124. Wong JB, Kaplan MM, Meyer KB, Pauker SG. Ablative radioactive iodine therapy for apparently localized thyroid carcinoma. A decision analytic perspective. Endocrinol Metabol Clin North Am 1990; 19:741-760.
125. Beierwaltes WH, Rabbani R, Dmuchowski C, Lloyd RV, Eyre P, Mallette S. An analysis of "ablation of thyroid remnants" with I-131 in 511 patients from 1947-1984:Experience at University of Michigan. J Nucl Med 1984; 25:1287-1293.
126. Goolden AWG. The indications for ablating normal thyroid tissue with 131-I in differentiated thyroid cancer. Clin Endocrinol 1985; 23:81-86.
127. Stael APM, Plukker JTM, Piers DA, Rouwé CW, Vermey A. Total thyroidectomy in the treatment of thyroid carcinoma in childhood. Br J Surg 1995; 82:1083-1085.
128. Mazzaferri EL. Thyroid remnant ^{131}I ablation for papillary and follicular thyroid carcioma. Thyroid 1997; 7:265-271.
129. DeGroot LJ, Reilly M. Comparison of 30- and 50-mCi doses of iodine-131 for thyroid ablation. Ann Intern Med 1982; 96:51-53.

130. Maxon HR, Englaro EE, Thomas SR, et al. Radioiodine-131 therapy for well-differentiated thyroid cancer -- a quantitative radiation dosimetric approach: outcome and validation in 85 patients. J Nucl Med 1992; 33:1132-1136.

131. Maxon HR, Thomas SR, Hertzberg VS, et al. Relation between effective radiation dose and outcome of radioiodine therapy for thyroid cancer. N Engl J Med 1983; 309:937-941.

132. Snyder J, Gorman C, Scanion P. Thyroid remnant ablation:Questionable pursuit of an ill-defined goal. J Nucl Med 1983; 24:659-665.

133. Kuni CC, Klingensmith WC. Failure of low doses of 131-I to ablate residual thyroid tissue following surgery for thyroid cancer. Radiology 1980; 137:773-774.

134. Siddiqui AR, Edmondson J, Wellman HN, et al. Feasibility of low doses of I-131 for thyroid ablation in postsurgical patients with thyroid carcinoma. Clin Nucl Med 1981; 6:158-161.

135. Ramanna L, Waxman AD, Brachman MB, Tanasescu DE, Sensel N, Braunstein GD. Evaluation of low-dose radioiodine ablation therapy in postsurgical thyroid cancer patients. Clin Nucl Med 1985; 10:791-795.

136. Johansen K, Woodhouse NJ, Odugbesan O. Comparison of 1073 MBq and 3700 MBq iodine-131 in postoperative ablation of residual thyroid tissue in patients with differentiated thyroid cancer. J Nucl Med 1991; 32:252-254.

137. Ozata M, Suzuki S, Miyamoto T, Liu RT, Fierro-Renoy F, DeGroot LJ. Serum thyroglobulin in the follow-up of patients with treated differentiated thyroid cancer. J Clin Endocrinol Metab 1994 ; 79:98-105.

138. Nêmec J, Zamrazil V, Pohunková D, Röhling S. Radioiodide treatment of pulmonary metastases of differentiated thyroid cancer. Results and prognostic factors. Nuklearmedizin 1979; 18:86-90.

139. McHenry C, Jarosz H, Davis M, Barbato AL, Lawrence AM, Paloyan E. Selective postoperative radioactive iodine treatment of thyroid carcinoma. Surgery 1989; 106:956-958.

140. Mazzaferri EL. Carcinoma of follicular epithelium: radiodine and other treatment outcomes. In: Braverman LE, Utiger RD, eds. The Thyroid: A Fundamental and Clinical Text. 7th ed. Philadelphia: Lippencott-Raven Pub., 1996; 922-945.

141. Mazzaferri EL. Impact of initial tumor features and treatment selected on the long-term course of differentiated thyroid cancer. Thyroid Today 1995; 18:1-13.

142. National Cancer Institute. Cancer Statistics Review 1973-87. Bethesda, MD: U.S. Department of Health and Human Service, Public Health Service, National Institutes of Health, 1991; I.39-III.36.

143. Gorlin JB, Sallan SE. Thyroid cancer in childhood. Endocrinol Metabol Clin North Am 1990; 19:649-662.

144. Buckwalter JA, Gurll NJ, Thomas CGJ. Cancer of the thyroid in youth. World J Surg 1981; 5:15-25.

145. La Quaglia MP, Corbally MT, Heller G, Exelby PR, Brennan MF. Recurrence and morbidity in differentiated thyroid carcinoma in children. Surgery 1988; 104:1149-1156.

146. Goepfert H, Dichtel WJ, Samaan NA. Thryoid cancer in children and teenagers. Arch Otolaryngol 1984; 110:72-75.

147. Harness JK, Thompson NW, McLeod MK, et al. Differentiated thyroid carcinoma in children and adolescents. World J Surg 1992; 16:547-554.

148. Dottorini ME, Vignati A, Mazzucchelli L, Lomuscio G, Colombo L. Differentiated thyroid carcinoma in children and adolescents: A 37-year experience in 85 patients. J Nucl Med 1997; 38:669-675.

12 RADIOIODINE AND EXTERNAL RADIATION THERAPY IN THE TREATMENT OF THYROID CANCER

James Brierley, M.D.
The Ontario Cancer Institute/Princess Margaret Hospital
Toronto, Canada

Harry R. Maxon, M.D.
University of Cincinnati
Cincinnati, Ohio

Radioiodine Therapy
Harry R. Maxon, M.D.

Historical Caveats

For over 50 years, radioiodine-131 has been used in the post surgical treatment of differentiated thyroid cancer (1). In 1957, workers at the University of Michigan popularized ^{131}I in an easy to use, empiric approach that recommended the administration of fixed activities of ^{131}I to patients who were allowed to become hypothyroid after their initial surgical therapy (2). It soon became evident that only about 70-80% of differentiated thyroid cancers would concentrate ^{131}I under these conditions (3). When patients whose recurrent/metastatic cancers could not be shown to concentrate ^{131}I on diagnostic ^{131}I scans were excluded, then ^{131}I therapy given to the point of "ablation" of ^{131}I uptake on subsequent diagnostic scans resulted in a significant improvement in mortality (4). The methods of patient preparation and treatment that were developed during the first 25 years of ^{131}I use have not been modified in most health care facilities. In part this has been due to a shift in physician training. During the first 25 years, about 80% of nuclear medicine physicians entered the field from backgrounds in internal medicine, resulting in interest and training both in diseases of the thyroid and in the use of radioactive medicine by radiologists who are interested primarily in image interpretation or by endocrinologists who are not broadly trained in the intricacies of the use of radioactive materials, both of which groups find the decades old empiric approaches convenient to use.

Many problems that were identified decades ago remain today. They include but are not limited to the following items that will be addressed:

1. Determination of who does and who does not need post operative ^{131}I therapy.

2. Patient preparation for therapy, including extent of initial surgery, elevation of TSH levels, low iodine diet, and lithium carbonate.

3. Acute and chronic side effects.

4. Benefits of therapy.

5. Treatment of children.

6. Diagnostic ^{131}I scans negative/Tg positive patients.

7. Choice of isotopes of iodine.

8. Selection of individually optimal activities of ^{131}I for therapy - risk vs. benefit.

9. Radiation safety considerations: outpatient vs. inpatient.

Definitions:

The phrase *radioiodine therapy* refers to the treatment of residual or recurrent thyroid cancer within the thyroid bed and to the treatment of metastatic thyroid cancer outside the thyroid bed. The use of radioactive iodine for the destruction of residual, macroscopically normal thyroid tissue following surgical thyroidectomy is referred to as *radioiodine ablation* of thyroid remnants.

   Differentiated thyroid cancer refers to papillary and to follicular carcinomas. The papillary carcinomas include so-called mixed papillary and follicular carcinomas.

   Microscopic residual disease indicates microscopic residual tumor at or within 2 mm of the surgical resection line, whereas *gross residual disease* is residual cancer evident to the surgeon.

   Recurrent disease refers to recurrence of cancer in the neck after a presumed disease-free interval.

   Nodal metastasis is used to indicate a focus of cancer in a lymph node in the cervical or supraclavicular chain in the neck.

   Distant metastasis refers to metastatic disease outside the confines of the neck.

   For the purpose of comparison with older papers, the administered activities of ^{131}I are given in millicuries (mCi) and radiation doses in rad. For conversions to international nomenclature, 30 mCi = 1.1 GBq; 100 mCi = 3.7 GBq; 150 mCi = 5.5 GBq; 1 rad = 1 cGy. In the section on external radiation in keeping with radiation oncology nomenclature, the Gray (Gy) will be used as the unit of absorbed dose of radiation, 1 Gy =100cGy = 100rads.

Selection of Patients for Radioiodine Therapy

Radioiodine therapy is given post operatively 1) to ablate thyroid residua in order to destroy occult microfoci that may remain; 2) to remove residual thyroid tissue that may be a source of thyroglobulin that can confound the use of that assay for follow-up; and 3) to permit predictively useful scanning using the large therapy administration to detect unsuspected metastases (5). Patients who are at low risk for recurrent or metastatic disease and who would not require ^{131}I therapy would be adults between the ages of 20 and 45 years at the time of diagnosis, with no past history of radiation to the thyroid gland, no family history or genetic evidence of familial thyroid cancer, and who have non-tall cell papillary thyroid cancer or minimally invasive well differentiated follicular cancer without vascular involvement that is completely intrathyroidal, unifocal, 1.5 cm or less in size, and not associated with any known local nodal or distant metastases (6).

All other patients with differentiated thyroid cancer are, in our opinion, candidates for post operative ^{131}I therapy. Such treatment has been associated with significant improvements in recurrence and in mortality (7,8). Given recent improvements in U.S. Nuclear Regulatory Commission Guidelines (9), patients may be treated as outpatients with much larger administered activities than were permitted previously, so long as meticulous attention is paid to careful measurements and documentation of such things as neck and whole body retention, the effective half-life of radioiodine in the body, the patient's living conditions, and time spent in proximity to other people. Patient instructions must be detailed and complete. However, when this is accomplished, then we calculate that up to 220 mCi of ^{131}I may be administered safely as an outpatient to many patients who have only post thyroidectomy residua that take up no more than 5% of the total activity. This removes most of the past economic and emotional pressure to treat patients with what may have been suboptimal activities in order to avoid hospitalization.

Pregnant or lactating women should never be treated with radioiodine.

Patient Preparation

Extent of Surgery

If a patient is considered to be a candidate for ^{131}I ablation, then that patient also should have undergone a total or near total thyroidectomy, leaving no more than about 2 grams of thyroid tissue(7,8). Response rates to thyroid ablative therapy with ^{131}I are significantly lower when patients have had less than a total or near total thyroidectomy or have a mass of residual thyroid tissue calculated to be more than 2 grams. The two most important factors in determining success are the mass of residual tissue and the effective half-time of ^{131}I in that tissue. The calculated instantaneous percent uptake of ^{131}I in the residual tissue is highly correlated with and unseparable from the mass of the residual tissue (10).

Thyroid Hormone Withdrawal

The ability of the pituitary gland to secrete TSH may require up to several months to recover after prolonged suppressive therapy with thyroid hormone (11). Traditionally, serum thyroxine containing medications have been stopped for 6 weeks prior to ^{131}I administration. Shorter acting L-triiodothyroxine (T3) has been administered for the first 3 weeks of the 6 week period to minimize potential stimulatory growth effects on the thyroid cancer as well as patient discomfort. The T3 administered is a total daily amount of no more than 0.3 micrograms per pound of body weight in divided doses. Following cessation of T3, there is a roughly exponential rise in serum TSH levels, with a peak at 3 weeks after cessation (12). Serum TSH concentrations of 30 μU/ml or more appear to be adequate for stimulation of uptake in iodine concentrating metastases (13). Mean neck and whole body radioiodine retention do not appear to be significantly different between 2 and 4 weeks off T3 (14). We routinely recommend the administration of T3 for the first 3 weeks after total thyroidectomy or after cessation of T4-containing preparations, followed by 3 weeks off all thyroid hormone. Using this approach, 90% of our patients have serum TSH concentrations of at least 30 μU/ml after 6 weeks. All of the 10% whose serum TSH level was less than 30 μU/ml by 6 weeks had unequivocal ^{131}I concentrating residual thyroid tissue or metastases (15).

Because clinical hypothyroidism that results from traditional thyroid hormone withdrawal is so unpleasant for patients, a reduced T4 dosage format for patient preparation has been proposed in which the patient's usual daily dose of L-thyroxine is changed to an every other day administration. When the patient's basal TSH was 1 μU/ml or greater (mean 2.9 ± 2.0 μU/ml), then 5/6 patients had a serum TSH of 25 μU/ml or greater after 5 weeks on protocol. When the basal TSH level was less than 1 μU/ml (mean 0.13 ± 0.17 μU/ml), then a serum TSH concentration of 25 μU/ml or greater could be achieved in 5/7 patients only after 8-12 weeks on protocol. The patient's symptoms of hypothyroidism were significantly better on the every other day protocol (16). In patients who are least likely to tolerate complete cessation and later restart-up of thyroid hormone (e.g. elderly patients with cardiac disease), this approach may prove to be quite useful so long as the patient's serum TSH levels are monitored sequentially to ensure adequate stimulation for ^{131}I scanning.

Exogenous TSH Stimulation

Bovine TSH was used for many years to stimulate radioiodine uptake, but it was associated with both allergic reactions and the development of neutralizing antibodies to both human and bovine TSH (17) and has been withdrawn from the U.S. market. Fortunately, recombinant human TSH (rhTSH) has been developed and currently is awaiting approval by the U.S. Food and Drug Administration. In a recent clinical trial (18), diagnostic ^{131}I scans were obtained both after traditional thyroid hormone withdrawal and after the administration of rhTSH while the patient was euthyroid. The two sets of scans were concordant in 106/127 (83%) patients. In 18/127 (14%) patients the scans after thyroid hormone withdrawal were thought to be superior, and in 8 of these 18 patients ^{131}I therapy was given based on the withdrawal scans. Thus, the diagnostic application of rhTSH may be most useful in patients who either have a low prescan likelihood of recurrent or metastatic disease, cannot respond to hormone withdrawal (e.g. hypopituitarism), or cannot tolerate hypothyroidism.

The kinetics of ^{131}I in euthyroid patients prepared with rhTSH are quite different from the kinetics of ^{131}I in hypothyroid patients. In hypothyroid patients renal function (19) and the renal clearance of iodine are markedly decreased (20), resulting in about a 50% decrease in renal clearance of ^{131}I and a 50% increase in bio-availability of ^{131}I as compared with euthyroid patients receiving rhTSH (20). This is especially important when considering ^{131}I therapy, and previous dogma regarding the activities of ^{131}I to be administered empirically to hypothyroid patients may not be applicable to patients prepared with rhTSH.

Iodine Depletion Regimens

The combination of a low iodine diet and a forced diuresis program resulted in a 2-3 fold increase in 24 hour radioiodine uptake in 16/25 (64%) patients with inoperable thyroid cancer (21). However, while such a combination may increase both uptake and retention by 146%, the iodine clearance may decrease by 56%, probably due to sodium and volume depletion, resulting in a 68% increase in total body radiation dose (22). Indeed, forced diuresis appears to be unnecessary, with a low iodine diet being able to approximately double the radiation dose to both cancer (23) and thyroid remnants (24). The effect of a low iodine regimen is not altered by the administration of T3 (25). Low iodine diets both in a food exchange formulation (24) and in a simplified format (25) have been published. We have used the exchange format diet for nearly two decades with success. Although patients do complain about its limitations, they tolerate it quite well. We institute the diet one week prior to the diagnostic ^{131}I scans and continue it until 3-24 hours after the therapy.

Medications such as amiodarone that are very high in iodine content will prohibit successful ^{131}I therapy. Other iodinated radiographic contrast media and antiseptics need to be stopped 2-12 weeks prior to initiation of the diagnostic ^{131}I scans (26).

Lithium Carbonate

The failure of ^{131}I in the treatment of thyroid cancer is often related to poor biologic retention of [131]I (15). When administered at pharmacological doses, lithium carbonate results in a significant decrease in radioiodine release from differentiated thyroid cancer, particularly when the tissue is damaged or inflamed by radiation.

Treatment of the patient with lithium carbonate prior to and during ^{131}I therapy may lead to a 4 fold decrease in the rate of ^{131}I release, resulting in an increase in radiation dose to the tumor of 50% when the biologic half-time of ^{131}I in tumor without lithium is 10 days and of 190% when it is only 2 days (27). The impact of lithium carbonate in lengthening the biological half-life of ^{131}I in metastatic tissue is greater than its effect on normal residual thyroid tissue (27,28). An administration of lithium carbonate (not sustained release) in a total daily dose of 10 mg/kg body weight, given in 3 divided portions daily with meals, appears to be adequate (28) and is tolerated by about 80% of patients in our experience. We initiate treatment with lithium at the same time as the low iodine diet and continue lithium for 5-7 days after the administration of [131]I. The patient must be closely monitored for lithium toxicity (29). The release of large amounts of radioiodinated thyroglobulin from large tumor masses in lithium treated patients may result in higher than anticipated radiation doses to the blood, with an associated dramatic bone marrow depression (27). We recommend quantitative blood dosimetry (see below) in all patients who are being prepared with lithium carbonate and closely monitor their complete blood counts for 6-10 weeks after ^{131}I therapy.

Gut Retention of Radioiodine

Radioiodine is found in tears, saliva, and gastric secretions and often is present in the bowel. In patients with normal kidneys, the whole body radiation dose from ^{131}I therapy reflects the effective whole body half-time of [131]I. In a review of 101 diagnostic ^{131}I studies on 64 patients, the effective whole body half-life of ^{131}I was greater in patients with large amounts of gut activity (mean 22.5 hours) than in those with very little gut activity (mean 14.5 hours, $p<0.05$) (30). We routinely insist that our patients have at least 1-2 bowel movements per day. If needed, a noniodine containing laxative (plain milk of magnesia), bowel stimulant (bisacodyl suppositories), and/or a lubricant (mineral oil enema) are prescribed.

Side Effects and Complications of Radioiodine Therapy

Acute/Subacute

Radiation Sickness. A syndrome consisting of headache, nausea, and occasional vomiting occurs in 60-70% of patients after the oral administration of about 200 mCi of ^{131}I for thyroid cancer (31,32). The symptoms begin 4-13 hours and usually resolve by 24-36 hours after the administration of [131]I (31). In our experience this syndrome is uncommon at administered activities of 100 mCi or less in adults. When it occurs, in its most severe form, supportive care with intravenous fluids and potent parenteral antiemetics such as ondansetron hydrochloride may be useful.

Salivary Gland Dysfunction. Radioiodine induced salivary gland inflammation and dysfunction has been recognized for over 40 years (33,34,35). Radiation doses to the salivary glands during the first 12 hours after a 100-200 mCi administration of ^{131}I may be as high as 700 rad (35). Symptoms such as parotid swelling, altered taste, and/or dry mouth are associated with a delayed peak uptake (15 hours vs. 3

hours), slower clearance, and higher radiation dose (3,000-30,000 rad vs. 300 rad or less) to the salivary glands than in patients without clinical evidence of sialoadenitis or salivary gland dysfunction (36). Clinical salivary gland problems rarely occur at administered activities below 70 mCi of ^{131}I but are common after administrations of 150 mCi or more (37). However, up to 70% of 21 asymptomatic patients treated with relatively large amounts of ^{131}I (mean 275 mCi) had salivary gland dysfunction as determined by ^{99m}TcO$_4^-$ uptake and excretion (38). Decreased quantity and quality of saliva in turn promote dental decay which can alter the integrity of the mandible (39).

The secretion of saliva and the composition of saliva are modulated by the parasympathetic and sympathetic systems respectively (40,41). Increasing salivary flow by having the patient suck on lemons the day of and for several days after ^{131}I therapy has been advocated as a means of decreasing the radiation dose to 1/5 - 1/10 by decreasing salivary gland retention time (42). Blocking norepinephrine receptors by the administration of reserpine 0.25 mg by mouth daily, beginning on the day of the diagnostic ^{131}I administration and continuing for one week after ^{131}I therapy, can significantly decrease parotid uptake of ^{131}I (43). Amifostine, a prodrug that is dephosphorylated in tissues to a pharmacologically active free thiol metabolite that can reduce the toxic effects of the chemotherapeutic agent, Cisplatin, has been shown to have a radioprotective effect on the salivary glands of rabbits treated with ^{131}I (44). Whether the drug can be used safely and effectively in humans for this purpose is unknown.

Peripheral Nerve Dysfunction. Two cases of vocal cord paralyses after ^{131}I therapy for thyroid cancer have been reported in patients with extensive disease. In one, the cancer was considered to be inoperable, and ^{131}I was used in an attempt to ablate the entire gland. In the other, extensive but incomplete surgery was performed with some cord dysfunction being noted immediately postoperatively that progressed to permanent paresis following ^{131}I to ablate residual tissue (45). Clearly this is an uncommon occurrence. Peripheral facial nerve paralysis after high activity ^{131}I therapy for papillary thyroid cancer also has been reported (46).

^{131}I Induced Edema in Central Nervous System Metastases. Brain metastases from differentiated thyroid cancer are relatively uncommon with a prevalence of only about 1-2%. They usually (about 80%) occur in the presence of other distant metastases, and most (about 80%) do not concentrate sufficient ^{131}I for therapy (47). When ^{131}I concentrating brain metastases are present, ^{131}I induced acute cerebral edema may occur. The use of dexamethasone, glycerol, or mannitol to prevent acute cerebral edema may be helpful (48). Spinal cord compression also may occur after ^{131}I therapy for metastases in or adjacent to the cord (49), and it would seem prudent to follow similar precautions in such cases. Pseudotumor cerebri has been reported in patients with thyroid cancer who are hypothyroid in preparation for ^{131}I administrations and must not be confused with metastatic disease (50).

Bone Marrow Depression. Bone marrow depression after ^{131}I therapy usually is maximal about 6 weeks after treatment. There is a rough correlation between administered activity and the incidence and severity of the resulting cytopenia. When careful whole blood dosimetry is performed, serious bone marrow depression is rare when the maximum dose to the whole blood from a single administration of ^{131}I is less than 200 rad (51,52). Current methodology allows useful predictive estimates of whole blood dose in hypothyroid patients undergoing diagnostic ^{131}I pretherapy studies using sequential external counting available in any nuclear medicine laboratory (53).

Although the determining factor in acute bone marrow depression is the whole blood dose from the immediate treatment, chronic bone marrow depression can be seen and is more related to the total cumulative administered activity. When the cumulative administered activity was less than 500 mCi, then clinically significant chronic bone marrow depression occurred in only 5/469 (1.1%) patients. When the cumulative activity administered was 500-1,000 mCi, the prevalence remained only 1/77 (1.3%), but at greater than 1,000 mCi total administered activity, 6/21 (28.6%) patients had significant chronic cytopenias (54).

Radiation Pneumonitis/Fibrosis. Acute radiation pneumonitis following ^{131}I therapy of pulmonary metastases has been reported, although it is rare when the patient's whole body retention of ^{131}I at 48 hours after the treatment is less than 70-80 mCi (51,52). Pulmonary fibrosis after ^{131}I treatment for lung metastases also is uncommon, having been reported in only 1/53 (1.9%) patients in one series (55).

Precipitation of Thyroid Storm by [131]I. Radioiodine induced inflammation can occur with releases of large amounts of stored thyroid hormone in some patients with very large functioning tumor burdens or large amounts of residual thyroid tissue. Such releases usually occur 2-10 days after the therapy and may result in thyroid storm and death (56,57). A clinical indication that such a situation might occur would be the failure of the patient to become hypothyroid during preparation for ^{131}I therapy.

Long Term Effects of 131I Therapy

Leukemia. Numerous case reports exist of acute myelogenous leukemia occurring after ^{131}I therapy (58). It usually has been associated with total cumulative administrations of more than 800 mCi and with intervals between treatments of less than 12 months, although that is not always the case (59). When outcomes analysis techniques were applied to a large number of patients with thyroid cancer in Sweden, there was a modest increase in the risk of leukemia that was attributable to the [131]I (2.4 excess cases/834 patients treated with an average of 123 mCi of ^{131}I) (60). We estimate that the lifetime risk of acute leukemia in ^{131}I treated thyroid cancer patients is about 3 to 22/cases/1000 patients, depending on the total cumulative administered activity (61).

Other Solid Cancers. Data regarding the risk of solid cancers after ^{131}I therapy for thyroid cancer are confounding. In one Japanese study, significantly elevated risks of developing central nervous system and respiratory organ malignancies were found in 3,321 thyroid cancer patients. However, there was no association between having received ^{131}I therapy and the elevated risk, suggesting that these were non ^{131}I related second primary neoplasms (62).

Three patients who received an average total of 1,055 mCi of ^{131}I resulting in 22,900 rad to the bladder were found to have developed bladder cancer, compared with only 0.5 cases expected in the general population. In that same study, six cases of breast cancer were observed in the 258 patients who had received ^{131}I for thyroid cancer, and only 2.5 cases were expected in the general population. Five of the women had sufficient data to calculate that their average total administered activity of ^{131}I was 960 mCi with an average dose to the breast of 2,200 rad (63). In a larger study of 834 thyroid cancer patients treated with an average of 123 mCi of ^{131}I in Sweden, only slight excesses of cancers of the kidneys, the stomach, the salivary glands, and female genitalia were noted, but no excess of breast or bladder cancers were evident (60). We estimate that ^{131}I therapy for thyroid cancer might result in at most a lifetime excess of 4-10 breast cancers in women and 23-62 excess bladder cancers for total administered activities between 300 and 800 mCi (61). An Italian study of 730 patients treated with a mean total cumulated activity of 276 mCi of ^{131}I and followed for not less than 3 years (mean 7.4 years) revealed a significant increase only in salivary gland cancers (standardized incidence ratio 60:1, 95% C.L. 12.38 - 175.34) (64).

Infertility and Gonadal Failure. The primary source of radiation to the gonads from ^{131}I therapy are circulating iodoproteins in the blood and ^{131}I in the bladder and gut.

In men, the testicular dose in a hypothyroid patient varies between 0.5 and 1.5 rad/mCi administered (65,66). Among 6 men who were evaluated with semen analyses after ^{131}I therapy, 2 were azoospermic after 350 and 400 mCi cumulative administrations respectively, and the other 4 had sperm counts of 11-32 million per ml after total administrations of 100-150 mCi of [131]I (66). Serial semen analyses in 2 of the men with severe spermatogenic depression revealed that 1 had recovered to normal sperm counts by 22 months post treatment and that the other showed progressive but incomplete recovery over the 26 months post treatment follow-up and remained infertile. Gonadal failure may occur in up to 12-13% of younger people after ^{131}I therapy for thyroid cancer (66), and such changes may be irreversible (65). Measurements of follicle stimulating hormone (FSH) and of testosterone in 103 males treated with ^{131}I for thyroid cancer were compared with similar measurements in 19 patients who did not receive [131]I. An abnormal increase in FSH after ^{131}I was noted in 37% of the ^{131}I treated patients. The pattern was variable: of 21 patients treated with ^{131}I and followed with sequential measurements, 6/21 (29%) had little or no change in FSH and 11/21 (52%) had transient increases in FSH at 6-12 months post ^{131}I that subsequently returned to normal, only to recur after additional therapy. A progressive increase in FSH which eventually become permanent was noted in 4/21 (19%) patients treated with multiple administrations of [131]I (67).

In the case of women, the gonadal radiation dose also can vary dramatically in patients with large metastatic deposits, varying from 0.1 rad/mCi in a patient with pulmonary metastases to 1.2 rad/mCi in a patient with a large sacral metastasis (68). Treatment with 140 mCi of ^{131}I to a 38 year old woman with a large pelvic metastasis was followed by ovarian failure (69).

In a 17 year follow-up of 35 women who had received [131]I (mean 149 mCi; range 77-250) at a mean age of 18 years (range 14-21), 3/35 (8.6%) were found after an extensive evaluation to be infertile. The remaining 32 patients had 69 pregnancies resulting in 60 term deliveries. One of the 32 was treated inadvertently with ^{131}I while pregnant, and another became pregnant within 6 months of ^{131}I therapy: both babies were born with subsequently fatal birth defects. All other pregnancies began more than 1 year after ^{131}I therapy, and none of the resulting children had birth defects. Of the 61 children alive for follow up, only 2 had asthma, and no other major health problems were identified. The risks of infertility and of birth defects were not different than those expected in the general public (70).

Dottorini and colleagues were unable to find significant decreases in the fertility rate or birth weight or increases in rate of prematurity of infants in 627 women of child bearing age who were treated with ^{131}I for thyroid cancer. They were compared with 187 women with thyroid cancer who did not receive ^{131}I therapy. The mean administered activity of ^{131}I was 145 mCi with a median of 100 mCi and a range of 46-1,200 mCi. The fertility rate was 23 live births per 1,000 fertile females per year in the ^{131}I treated group and 19 in the non-^{131}I treated group (64).

Another European study evaluated 2,113 pregnancies in women exposed to ^{131}I during thyroid cancer treatment. The prevalence of miscarriages was 11% before thyroid cancer, increased to 20% after thyroid surgery, and remained 20% after ^{131}I therapy. The prevalence did not vary with cumulative exposure to ^{131}I, and ^{131}I therapy did not significantly alter the likelihood of preterm birth, still birth, low birth weight, congenital malformations, thyroid disease, death in the first year of life, or the risk of non-thyroidal malignancies. There were 10 women who became pregnant within 1 year of treatment with [131]I (mean: 108 mCi), and 4/10 (40%) experienced miscarriages (71).

In the case of a 28 year old woman who was treated twice with 100 mCi of ^{131}I, during the second and twenty second weeks of pregnancy, a decision was made to terminate the pregnancy. The fetal thyroid dose was calculated to have been between 9,000 and 90,000 rad from the second treatment, and the most evident changes at the autopsy of the fetus were in the thyroid. Necrosis of follicular epithelial cells, interstitial fibrosis, sclerosis, and atrophy all were present in the fetal thyroid. No chromosomal aberrations were noted in cultures of dermal fibroblasts (72). In another case report of an 18 year old woman treated with 99 mCi of ^{131}I midway into the first trimester, the resultant infant had both cretinism and an increased number of chromosomal breakages when compared to controls (73).

Chromosomal aberrations in the peripheral lymphocytes of patients treated with ^{131}I are relatively common but have not been associated clearly with ill effects on the patient's health. Chromosomal aberrations in peripheral lymphocytes of 10 patients treated with an average of 91 mCi of ^{131}I for ablation of thyroid remnants increased from 2% prior to treatment to 3.7% after treatment (p<0.05). Such aberrations were noted in 4.7% of lymphocytes in patients who previously had received a mean of 602 mCi of ^{131}I, with an increase to 9.0% following an average additional administration of 175 mCi (p<0.01) (74). In a separate evaluation of the presence of micronuclei in binucleated peripheral blood lymphocytes in 22 women who were treated with ^{131}I for thyroid cancer, no significant increases in the frequency of micronuclei were noted. The ^{131}I therapies had been given 1-5 years earlier, suggesting that at least some of the apparent genetic damage to peripheral lymphocytes may not be permanent (75).

Benefits of Radioiodine Therapy

Adults

Therapeutic outcomes are reviewed extensively in Chapter 11. In brief, the post thyroidectomy ablation of thyroid remnants in patients with non-invasive papillary cancer is associated with a significant decrease in the risk of recurrence (p<0.01) or of death (p<0.05) (7). Such treatment of papillary and follicular carcinoma resulted in lower recurrence (p<0.001) and in lower cancer specific mortality (p<0.001) rates in patients without obvious residual cancer after initial surgery (8).

In a series of 1,599 patients who were treated for differentiated thyroid cancer at the M.D. Anderson Cancer Center with post operative ablation of thyroid remnants using 100 mCi of ^{131}I, followed by sequential 150 mCi administrations for metastatic disease until either a complete response was evident or the total cumulative administered activity reached 500 mCi, patients classified as "low risk" had significant reductions in the likelihood of either recurrence or death (p<0.001) when they received ^{131}I therapy. With high risk patients, the benefits of ^{131}I therapy were less apparent (76).

We have completed our preliminary analysis of outcome of therapy in high risk patients with papillary and non-Hurthle follicular carcinomas. Patients were prospectively enrolled in the National Cooperative Thyroid Cancer Treatment Study Registry from 14 participating medical centers, stratified using common criteria, and followed for outcome by therapy between January, 1987 and September, 1995. Post operative radioiodine-131 therapy was associated with improvements both in progression and in cancer specific mortality in patients with papillary carcinoma; patients in a small subgroup of tall cell variant accounted for much of the benefit. In the case of non-Hurthle follicular carcinomas, radioiodine-131 therapy had significant beneficial impacts on cancer specific mortality, progression, and disease free survival (77).

Children

Children with differentiated thyroid cancer often present with more advanced disease than their adult counterparts and have a higher likelihood of presenting with nodal (about 70-80%) or distant (about 10-20%) metastases. Although they tend to tolerate their disease better than do adults, their disease can be fatal (78,79,80).

Experience with ^{131}I therapy in children is somewhat limited, although it appears to be effective in about 70-80% of nodal metastases and 20-80% of lung metastases, with only a small increase in the risk of the development of second primary cancers (79,81-84). When ^{131}I therapy is elected, the choice of the amount to be administered can be problematic in children. Reynolds has shown that the amount of ^{131}I that will result in the same absorbed dose to a child as 1 mCi administered to an adult is linearly related to body weight and to body surface area (85). This permits one to calculate the "relative" amount of ^{131}I to be administered to children as compared with an adult (Table 1). For example, if a child with a normal habitus and normal renal function had a body weight of 25 kg, then, if the desired administration to an adult for the same condition were 100 mCi, the child could be treated with 40 mCi (0.4 x 100) of ^{131}I to attain approximately similar risks and benefits.

TABLE 1

Modification Factors for the Treatment of Children with ^{131}I for Thyroid Cancer

Factor	Body Weight (kg)	Body Surface Area (m²)*
0.2	10	0.4
0.4	25	0.8
0.6	40	1.2
0.8	55	1.4
1.0	70	1.7

* BSA = 0.1 x $W^{0.67}$ where W = weight in kg.
  Derived from Reynolds (85).

Isolated Serum Thyroglobulin Elevations

In general, in athyrotic patients without anti-thyroglobulin antibodies, serum thyroglobulin (Tg) levels are positively correlated with synthesis of thyroglobulin by their thyroid cancer. However, the presence of circulating thyroglobulin is not always correlated with ^{131}I uptake by the cancer because, in some cases, almost no thyroglobulin is present within the tumor follicles (86). In other instances, thyroglobulin may be present but either in reduced amounts or with a decreased concentration of iodine (87). When circulating antibodies to thyroglobulin are present, the utility of thyroglobulin measurements in that individual is decreased.

The subsequent disappearance of the antibodies may be associated with a good prognosis, whereas about 25% of patients in whom antibodies persisted in one series progressed or relapsed (88).

Since thyroglobulin is produced only by thyroid tissue or thyroid cancer, then the presence of measurable thyroglobulin in the serum in athyrotic patients should indicate the presence of residual or recurrent thyroid cancer. Therefore, some workers have advocated ^{131}I therapy in patients with elevated serum Tg levels even when they have no other evidence of disease (87-91). When such patients are treated with ^{131}I, scans obtained a few days after the treatment reveal ^{131}I concentrating tissue in the thyroid bed about 25% of the time, in neck or mediastinal lymph nodes in about 25% of cases, and in lung metastases about 34% of the time. In 16% of the patients, post therapy scans will be negative, but, in the majority of those patients, non ^{131}I concentrating lung metastases became apparent within 5 years (89-91). A positive response to therapy with ^{131}I has been noted in two reports (90,91). In one series 8/16 patients with positive post therapy scans demonstrated a decrease in their TSH stimulated serum thyroglobulin to less than 5 ng/ml and 8/16 demonstrated resolution of abnormal uptake on post therapy scans (90). In the other report, 15 patients were found to have positive post therapy scans for lung metastases. After ^{131}I therapy, 14/15 subsequently developed negative post therapy scans; 9/15 showed a decrease in TSH stimulated thyroglobulin levels to less than 5 ng/ml; 6/8 experienced normalization of radiographic CT scans; and 2/2 had negative lung biopsies (91).

There are insufficient data to determine the impact, if any, of ^{131}I therapy of thyroglobulin positive/^{131}I scan negative patients on long term outcome. However, an additional argument for at least one treatment in such patients is that the post therapy scan may identify foci of disease that then can be watched carefully and, depending on their location, treated as needed with other modalities such as surgery for nodal metastases (91). There is far from uniform agreement on this issue (92).

The level of serum thyroglobulin in a TSH stimulated patient that may trigger consideration of ^{131}I therapy is not well defined. Of the two groups that have reported some benefit to this approach, both advocate a threshold of 10 ng/ml below which they do not treat the patient (29,90,91). This obviously will vary with the thyroglobulin assay being used and must be validated in each center.

Choice of Iodine Isotopes For Therapy

Radioiodine-131 has been the mainstay of radionuclide therapy for differentiated thyroid cancer and remains the isotope of choice when disease is clearly defined on diagnostic studies. However, when micrometastases are evident only on radioiodine scans (such as positive post therapy diffuse lung uptake in thyroglobulin positive/scan negative patients), then this may not be the case.

Given a 2 mm resolution of many radiographic CT units, a lung metastasis that is below detectability with such a unit would be 1.9 mm in diameter or less and would weigh 3.6 mg or less. Most differentiated thyroid cancers concentrate and retain radioiodine within a follicular space, the sizes and distributions of which are highly variable (93), ranging from 0.01 to 1.0 mm. For this reason, emissions with a shorter average path length than those from ^{131}I might be more desirable for very small lesions.

High specific activity ^{125}I can be manufactured at a cost about 50% greater than that of ^{131}I. With a 60 day physical half life, it has a long enough shelf life to permit regularly scheduled shipments to large thyroid cancer centers. The average path length in soft tissue of particulate emissions from ^{125}I (which account for 73% of the radiation dose) is only 0.012 mm, or about 1/30 that of ^{131}I. Given an observed biologic half time of radioiodine in metastatic thyroid cancer of 5.6 days, the calculated effective half life of ^{125}I in thyroid cancer is 5.1 days as compared to 3.3 days for ^{131}I. Assuming the same absolute uptake of radioiodine uniformly in a spherical lesion, we calculated the various radiation doses that would be delivered by each isotope (^{125}I and ^{131}I) to different sized lesions. In lesions > 0.1 mm in diameter, ^{125}I was significantly less efficient in delivering radiation to the tumor than was ^{131}I. For lesions 0.05 mm in diameter the two isotopes were equally efficient. However, ^{125}I resulted in a 5 to 8 fold increase in radiation dose to lesions between 0.01 and 0.02 mm in diameter (93).

Amount of ^{131}I For Therapy

Empiric, Fixed Activities

This approach advocates the administration of a fixed amount of ^{131}I based on what is being treated. Typically, 75-125 mCi are given to ablate thyroid remnants; 150-175 mCi for residual cancer in the neck and/or cervical nodal metastases; and 200 mCi or more for distant metastases (94). The use of 30 mCi to ablate thyroid remnants, once popular as a way to avoid hospitalization of the patient, is no longer necessary because of recent changes in federal regulations (9). A 100 mCi dosage of ^{131}I will successfully ablate small thyroid remnants about 80-90% of the time as compared with a 56% success rate after 30 mCi (10). Based on a review of their own experience and of 14 published reports, workers at the University of Michigan found that empiric ^{131}I therapy had resulted in both radiographic and ^{131}I scintigraphic resolution of micronodular lung metastases in 176/420 (42%) patients. Nodal metastases will respond to empiric ^{131}I therapy about 68% of the time, while only about 7% of non-pulmonary distant metastases respond (58).

Menzel and colleagues reported outcomes after a relatively aggressive "high dose" approach with sequential empiric administration of ^{131}I to 26 patients with metastatic differentiated thyroid cancer (96). Treatments were given at 3 month intervals and consisted of 50-150 mCi administrations to ablate thyroid remnants (84 treatments), 200 mCi for rising thyroglobulin alone (5 treatments), and 300 mCi for metastatic disease visible on 5 mCi ^{131}I diagnostic scans (78 administrations). At least one administration of 300 mCi was given to 25 patients, and 3 patients experienced moderate to severe hematopoietic toxicity after 2, 3, and 4 such administrations. None died of bone marrow suppression, but one had to discontinue further ^{131}I therapy. Of patients who had metastatic disease involving only the lungs with or without neck or mediastinal node involvement, 7/10 (70%) demonstrated a complete response to treatment with an average (± 1 SD) total administered activity of 1,020 ± 287 mCi of ^{131}I. None of an additional 7 patients who had lung involvement plus either local recurrence in the neck or other non-nodal distant metastases experienced a complete remission. The average administered activity to the less than complete responders was 1,508 mCi. The mean follow-up period following the diagnosis of metastatic disease was 4 years.

Upper Bound Limits Set By Blood Dosimetry

Whole blood dosimetry may be used to set an upper bound limit on the amount of ^{131}I that may be given safely. In general, we use the 200 rad whole blood dose from a single administration as the limiting factor (51,52,53). However, we have observed several patients in whom sequential treatments, totaling over 1,000 mCi of ^{131}I given in such a way that each administration resulted in about 200 rad to the whole blood, failed to destroy radioiodine concentrating, thyroglobulin producing metastases. In such patients larger activities exceeding the tolerable blood dose limits followed by bone marrow rescue might be useful, but very close hematologic follow-up and support would be mandatory.

Quantitative Tumor Dosimetry

In 1983, we demonstrated (15) a radiation dose response in the ablation of thyroid remnants with ^{131}I: 22/23 patients had successful ablations when the dose to their thyroid remnants was 30,000 rad or more, but only 3/7 patients whose remnants received less than that dose responded (p<0.05). We then evaluated prospectively the efficacy of using these dosimetric criteria to determine therapy in a separate group of 70 patients (10) whose ^{131}I treatment was projected to deliver at least 30,000 rad to their thyroid residua. There were 142 thyroid remnants found in these 70 patients; 86% of the remnants and 81% of patients were successfully ablated. The administered activities ranged between 25.8 and 246.3 mCi (mean 86.8 mCi), and almost half of the patients received less than 50 mCi. There was no apparent gain from using radiation doses > 30,000 rad. Response rates were significantly lower when patients had less than a total or near total thyroidectomy (p<0.001) prior to ^{131}I ablation or had a mass of thyroid residua calculated to be more than 2 grams (p<0.01). The two most important factors in determining success were the mass of residual tissue (p<0.001) and the effective half time of ^{131}I in that tissue (p<0.05). The calculated instantaneous percent uptake of ^{131}I in the residual tissue was highly correlated with and inseparable from the mass of residual tissue (r=0.63, p<0.001). In a separate prospective trial in India, patients were randomized to receive post surgical activities of 25-35 (mean 30.0), 35-64 (mean 50.6), 65-119 (mean 88.6), or 120-200 (mean 155.0) mCi of ^{131}I. Their optimal success rate of 78% was achieved in the group receiving an average of 50.6 mCi estimated to have delivered about 31,000 rad to the thyroid residua. They found no apparent increase in efficacy as the administered activities and estimated radiation doses increased further (97).

As a way of predicting the outcome of initial post surgical ^{131}I therapy, Muratet et al suggest that a 7-8 fold increase in serum thyroglobulin levels 5 days after the initial ^{131}I therapy may be a useful positive predictor of success. In contrast, at least a doubling of serum thyroglobulin levels 9 days after a 3 mCi ^{131}I diagnostic scan was associated with failure of subsequent ^{131}I ablative therapy, presumably due to radiation thyroiditis and "stunning" (98).

These reports on the success of ^{131}I therapy refer to the ablation of thyroid remnants following thyroidectomy in patients who were prepared by withholding thyroid hormone replacement. Although quantitative radiation dosimetric methods would be expected to be applicable regardless of patient preparation, previously derived empiric approaches that administer fixed activities to patients (e.g. 30 mCi, 50 mCi, 100 mCi) may not be transferable to patients who are not hypothyroid but who have been prepared for radioiodine therapy using recombinant human TSH (18,19).

The conjugate view method of determining in vivo the amount of ^{131}I and the effective half life of ^{131}I in thyroid residua and metastatic lesions was described by us two decades ago (99). We used a 2 mCi administered activity for the pre-therapy quantitative study and projected that the diagnostic results might overestimate the actual therapeutic dose by 10-15% (100). Eight years later, Hadjieva (101) evaluated 30 patients with 0.2 - 2.0 mCi ^{131}I diagnostic studies before ablation and also obtained post ablation dosimetric calculations. In 64% of patients the two calculations agreed, but in 36% the actual radiation dose was less than predicted due to more rapid clearance of the therapeutic activity. Jeevanram et al (102) found that, when radiation doses to thyroid remnants from diagnostic studies were less than about 1,800 rad (approximately the dose from a 2 mCi diagnostic administration to a 2 g remnant with 2% uptake), then the subsequent uptake of the therapeutic administration was 76% of that predicted by the diagnostic study. When the diagnostic radiation dose was greater than 3,500 rad, then the subsequent uptake of the therapeutic administration was only about 25% of the predicted value. Similarly, Hurley and Becker (26) found that the mean radiation dose actually delivered for ablation of remnants in 30 patients was about 80% of that predicted by a 2 mCi diagnostic ^{131}I study. This appeared to be due largely to accelerated release of ^{131}I post therapy. Therefore, actual radiation doses delivered to thyroid remnants may be only about 80% of those projected from 2 mCi ^{131}I diagnostic studies due to decreased uptake and retention of ^{131}I secondary to radiation damage.

Post surgical thyroid remnants in most thyroid cancer patients are composed largely of non-malignant thyroid tissue. The average path length of the particulate radiation that accounts for 94% of the radiation dose from ^{131}I in soft tissue is 0.36 mm. Therefore, in the case of post surgical thyroid remnants of about 2 grams in size and from which any grossly abnormal thyroid tissue has been removed, penetration of the remnant by particulate radiation from ^{131}I would be fairly uniform.

The determination of the size of the thyroid remnant also is important and problematic. In our laboratory we always review the operative notes of the surgeon and the pathology report to determine what percent of the thyroid gland was left behind and in what location. We then discuss the case with the surgeon to get his/her opinion of how much thyroid tissue was left behind.

Since we consider the indications for ^{131}I ablation to be the same as those for a total/near total thyroidectomy, the majority of our patients (87%) have undergone total/near total thyroidectomies prior to ablation (10). In such cases, the surgeons have removed all grossly visible thyroid tissue, so we determine the mass by assuming a thickness of 2 mm and by determining the surface area of the remnant from an anterior gamma camera image of the neck using a flat field collimator suitable for ^{131}I and an isocontour edge tracking program.

In the particular program that we use (MEDASYS® Ann Arbor, Michigan), we initially define a large square or rectangular region of interest that includes the thyroid residua and a similarly large surrounding background region. From this we determine the maximum pixel count value (MAX) and the average background count per pixel (BKG). We then define the isocontours at the following percentage level:

$$\frac{\text{greater of either (2 X BKG) or (BKG} + 3\ \sqrt{\text{BKG}})}{\text{MAX}} \quad \text{X} \quad 100$$

The mass in grams then is estimated to be:

$$\begin{array}{l}\text{\# pixels of uptake in} \\ \text{(thyroid residua as determined by} -10) \times (0.09\ \text{cm}^2/\text{pixel}) \times (0.2\ \text{cm thickness}) \\ \text{the isocontour program}\end{array}$$

where the subtraction of 10 pixels adjusts for system blurring.

When amounts of thyroid tissue remain that are grossly visible to the surgeon, then we define the isocontour percent to be half-way between BKG and MAX as:

$$\frac{\text{MAX} + \text{BKG}}{2\ \text{MAX}} \quad \text{X} \quad 100$$

We then calculate volume using a spherical model where mass (gm) $= 4/3\pi r^3$ and

$$r \quad = \quad \sqrt{\frac{(\text{\#pixels}-10) \times 0.09}{\pi}}$$

This is cross checked with estimates of the mass of residua based on operative notes and pathology reports and the fact that the average normal adult gland in Cincinnati weighs 18 grams. In cases where the lesion is more oval, the formula is modified for other ellipsoids. If the lesion is too small to permit a determination of mass as noted above, then a default value of 150 mg is used.

Other approaches that have been used to determine mass include planimetric techniques and rectilinear scans (103) or computerized gamma camera images (104). When a 5% isocontour planar image was obtained from an anterior view and the volume was calculated using a formula described in 1968 by Stamstrong in Sweden (volume = area x 0.75 x width of the remnant), then the mean relative error between actual and calculated volumes based on phantom studies was only 12.3 ± 3.7% (105). Using the same mathematical formula, other workers have used ultrasound to determine input parameters for the volume calculations (106).

For the treatment of discrete foci of metastatic disease that are well defined on diagnostic ^{131}I scans, we calculate mass using the same nuclear medicine techniques described above, assuming a spherical mass. Whenever possible, the mass also is determined by ultrasound, radiographic CT, or MRI studies (see Chapter 9), and we combine the results to give us our "best working estimate" of mass. Our earlier work indicating that radiation doses of 8,000 rad were highly effective in ablating nodal metastases whereas doses less than 4,000 rad were almost always unsuccessful (15) has been confirmed in several subsequent studies (10,107,108). Thus, we routinely attempt to deliver 10,000 ± 2,000 rad to nodal metastases. If the projected dose to tumor from an amount of ^{131}I that would deliver 200 rad to the whole blood is less than 3,000-4,000 rad, then we recommend surgical and/or external radiation therapy.

When discrete metastases cannot be visualized, as is the case in some pulmonary metastases, Hurley and Becker (26) consider the tumor mass to be 10 grams when the metastases are not visible on standard chest radiographs and to be 50 grams when they are distinguishable but not well delineated. We have estimated that chest x-ray negative/CT scan negative pulmonary metastases would weigh no more than 3.6 mg and that 2,780 such lesions would be required to attain a total cancer mass of 10 grams (93).

Our current recommendations for radioiodine therapy are summarized in Table 2.

Radiation Safety Considerations

The careful determination of the effective whole body half life of ^{131}I and of uptake and retention in selected sites for each patient, coupled with recent changes in federal regulations (9), permit many more patients to be treated as outpatients. Meticulous attention must be paid to individual patient calculations and instruction, and close interaction with the radiation safety office is mandatory. Nonetheless, the result has been much more cost effective and emotionally acceptable (to both patients and physicians) therapy.

TABLE 2

Therapy Based on Quantitative ^{131}I Dosimetry:
Current Recommendations in Adults

Ablation of Thyroid Remnants	• 30,000 rad • 80% complete response
Treatment of Nodal or Discrete Soft Tissue Metastases	• 10,000 ± 2,000 rad • 80% complete response • If less than 3,000 - 4,000 rad use surgery and/or external radiation
Pulmonary Metastases	• Give that amount which will deliver 200 rad to whole blood with no more than 80 mCi whole body retention at 48 hours • Up to 50% complete response if microscopic
Skeletal Metastases or Distant Metastases Other Than Lymph Nodes or Lung	• Give that amount which will deliver 200 rad to whole blood with no more than 120 mCi whole body retention at 48 hours if no lung uptake is present • May require surgery and/or external radiation since relatively few respond to ^{131}I alone
Isolated Serum Thyroglobulin Elevation	• Treat only patients at high risk for recurrence or metastases. • Follow pulmonary metastases treatment protocol • Consider using a mixture of ^{131}I and ^{125}I

For those centers that are not regulated by the U.S. Nuclear Regulatory Commission, several excellent discussions of radiation safety considerations in the ^{131}I treatment of thyroid cancer are recommended (109,110). Castronovo et al have specifically addressed the problem of radiation exposures attendant to caring for hospitalized ^{131}I therapy patients (111).

Summary

Radioiodine-131 is one of the safest and most effective methods of treating differentiated thyroid cancer. However, careful patient selection and preparation followed by individually determined therapy and safety precautions are mandatory if its full potential is to be realized.

External Radiation Therapy
James Brierley, M.D.

Historical Caveat

External radiation therapy has been used in the treatment of malignancy since the turn of the century. In 1966 Sheline et al published the results of the experience at the University of San Francisco of the role of external radiation in the management of patients with persistent thyroid cancer, treated over a thirty year period (1935-1964) (112). They demonstrated not only that external radiation could control gross residual disease in the neck in patients with papillary and follicular thyroid cancer but that it may also have a role in the adjuvant setting in patients with microscopic residual disease. Despite this the role of external radiation in the management of thyroid malignancy remains controversial.

The following items will be addressed:

1. The difference between external radiation and radiation from [131]I.

2. The role of external radiation as adjuvant therapy in differentiated thyroid cancer.

3. The role of external radiation as definitive treatment of differentiated thyroid cancer.

4. The role of external radiation in the management of metastatic differentiated thyroid cancer

5. The role of external radiation as adjuvant therapy in medullary thyroid cancer.

6. The role of external radiation as definitive treatment of medullary thyroid cancer.

7. The role of external radiation in the management of anaplastic thyroid cancer

External Radiation

Radiation therapy delivered by external beam radiation differs from radiation delivered by an unsealed source such as ^{131}I in its production and its method of delivery, but the mechanism of action on the cell is the same. External radiation can be in the form of photons; X-rays produced by accelerated electrons hitting a target, as in a linear accelerator, or γ–rays produced by radioactive decay of a cobalt source. The photons produced by these methods have a higher energy than those from ^{131}I decay, usually in the range of 4 MeV to 25 MeV for a linear accelerator and an average energy of 1.25 MeV for cobalt, in contrast to an average energy of 0.36 MeV for γ–rays from decay of [131]I. An alternative form of external radiation is electron therapy. Typically electron energy ranges from 12 to 20Me. This contrasts with the lower energy electrons produced from ^{131}I decay of 0.25 – 0.61 MeV. External radiation, unlike ^{131}I therapy is not dependent on the tumor cells ability to take it up or on its distribution by the blood stream.

External radiation is given as a fractionated course of treatment, typically over a four to six week course of daily treatments. The biological effectiveness of a course of radiation is determined not only by the total dose of radiation, but also by the size of the daily dose and the overall treatment time. Therefore the biological effectiveness of 60 Gy given over six weeks, with 2 Gy daily fractions five days a week for 30 fractions is approximately equivalent to 50 Gy given over four weeks, with 2.5 Gy fractions, five days a week for 20 fractions.

Differentiated Thyroid Cancer

Adjuvant Therapy

As has been discussed earlier, the usual therapy in the management of differentiated thyroid cancer is surgical excision followed by radioactive iodine and TSH suppression. Despite the general excellent results from this treatment philosophy, there is a subgroup of patients whose outcome is poor. In a retrospective series of 1,012 patients with differentiated thyroid cancer treated by surgical excision at Memorial Sloan-Kettering, 79 (8%) were identified as having extrathyroidal extension of the tumor (113). The 30 year disease free survival for patients without extrathyroidal extension was 87%, but only 29% with extrathyroidal extension (p<0.0001). However, this marked effect on prognosis of extrathyroidal extension was seen only in patients over the age of 45 years. In patients under 45 with negative surgical margins and extrathyroidal extension, the 30 year disease free survival was no different from other patients under the age of 45 without extrathyroidal extension. The deleterious effect of extrathyroidal extension also has been shown in a study from M.D. Anderson reported by Vassilopoulou-Sellin et al (114). From their data base of 1673 patients with differentiated thyroid cancer, they identified 65 cases of papillary thyroid cancer treated by surgical excision and ^{131}I in whom disease recurred. In 40 of the 65 patients there was failure to take up ^{131}I in the recurrence. This was most marked in patients who presented with extrathyroidal extension (14 out of 15 failed to take up ^{131}I). Patients with extrathyroidal extension were more likely to die from their disease than patients without. They also noted that, unless the residual disease after surgical excision is very limited, postoperative ^{131}I may fail to ablate potential extrathyroidal extension.

These two studies suggest that patients over the age of 45 with extrathyroidal extension are more likely to die from their disease than patients without and that ^{131}I postoperatively may be insufficient therapy to eliminate potential residual thyroid cancer in the thyroid bed. Therefore it is in these patients that there may be a role for external radiation as adjuvant to surgical excision and ^{131}I therapy. There have been many studies that report on the role of external radiation in differentiated thyroid cancer, however they are all retrospective and result in conflicting conclusions. Conclusions have varied from Mazzaferri and Young (115) who concluded that "external radiation used as initial adjunctive therapy adversely influenced outcome" to Simpson et al who stated that they "provide convincing data concerning the effectiveness of external radiation and of radioiodine in the adjuvant treatment of papillary and follicular cancer patients..." (116). In addition to the usual problems of all retrospective reports those describing external radiation in differentiated thyroid cancer invariably include patients at low risk who would not necessarily benefit from external radiation as defined above. Particularly in the earlier studies, the patients may not have all been treated with what would now be considered to be standard therapy in high risk patients, namely adequate surgery, ^{131}I, and TSH suppression.

Two reports that support the use of external radiation illustrate the problems of retrospective reports. In a study from China, Wu et al report on 405 patients with thyroid cancer treated by surgery with or without postoperative external radiation (117). Two hundred and thirty-eight patients had complete surgical excision. The 5 year survival for patients not given external radiation was 98%, but in patients given external radiation it was only 78%, suggesting a deleterious effect of external radiation after complete excision. In 108 patients with presumed microscopic residual disease, the converse was found, the 5 year survival was 33% without external radiation and 71% with external radiation. Although no patients were given ^{131}I and all thyroid histologies were included, the main problem with this study is that the decision to give external radiation or not was not dependent on the extent of the disease, or the completeness of the surgery, but the treatment policy of the surgeon. Some surgeons referred all patients for external radiation; some referred none. This made it impossible to compare meaningfully the two groups. From Hungary, Esik et al described significantly improved local relapse free survival (p=0.001) and cause-specific survival (p=0.001) in patients treated with an adequate dose of adjuvant external radiation after resection of all gross disease, compared to an inadequate dose (118). Patients in this study were not given [131]I. More recently the same group have reported that the dose of external radiation was a statistically significant independent prognostic factor in a multivariate analysis for cause specific survival, along with age, distant metastases at presentation, extent of surgery, primary tumor size, extrathyroidal extension, and degree of TSH suppression (119). Only 17% of the patients had [131]I. Therefore it is difficult to extrapolate from this data what the effect of external radiation would have been in a similar population of patients who would in the standard North American setting have been given [131]I.

Philips et al reported a small series of 113 patients, all of whom received ^{131}I after surgery; 38 also had external radiation (120). The overall survival was identical for those given external radiation and those not treated with external radiation. Despite having worse disease (either microscopic or minimal residual disease, or positive lymph node involvement with extracapsular extension) the local relapse rate was 3% for those who received external radiation but only 21% for those who did not and in whom a lower relapse rate would have been expected. This study does suggest a role for external radiation in addition to ^{131}I in improving local control in a selected group of high risk patients with locally advanced papillary or follicular thyroid cancer with extrathyroidal extension. In young patients (under the age of 38) without gross residual disease after surgery, they reported no benefit from external radiation. In all other patients, local regional control was improved after external radiation (89% v 60%). In 26 patients over the age of 38 with macroscopic complete resection treated with ^{131}I and external radiation the local regional control rate was 97%. One patient died from progressive local disease. The authors comment that older patients with extrathyroidal extension and younger patients with extensive extrathyroidal extension are treated at the center with external radiation in addition to surgery, ^{131}I, and TSH suppression.

In a report from Essen on the role of adjuvant external radiation, Benker et al concluded that even in a subgroup of patients with extrathyroidal extension over the age of 40, external radiation did not result in improved survival (58% 10 year survival) compared to patients not given external radiation (48% 10 year survival, p=0.09) (121). More recently Farahati et al from Essen have reported on patients over the age of 40 with extrathyroidal extension (122). All patients had standard therapy of total thyroidectomy, ^{131}I, and TSH suppression. Patients were given radiation to the thyroid bed, cervical and upper mediastinal nodes to a dose of 50 to 60 Gy. Eighty-five patients received external radiation and 52 did not. They reported external radiation was a predictive factor for improvement in time to locoregional recurrence (p<0.01).

In the review of patients with differentiated thyroid cancer treated at Princess Margaret Hospital, we identified a cohort of patients considered to be at significant risk of relapse in the thyroid bed (123). These were patients over the age of 45 who had microscopic residual disease (patients in whom there was evidence of disease at or within 2 mm of the resection margin or in whom the tumor was shaved off adjacent structures in the neck, i.e. trachea, recurrent laryngeal nerve or esophagus). All patients had standard therapy of total thyroidectomy, ^{131}I, and TSH suppression. Fifty two patients with residual microscopic follicular cancer did not benefit from external radiation. One hundred and fifty-five patients were identified as having microscopic residual papillary thyroid cancer after surgical excision. In addition to surgery and TSH suppression, 27 received external radiation, 30 had ^{131}I, 63 had both ^{131}I and external radiation, and 35 had neither. Both the 10 year cause-specific survival (100% v 95%, p=0.04) and the local relapse free rate (93% v 78%, p=0.01) were greater in patients given external radiation than in those patients not given external radiation. Neither extent of surgery or the use of ^{131}I had a statistically significant effect on cause specific survival or locoregional failure in this group. Unfortunately not all patients were treated in a uniform manner in that not all patients had ^{131}I. The only way to prove a role for adjuvant external radiation would be from a randomized controlled study. In the absence of one, at Princess Margaret Hospital we advise external radiation after total or near total thyroidectomy and ^{131}I ablation in all patients over the age of 45 with extrathyroidal extension. Patients in whom extrathroid extension is only diagnosed microscopicaly on pathological review are excluded. The dose of external radiation prescribed is usually 40.05 Gy in 15 fractions, 2.67 Gy per fraction over 3 weeks to the thyroid bed.

Definitive Radiation

In patients who have unresectable disease, it is possible to treat the patient with radical radiation. Sheline et al (112) in an early study reported on patients with thyroid cancer of various histologies treated with external radiation. Fifteen patients had papillary tumors and gross residual disease after surgery. Following external radiation, 8 were alive and well, free from disease. O'Connell et al have reported the Royal Marsden Hospital experience of treating patients with differentiated thyroid carcinoma with radical external radiation giving a minimum of 60 Gy in 30 fractions (124). Thirty-two patients with gross residual disease had a complete regression rate of 37%. At Princess Margaret Hospital, we identified 33 patients with gross residual disease following attempted resection who were treated with a radical course of external radiation (123). The actuarial local control rate was 62% at 5 years. Glatzman and Lutolf reported that, in older patients with gross residual disease, the complete response rate was 43% (6 out of 14) with external radiation (125). They also report that 10 patients were treated with ^{131}I alone, one who had tracheal infiltration, remain alive and well without evidence of disease. These studies all show that long term control is possible in patients with differentiated thyroid cancer which is surgically unresectable or in whom there is gross residual disease after attempted resection. At Princess Margaret Hospital we recommend a radical course of radiation to the thyroid bed and area of gross disease, without attempting to include all regional lymph nodes. Fifty gray in 20 fractions 2.5 Gy per fraction over 4 weeks is usually prescribed. If a thyroidectomy has been performed we will also give a therapeutic administration of [131]I.

External Beam Radiation for Metastases

As discussed above, the major modality of treatment of differentiated thyroid cancer metastasis is ^{131}I therapy. Although often effective in treating lung metastasis, ^{131}I therapy is of limited effectiveness in the management of bone metastasis. This is illustrated by a report from Brown et al who had no 10 year survivors in a group of patients with bone metastases treated by ^{131}I but who had a 54% 10 year survival in patients with lung metastasis (126). In patients with both, the lung metastasis responded to therapy but the bone secondaries did not. Similarly, Casara et al (127) found that 60% of patients with bone metastases took up ^{131}I but only 3% were considered to have achieved a complete response following therapy. This failure of ^{131}I therapy in bone metastases has lead to an aggressive surgical approach being advocated (128-129). However, not all bone metastasis are resectable, either because of their site or their number. In the situation of a metastasis in an unresectable site, we give external radiation in addition to [131]I. For solitary metastases 50 Gy in 25 fractions is usually given, but in the presence of multiple secondaries we usually prescribe 30 Gy in 10 fractions or 20 Gy in 5 fractions. Because of the limited radiation tolerance of the lung, external radiation is used only rarely for pulmonary metastases. Although whole brain irradiation is a common therapeutic procedure in the management of brain metastasis from all sites, in a recent review of 47 patients with brain metastases from thyroid cancer of all histologies, Chiu et al reported no survival advantage from the use of ^{131}I, chemotherapy, or external radiation (130). They did suggest that there was a survival benefit to surgical resection. In patients with unresectable brain metastases either because of site, number, or performance status we would suggest palliative whole brain external radiation.

Anaplastic Thyroid Cancer

Survival following the diagnosis of anaplastic thyroid cancer is invariably poor. Complete surgical resection gives the best chance of cure, however this is only possible in a minority of patients. Anaplastic thyroid cancer does not concentrate ^{131}I so radiation is usually given in the form of external radiation, with the aim of improving local control.

Junor et al reported on the use of radiation following surgery in 91 patients. In 33 patients an attempt at surgical excision was made; in the other 58, biopsy only was performed (131). The overall survival was 11% at three years with a median survival of 21 months. external radiation was given to 86 patients. Even after external beam radiation, local control was a major problem, but in patients in whom local control was achieved, death still occurred from distant metastatic disease. The main aim for local therapy in a cancer such as anaplastic thyroid cancer where distant metastatic disease is such a problem is to control the extent of disease in the neck and prevent the distress to patient and family of death from uncontrolled disease resulting in esophageal or tracheal obstruction or tumor breakdown through the skin.

The ineffectiveness of radiation alone in this disease has lead to the development of both novel fractionation schedules and concurrent chemotherapy. Because anaplastic thyroid cancer grows quickly, hyperfractionated and accelerated radiation has been used. It has been suggested in the treatment of other cancer types that, if the tumor is growing quickly, it is important to give the radiation treatment over a short time using accelerated radiation. The most successful regime in obtaining local control is that described by Tennvall et al (132). Combined hyperfractionated radiation and concurrent chemotherapy are given preoperatively followed by surgical resection. After resection, further radiation and chemotherapy are given. Thirty-three patients were treated with this regime, and debulking surgery was possible in 23 (70%). Local control was achieved in 48%, with death being attributed to local disease in only 8 patients. Despite this local control rate, only 4 patients lived for two years or more.

The aim of giving chemotherapy with radiation concurrently is to act as a radiation sensitizer to make the radiation more effective and thereby improve local control. Even if this were effective, and local control had been achieved, the problem of the high metastatic rate remains. Giving chemotherapy beyond the course of radiation may improve survival if it eliminates micrometastatic disease. Schlumberger et al gave doxorubicin every four weeks for up to 9 courses, in addition to radiation, and achieved only 15% survival at 20 months (133). Currently at Princess Margaret Hospital, in good performance status patients, we give accelerated hyperfractionated radiation: 60 Gy in 40 fraction over 4 weeks, with two fraction of 1.5 Gy per day. For patients with poor performance status, we give palliative radiation only. Anaplastic thyroid cancer remains an extremely lethal disease, and innovative approaches are needed because presently available therapies are ineffective.

Medullary Thyroid Cancer

The mainstay of therapy in MTC is surgery. It has been stated that "radiotherapy has little effect on medullary thyroid cancer"(134). However there is increasing evidence of a role of adjuvant XRT as well as definitive treatment in unresectable disease.

Adjuvant External Radiation

In a group of 59 high risk patients, Nguyen et al reported that the local control rate after radiation was 70% (135). Fife et al, in a series of 51 patients given XRT, reported a 100% local control rate in patients with no residual disease and 65% for patients with microscopic disease after surgical resection (137). Mak et al reported a study of patients with regional nodal disease (137). Thirty-nine patients were treated by surgery alone, and 23 patients with surgery and radiation therapy. This latter group had more extensive disease. The actuarial local/regional control rate for patients treated by surgery only was 13% at 15 years compared to 84% at 15 years for the surgery and radiation group (p=0.0004), however there was no difference in survival. At Princess Margaret Hospital, we have reviewed 73 patients with medullary thyroid cancer who were referred to PMH on initial diagnosis (138). Forty patients had definite microscopic residual or presumed microscopic residual disease or lymph node involvement and were considered to be at high risk of local-regional relapse. Twenty-five patients were irradiated with a 10 year regional control rate of 86% in contrast to a rate of 52% for 15 patients who did not receive radiation. The difference was statistically significant, (p=0.049), but there was no demonstrable improvement in survival. Despite the failure to improve survival, presumably because of microscopic metastatic disease beyond the neck and upper mediastinum, locoregional control is important since cervical relapse can have a deleterious impact on the patient's quality of life, even if it does not affect survival. We therefore recommend adjuvant external radiation in patients at high risk of local regional relapse. We usualy prescribe 40 in 2 Gy fractions to a large volume to the neck and upper mediastinum and a boost to the thyroid bed to a total of 50Gy in 25 fractions over 5 weeks

Definitive Treatment

In the series from Princess Margaret Hospital, 29 patients had gross residual disease after surgery (138). Of these, 21 were given external radiation. The local control rate was 20%. Similarly, Fife et al reported a 24% 5 year survival in patients with gross residual disease (136). Therefore, when complete surgical resection is not possible, we recommend external radiation for long term local control.

Summary

In patients with unresectable tumors or gross residual disease following attempted surgical resection, external radiation has a definite role in improving local control. In differentiated thyroid carcinoma following thyroidectomy it should be combined with ^{131}I therapy. For patients with differentiated thyroid cancer or medullary thyroid cancer at high risk of local relapse, external radiation probably improves local control, but in the absence of any data from a randomized controlled trial this remains controversial.

References

1. Seidlin SM, Marinelli L, Oshry E. Radioactive iodine therapy effect on functioning metastases of adenocarcinoma of the thyroid. JAMA 1946; 132:838-847.
2. Beierwaltes WH, Johnson PC, Solari AJ: Clinical use of radioisotopes. Sanders, Philadelphia, 1957.
3. Pochin E.E. Prospects from the treatment of thyroid carcinoma with radioiodine. Clin Radiol 1967; 18: 113-125.
4. Varma VM, Beierwaltes WH, Nofal MH, et al. Treatment of thyroid cancer: death rates after surgery and after surgery followed by [131]I. JAMA 1970; 214:1437-1442.
5. Schlumberger MJ. Papillary and follicular thyroid carcinoma. NEJM 1998; 338: 297-306.
6. Mazzaferri EL. Treating differentiated thyroid carcinoma: Where do we draw the line? Mayo Clin Proc 1991; 66: 105-111.
7. DeGroot LJ, Kaplan EL, McCormick M, Straus FH. Natural history, treatment, and course of papillary thyroid carcinoma. J Clin Endocinol Metab 1990; 71: 414-424,.
8. Mazzaferri EL, Jhiang SM. Long-term impact of initial surgical and medical therapy on papillary and follicular thyroid cancer. Am J Med 1994; 97: 418-428 and Erratum Am J Med 1995; 98: 215,.
9. Regulatory Guide 8.39 Release of patients administered radioactive material. U.S. Nuclear Regulatory Commission, Washington, D.C. April, 1997.
10. Maxon HR, Englaro EE, Thomas SR, et al. Radioiodine-131 therapy for well differentiated thyroid cancer - A quantitative radiation dosimetric approach: Outcome and validation in 85 patients. J Nucl Med 1992; 33:1132-1136.
11. Krugman LG, Hershman JM, Chopra IJ, et al. Patterns of recovery of the hypothalamic- pituitary-thyroid axis in patients taken off chronic thyroid therapy. J Clin Endocrinol Metab 1975; 41: 70-80.
12. Hilts SV, Hellman D, Anderson J, et al. Serial TSH determination after T3 withdrawal or thyroidectomy in the therapy of thyroid carcinoma. J Nucl Med 1979; 20: 928-932.
13. Edmonds CJ, Hayes S, Kermode JC, et al. Measurement of serum TSH and thyroid hormones in the management of treatment of thyroid carcinoma with radioiodine. Br J Radiol 1977; 50: 799-807.
14. Goldman JM, Line BR, Aamodt RL, et al. Influence of triiodothyroxine withdrawal time on I-131 uptake post-thyroidectomy for thyroid cancer. J Clin Endocrinol Metab 1980; 50: 734-739.
15. Maxon HR, Thomas SR, Hertzberg VS, et al. Relation between effective radiation

dose and outcome of radioiodine therapy for thyroid cancer. NEJM 1983; 309: 937-941.

16. Guimaraes V, Degroot LJ. Moderate hypothyroidism as preparation for whole body ^{131}I scintiscans and thyroglobulin testing. Thyroid 1996; 6: 69-73.

17. Hays MT, Solomon DH, Beall GN. Suppression of human thyroid function by antibodies to bovine thyrotropin. J Clin Endocrinol 1967; 27: 1540-1549.

18. Ladenson PW, Braverman LE, Mazzaferri EL, et al. Comparison of administration of recombinant human thyrotropin with withdrawal of thyroid hormone for radioactive iodine scanning in patients with thyroid carcinoma. NEJM 1997; 337: 888-896.

19. Park SG, Reynolds JC, Brucker-Davis E, et al. Iodine kinetics during ^{131}I scanning in patients with thyroid cancer: comparison of studies with recombinant human TSH (rhTSH) vs. hypothyroidism. J Nucl Med 1996; 37: 15P, (abstract).

20. Montenegro J, Gonzalez O, Saracho R, et al. Changes in renal function in primary hypothyroidism. Am J Kidney Dis 1996; 27: 195-198.

21. Hamburger JI. Diuretic augmentation of ^{131}I uptake in inoperable thyroid cancer. NEJM 1969; 280: 1091-1094.

22. Maruca J, Santner S, Miller K, et al. Prolonged iodine clearance with a depletion regimen for thyroid carcinoma: concise communication. J Nucl Med 1984; 25: 1089-1093.

23. Goslings BM. Effect of a low iodine diet on ^{131}I therapy in follicular carcinomata. J Clin Endocrinol 1975; 64: 30P, (abstract).

24. Maxon HR, Thomas SR, Boehringer A, et al. Low iodine diet in ^{131}I ablation of thyroid remnants. Clin Nucl Med 1983; 8: 123-126.

25. Lakshmanan M, Schaffer A, Robbins J, et al. A simplified low iodine diet in ^{131}I scanning and therapy of thyroid cancer. Clin Nucl Med 1988; 13: 866-868.

26. Hurley JR, Becker DV. Treatment of thyroid carcinoma with radioiodine. In Gottschack A, Hoffer PB, Potchen EJ and Berger HJ (eds). Diagnostic Nuclear Medicine. Second edition. Williams & Wilkins, Baltimore, 1988, pp 792-814.

27. Robbins J. The role of TRH and lithium in the management of thyroid cancer. In Andreoli M, Monaco F, Robbins J (eds): Advances in Thyroid Neoplasia. Field Educational Italia, Rome, 1981, p 233.

28. Pons F, Carrio I, Estorch M, et al. Lithium as an adjuvant of iodine-131 uptake when treating patients with well differentiated thyroid carcinoma. Clin Nucl Med 1987; 12: 644-647.

29. Reynolds JC, Robbins J. The changing role of radioiodine in the management of differentiated thyroid cancer. Sem Nucl Med 1997; 27: 152-164.

30. Maxon R, Thomas SR, Maxon H. Effect of gut retention on the effective whole body half-time of iodine-131 in thyroid cancer patients. J Nucl Med Tech 1987; 15: 13-15.

31. Abbatt JD, Brown WMC, Farran HEA. Radiation sickness in man following the administration of therapeutic radioiodine: relationship between latent period, dose rate, and body size. Br J Radiol 1955; 28: 358-363.

32. Van Nostrand D, Neutze J, Atkins F. Side effects of "rational dose" iodine-131 therapy for metastatic well-differentiated thyroid carcinoma. J Nucl Med 1986; 27: 1519-1527.

33. Rigler RG, Scanlon PW. Radiation parotitis from radioactive iodine therapy. Proc Staff Meetings Mayo Clinic 1955; 30: 149-153.

34. Schneyer LH. Effect of administration of radioactive iodine on human salivary gland dysfunction. J Dent Res 1953; 32: 146 (abstract).

35. Goolden AWG, Mallard JR, Farran HEA. Radiation sialitis following radioiodine therapy. Br J Radiol 1957; 30: 210-212.

36. Imbriaco M, Furhang EE, Humm JL, et al. Radiation dose to the salivary glands during ^{131}I treatment of thyroid cancer: correlation with clinical findings. J Nucl Med

1997; 38: 230P (abstract).

37. Delprat CC, Hoefnagel CA, Marcuse HR. The influence of ^{131}I therapy in thyroid cancer on the function of salivary glands. Acta Endocrinologica 1983; 252 (suppl): 73-74,.

38. Malpani BL, Samuel AM, Ray S. Quantification of salivary gland function in thyroid cancer patients treated with radioioidine. Int J Radiation Oncol Biol Phys 1996; 35: 535-540.

39. Cooper JS, Fu K, Marks J, Silverman S. Late effects of radiation therapy in the head and neck region. Int J Radiat Oncol Biol Phys 1995; 31: 1141-1164.

40. Lee CM, Javitch JA, Snyder SH. Recognition sites for norepinephrine uptake: regulation by neurotransmitter. Science 1983; 220: 626-629.

41. Abe K, Yoneda K, Fujita R, et al. The effects of epinephrine, norepinephrine, and phenylephrine on the types of proteins secreted by rat salivary glands. J Dent Res 1980; 59: 1627-1634.

42. Creutzig H. Sialadenitis following iodine-131 therapy for thyroid carcinoma [letter] J Nucl Med 1985; 26: 817.

43. Levy HA & Park CH. Effect of reserpine on salivary gland radioioidine uptake in thyroid cancer. Clin Nucl Med 1987; 12: 303-307.

44. Bohuslavizki KH, Brenner W, Hhbner R, et al. Protective effect of Amifostine on salivary glands of rabbits treated with high dose iodine-131. J Nucl Med 1997; 5: 223P (abstract).

45. Lee TC, Harbert JC, Dejter SW, et al. Vocal cord paralysis following ^{131}I ablation of a postthyroidectomy remnant. J Nucl Med 1985; 26: 49-50.

46. Levenson D, Gulec S, Sonenberg M, et al. Peripheral facial nerve palsy after high-dose radioioidine therapy in patients with papillary thyroid carcinoma. Ann Intern Med 1994; 120: 576-578.

47. Samuel AM & Shah DH. Brain metastasis in well differentiated carcinoma of the thyroid. Tumori 1997; 83: 608-610.

48. Datz FL. Cerebral edema following iodine-131 therapy for thyroid carcinoma metastatic to the brain. J Nucl Med 1986; 27: 637-640.

49. Ginsberg J, Pedersen JD, Von Westarp C, et al. Cervical cord compression due to extension of a papillary thyroid carcinoma. Am J Med 1987; 82: 156-158.

50. Panza N, DeRosa M, Lombardi G, et al. Pseudotumor cerebri and thyroid replacement therapy in patients affected by differentiated thyroid carcinoma. J Endocrinol Invest 1985; 8: 357-358.

51. Benua RS, Cicale NR, Sonenberg M, et al. The relation of radioioidine dosimetry to results and complications in the treatment of metastatic thyroid cancer. Am J Radiol 1962; 87: 171-182.

52. Leeper RD & Shimaoka K. Treatment of metastatic thyroid cancer. Clin Endocrinol Metab 1980; 9: 383-404.

53. Thomas SR, Samaratunga RC, Sperling M, Maxon HR. Predictive estimate of blood dose from external counting data preceding radioioidine therapy for thyroid cancer. Nucl Med Biol 1993; 20: 157-162.

54. Grunwald F, Schomburg A, Menzel C, et al. Changes in the blood picture after radioioidine therapy of thyroid cancer. Med Klin 1994; 10: 522-528.

55. Maheshwari YK, Hill CS Jr., Haynie TP III, et al. ^{131}I therapy in differentiated thyroid carcinoma: M.D. Anderson Hospital experience. Cancer 1981; 47: 664-671.

56. Cerletty JM & Listwan WJ. Hyperthyroidism due to functioning metastatic thyroid carcinoma: precipitation of thyroid storm with therapeutic radioactive iodine. JAMA 1979; 242: 269-270.

57. Smith R, Blum C, Benua RS, et al. Radioactive iodine treatment of metastatic thyroid carcinoma with clinical thyrotoxicosis. Clin Nucl Med 1985; 10: 874-875.

58.   Maxon HR & Smith HS.   Radioiodine-131 in the diagnosis and treatment of metastatic well differentiated thyroid cancer. Endo Metab Clin N Am 1990; 19: 685-718.

59.   Bitton R, Sachmechi I, Benegalrao Y, Schneider BS. Leukemia after a small dose of radioiodine for metastatic thyroid cancer. J Clin Endocrinol Metab 1993; 77: 1423-1426.

60.   Hall P, Holm LE, Lundell G, et al. Cancer risks in thyroid cancer patients. Br J Cancer 1991; 64: 159-163.

61.   Maxon HR. The role of ^{131}I in the treatment of thyroid cancer. Thyroid Today, Vol 16, #2, 1993.

62.   Ishikawa K, Noguchi S, Tanaka K, et al. Second primary neoplasms in thyroid cancer patients. Jpn J Cancer Res 1996; 87: 232-239.

63.   Edmonds CJ, Smith T. The long term hazards of the treatment of thyroid cancer with radioiodine. Br J Radiol 1986; 59: 45-51.

64.   Dottorini ME, Lomuscio G, Mazzucchelli L, et al. Assessment of female fertility and carcinogenesis after iodine-131 therapy for differentiated thyroid cancer. J Nucl Med 1995; 36: 21-27.

65.   Ahmed SR & Shalet SM. Gonadal damage due to radioactive iodine I^{131} treatment for thyroid carcinoma. Post Grad Med J 1985; 61: 361-362.

66.   Handelsman DJ & Turtle JR. Testicular damage after radioactive iodine (I-131) therapy for thyroid cancer. Clin Endocrinol 1983; 18: 465-472.

67.   Pacini F, Gasperi M, Fugazzola L, et al. Testicular function in patients with differentiated thyroid carcinoma treated with radioiodine. J Nucl Med 1994; 35: 1418-1422.

68.   Briere J & Philippon B. Absorbed dose to ovaries or uterus during a ^{131}I therapeutic of cancer or hyperthyroidism: comparison between in vivo measurements by TLD and calculations. Interntl J Applied Radiation and Isotopes 1979; 30: 643-650.

69.   Dobyns BM & Maloof F. The study and treatment of 119 cases of carcinoma of the thyroid with radioactive iodine. J Clin Endocrinol 1951; 11: 1323-1360.

70.   Smith MB, Xue H, Takahashi H, et al. Iodine 131 thyroid ablation in female children and adolescents: long term risk of infertility and birth defects. Ann Surg Oncol 1994; 1: 128-131.

71.   Schlumberger M, deVathaine F, Ceccarelli C, et al. Exposure to radioactive iodine for scintigraphy or therapy does not preclude pregnancy in thyroid cancer. J Nucl Med 1996; 37: 606-612.

72.   Arndt D, Mehnert WH, Franke WG, et al. Radioiodine therapy during an unknown pregnancy and radiation exposure of the fetus. A case report. Strahlenther Onkol 1994; 170: 408-414.

73.   Goh K. Radioiodine treatment during pregnancy: chromosomal aberrations and cretinism associated with maternal iodine-131 treatment. J Am Med Wom Assoc 1981; 36: 262-265.

74.   Ardito G, Lamberti L, Bigatti P, et al. Comparison of chromosome aberration frequency before and after administration of ^{131}I in two groups of thyroid cancer patients. Tumori 1987; 73: 257-262.

75.   Gutierrez S, Carbonell E, Galofrea P, et al. A cytogenetic follow-up study of thyroid cancer patients treated with ^{131}I. Cancer Lett 1995; 91: 199-204.

76.   Samaan NA, Schultz PN, Hickey RC, et al. Well differentiated thyroid carcinoma and the results of various modalities of treatment. A retrospective review of 1599 patients. J Clin Endocrinol Metab 1992; 75: 714-720.

77.   Taylor T, Specker B, Robbins J, et al. Multicenter prospective study of outcome following treatment of high risk papillary and non-Hurthle follicular thyroid carcinoma. Ann Intern Med - 1998, under revision.

78.   Winship T & Rosvoll RV. Thyroid carcinoma in childhood: final report on a 20 year

study. Clin Proc Children's Hospital 1970; 26: 327-348.

79. Schlumberger M, deVathaine F, Travagli JP, et al. Differentiated thyroid carcinoma in childhood: long term follow-up of 72 patients. J Clin Endocrinol Metab 1987; 65: 1088-1094.

80. Zimmerman D, Hay ID, Gough IR, et al. Papillary thyroid carcinoma in children and adults: long term follow up of 1039 patients conservatively treated at one institution during three decades. Surgery 1988; 104: 1157-1168.

81. Ceccarelli C, Pacini F, Lippi F, et al. Thyroid cancer in children and adolescents. Surgery 1988; 104: 1143-1148.

82. LaQuaglia MP, Corbally MT, Heller G, et al. Recurrence and morbidity in differentiated thyroid carcinoma in children. Surgery 1988; 104: 1149-1156.

83. Samuel AM & Sharma SM. Differentiated thyroid carcinomas in children and adolescents. Cancer 1991; 67: 2186-2190.

84. Dottorini M, Vignati A, Mazzucchelli G, et al. Differentiated thyroid carcinoma in children and adolescents: A 37-year experience in 85 patients. J Nucl Med 1997; 38: 669-675.

85. Reynolds JC. Comparison of I-131 absorbed radiation doses in children and adults: a tool for estimating therapeutic I-131 doses in children, in Robbins J (ed) Treatment of Thyroid Cancer in Childhood, DOE/EH-0406, US Department of Commerce, Technology Administration, National Technical Information Service, Springfield, Virginia 22161. September, 1994, pages 127-135.

86. Dralle H, Schwarzrock R, B`cker W, et al. Thyroglobulin synthesis and radioiodine uptake in differentiated thyroid carcinomas. ACTA Endocinol (suppl) 252: 45-46, 1983.

87. Valenta L, Lissitzky S, Aquaron R. Thyroglobulin-iodine in thyroid tumors. J Clin Endocrinol Metab 1968; 28: 437-441.

88. Rubello D, Casara D, Girelli ME, et al. Clinical meaning of circulating antithyroglobulin antibodies in differentiated thyroid cancer: a prospective study. J Nucl Med 1992; 33: 1478-1480.

89. Pacini F, Lippi F, Formica N, et al. Therapeutic doses of iodine-131 reveal undiagnosed metastases in thyroid cancer patients with detectable serum thyroglobulin levels. J Nucl Med 1987; 28: 1888-1891.

90. Pineda JD, Lee T, Ain K, et al. Iodine-131 therapy for thyroid cancer patients who have positive serum thyroglobulin levels and negative radioiodine scans. J Clin Endocrinol Metab 1995; 80: 1488-1492.

91. Schlumberger M, Mancusi F, Baudin E, Pacini F. [131]I therapy for elevated thyroglobulin levels. Thyroid 1997; 7: 273-276.

92. McDougall IR. [131]I treatment of ^{131}I negative whole body scan and positive thyroglobulin in differentiated thyroid carcinoma: what is being treated? Thyroid 1997; 7: 669-672.

93. Maxon HR, Thomas SR, Samaratunga RC. Dosimetric considerations in the radioiodine treatment of macrometastases and micrometastases from differentiated thyroid cancer. Thyroid 1997; 7: 183-187.

94. Nusynowitz ML. Differentiated thyroid cancer: current concepts and management. New perspectives in cancer diagnosis and management. 1997; 4: 49-57.

95. Sisson JC, Giordano TJ, Jamadar DA, et al. [131]I treatment for micronodular pulmonary metastases from papillary thyroid carcinoma. Cancer 1996; 78: 2184-2192.

96. Menzel C, Grunwald F, Schomburg A, et al. "High dose" radioiodine therapy in advanced differentiated thyroid carcinoma. J Nucl Med 1996; 37: 1496-1503.

97. Bal C, Padhy AK, Jana S, et al. Prospective, randomized clinical trial to evaluate the optimal dose of ^{131}I for remnant ablation in patients with differentiated thyroid carcinoma. Cancer 1996; 77: 2574-2580.

98. Muratet J-P, Giraud P, Dauer A, et al. Predicting the efficacy of first iodine-131 treatment in differentiated thyroid carcinoma. J Nucl Med 1997; 38: 1362-1368.

99. Thomas SR, Maxon HR, Kereiakes JG. In vivo quantitation of lesion radioactivity using external counting. Med Phys 1976; 3: 253-255.

100. Thomas SR, Maxon HR, Kereiakes JG, Saenger EL. Quantitative external counting techniques enabling improved diagnostic and therapeutic decisions in patients with well-differentiated thyroid cancer. Radiology 1977; 122: 731-737.

101. Hadjieva T. Quantitative approach to radioiodine ablation of thyroid remnants following surgery for thyroid cancer. Radiobiol radiother 1985; 26: 819-823.

102. Jeevanram RK, Shah DH, Sharma SM, Ganatra RD. Influence of initial large dose on subsequent uptake of therapeutic radioiodine in thyroid cancer patients. Nucl Med Biol 1986; 13: 277-279.

103. Goodwin WE, Cassen B, Bauer FK. Thyroid gland weight determination from thyroid scintigrams with postmortem verification. Radiology 1963; 61: 88-92.

104. Olsen KJ. Scintigraphic estimation of thyroid volume and dose distribution at treatment with ^{131}I. ACTA Radiologica Oncology 1978; 17: 74-80.

105. Zaidi H. Comparative methods for quantifying thyroid volume using planar imaging and SPECT. J Nucl Med 1996; 37: 1421-1426.

106. Szebeni A & Beleznay E. New simple method for thyroid volume determination by ultrasonography. J Clin Ultrasound 1992; 20: 329-337.

107. Kimmig B & Hermann HJ. Measurement of dose during radioiodine treatment of thyroid cancer. ACTA Endo 1983; 252 (S): 72.

108. Flower MA, Schlesinger T, Hinton PJ, et al. Radiation dose assessment in radioiodine therapy. Practical implementation using quantitative scanning and PET, with initial results in thyroid carcinoma. Radiother Oncol 1989; 15: 345-357.

109. Zanzonico PB. Radiation dose to patients and relatives incident to ^{131}I therapy. Thyroid 1997; 7: 199-204.

110. Beckers C. Regulations and policies on radioiodine ^{131}I therapy in Europe. Thyroid 1997; 7: 221-224.

111. Castronovo FP, Jr., Beh RA, Veilleux NM. Dosimetric considerations while attending hospitalized I-131 therapy patients. J Nucl Med Technology 1982; 10: 157-160.

112. Sheline GE, Galante M, Lindsay S. Radiation therapy in the control of persistent thyroid cancer. American Journal of Roentgenol, Radium Therapeutic and Nuclear Medicine 1966; 97: 923-930.

113. Anderson P, Kinsella J, Loree, et al. Differentiated carcinoma of the thyroid with extrathyroid extension. American J of Surgery 1995; 170: 467-470.

114. Vassilopoulou-Sellin, Schultz P, Haynie T. Clinical outcome of patients with papillary thyroid carcinoma who have recurrence after initial radioactive iodine therapy. Cancer 1996; 78: 493-501.

115. Mazzaferri EL, Young RL. Papillary thyroid carcinoma: A 10 year follow-up report of the impact of therapy in 576 patients. American Journal of Medicine 1981; 70: 511-517.

116. Simpson WJ, Panzarella T, Carruthers J et al. Papillary and follicular thyroid cancer: Impact of treatment in 1578 patients. International Journal of Radiation Oncology, Biology, Physics 1988; 14: 1063-1075.

117. Wu XL, Hu YH, Li QH, et al. Value of postoperative radiotherapy for thyroid cancer. Head and Neck Surgery 1987; 10: 107-112.

118. Esik O, Nemeth G, Eller J. Prophylactic external irradiation in differentiated thyroid cancer: a retrospective study over a 30 year observation period. Oncology. 1994; 51: 372-379.

119. Esik O, Tusnady G, Daudner K, et al. Survival chance in papillary thyroid cancer in Hungary: individual survival probability estimation using the Markov method.

Radiotherapy and Oncology 1997; 44: 203-212.

120. Phlips P, Hanzen C, Andry G, et al. Postoperative irradiation for thyroid cancer. European Journal of Surgical Oncology 1993; 19:399-404.

121. Benker G, Olbricht T, Reinwein D, et al. Survival rates in patients with differentiated thyroid carcinoma: influence of postoperative external radiotherapy. Cancer 1990; 65:1517-1520.

122. Farahati J, Reiners C, Stuschke M, et al. Differentiated thyroid cancer impact of adjuvant external radiotherapy. Cancer 1996; 77: 172-180.

123. Tsang R, Brierley J, Simpson W, et al. The effect of surgery, radiactive iodineand external radiation on the outcome of differentiated thyroid cancer. Cancer 1998; 82: 375-388.

124. O' Connell MEA, A'Hern RP, Harmer CL. Results of external beam radiotherapy in differentiated thyroid carcinoma: a retrospective study from the Royal Marsden Hospital. European Journal of Cancer 1994; 30A: 733-739.

125. Glanzmann C, Lutolf UM. Long-term follow-up of 92 patients with locally advanced follicular or papillary thyroid cancer after combined treatment. Strahlenther Onkol 1992; 168: 260-269.

126. Brown A, Greening W, McCready et al. Radioiodine trearment of metastatic thyroid carcinma. Br J Radiol 1984; 57: 323-327.

127. Casara D, Rubello D, Saladini G, et al. Distant metastases in diffentiated thyroid cancer: longterm results of radioiodine treatment. Tumori 1991; 77: 432-436.

128. Proye C, Dromer M, Carnaille B et al. Is it worthwhile to treat bone metastases from differentiated thyroid carcinoma with radioactive iodine. World J. Surg 1992; 16: 640-646.

129. Niederle B, Roka R, Schemper M, et al. Surgical treatment of distant metastases in differentiated thyroid cancer: indications and results. Surgery 1986; 100: 1088-1097.

130. Chu A, Delpassand, Sherman S. Prognosis and treatment of brain metastases in thyroid carcinoma. J Clin Endocrinol Metab 1997; 82: 3637-3642.

131. Junor E, Paul J, Reed N. Anaplastic thyroid carcinoma: 91 patients treated by surgery and radiotherapy. European Journal of Surgery 1992; 18: 83-88.

132. Tennvall J, Lundell G, A H. Combined doxorubicin, hyperfractionated radiotherapy, and surgery in anaplastic thyroid carcinoma. Cancer 1994; 74: 1348-1354.

133. Schlumberger M, Parmentier C, Delisl M. Combination therapy for anaplastic giant cell thyroid carcinoma. Cancer 1991; 67: 564-566.

134. Samaan N, Schultz P, Hickey R. Medullary thyroid carcinoma: prognosis of familial versus sporadic disease and the role of radiotherapy. Medicine 1988; 67: 801-805.

135. Nguyen T, Chassord J, Lagarede P. Results of postoperative radiation therapy in medullary carcinoma of the thyroid. Radiotherapy and Oncology 1992; 23: 1-5.

136. Fife KM, Bower M, Harmer CL. Medullary thyroid cancer: the role of radiotherapy in local control. Eur J Surg Oncol 1996; 22: 588-591.

137. Mak A, Morrison W, Garden A, Ordonez N, Weber R, Peters L. The value of postoperative radiotherapy for regional medullary carcinoma of the thyroid. International Journal of Radiation Oncology, Biology, Physics 1994; 30: 234.

138. Brierley J, Tsang R, Gospodarowicz M, et al. Medullary thyroid cancer analyses of survival and prognostic factors and the role of radiation therapy. Thyroid 1996; 6: 375-388.

13 RARE FORMS OF THYROID CANCER

Kenneth B. Ain, M.D.
University of Kentucky Medical Center
Lexington, KY

The majority of thyroid carcinomas present rather well-defined clinical challenges and therapeutic options. Rare forms of thyroid cancer are generally unfamiliar to clinicians and require creative approaches. This chapter attempts to introduce unusual variants of differentiated epithelial thyroid carcinoma, undifferentiated thyroid cancers, and extraordinary primary thyroid cancers with limited clinical epidemiology. The initial sections will discuss the presentation and clinicopathologic features of these neoplasms, many of which are controversial. The final section will suggest strategies for therapeutic management.

Variants of differentiated epithelial thyroid carcinoma

In recent years, unusual variants of papillary thyroid carcinomas have been described which express distinct clinical outcomes (1). These include the tall-cell, columnar cell, Hürthle-cell (oxyphilic), diffuse sclerosing, and diffuse follicular variants (see also Chapter 5). All constitute a distinct minority of incident thyroid cancers and some are too infrequent to accurately quantitate. Variants with uncertain clinical significance, such as clear cell, trabecular, and lipomatous, are omitted. Not all pathologists are equally capable of recognizing papillary cancer subtypes and, even among pathologists skilled in thyroid histopathology, there is poor agreement in pathological designations (2). For this reason, there is frequently a need for additional pathology consultations in difficult cases.

Tall-cell variant papillary thyroid carcinoma

Although Hawk and Hazard (3), in 1976, were the first to describe the unique clinicopathologic features of this papillary carcinoma variant, it has not been widely appreciated as having prognostic significance until the last several years. Patients with this cancer seemed to present with large, invasive tumors and exhibit a particularly aggressive clinical course (4). The cells of this cancer are tall and columnar with heights at least twice their widths and strikingly oxyphilic. Tall-cell cancers constitute from 3 to 12% of papillary carcinomas (3,5-11). These primary tumors frequently present at a larger size than typical papillary cancers (3,9,12), are more likely to be locally invasive into extrathyroidal tissues (1,6-9,11,12), and have greater inclination for distant metastasis (1,7,8). Some investigators find this tumor more often in patients older than 50 years (3,6,12) with increased clinical aggressiveness in older patients (9); however we have observed similar aggressive features in patients under 40 years of age (28% of patients with this cancer phenotype) (1). Tall-cell variant carcinoma patients have been reported to have a 16 to 25% mortality despite short follow-up periods ranging from 1-7 years (1,3,6,7).

These cancers, presenting as thyroid masses, are not distinctly discernible as tall-cell variant using fine needle aspiration cytology (13,14). Gamboa-Domínguez et al (10) report that cytologic findings of non-cohesive cells with a tadpole shape and a respiratory epithelium-like arrangement are suggestive of the tall-cell variant. Definitive diagnosis relies upon surgical histology after thyroid resection. Immunohistochemistry of tall-cell variant differs from usual papillary carcinoma in that it demonstrates unique reactivity to Leu M1, a myelomonocytic antigen, and with ZC-23, an antibody to carcinoembryonic antigen which is cross-reactive to both biliary glycoprotein and an uncharacterized non-specific antigen (11). Positive immunostaining for the product of the mutated p53 gene is more frequent (61%) in tall-cell variant than in usual papillary cancers (11%), although such staining was not statistically significant as a prognostic indicator of survival (15). There are no clear differences in DNA ploidy or nuclear morphometry between tall-cell variant and usual papillary carcinomas (16).

The reasons for the aggressive clinical behavior of tall-cell variant cancers are not clear; however foci of anaplastic carcinoma transformation with spindle and squamoid cells can be seen within the tall-cell tumors (17). This may provide an explanation for metastatic behavior and loss of iodine uptake which is seen in 20 to 50% of cases (1,8). Ozaki et al (5) have recently described a less aggressive population of tall-cell variant cancers with extensive lymphocyte and plasma cell infiltration. This report should be interpreted with caution considering that oxyphilic changes associated with autoimmune thyroiditis could modify the appearance of usual papillary cancers and cause confusion in classification.

Columnar cell variant papillary carcinoma

Only ten cases of columnar cell variant of papillary carcinoma had been reported until this year (18-24). This rare variant was described by Evans in 1986 (21) as a tumor with papillary architecture containing tall, columnar cells with nuclear stratification and areas of solid growth with spindle-cell features. Of earlier reported cases with sufficient clinical information, 80% had distant metastases and the disease-specific mortality was 75%. It is difficult to estimate the incidence of this rare tumor; however, in a series of 1500 cases of papillary carcinoma seen at the

Mayo Clinic, only three patients with columnar cell variant cancer were identified (22). Two of the reported cases had features of both tall-cell and columnar cell variant carcinoma (19,24), suggesting that these cancers are closely related and may be modifications of the same papillary carcinoma variant.

A recent report by Wenig *et al* (25) added 16 additional cases of columnar cell variant cancer, derived from analysis of more than ten thousand papillary carcinomas, suggesting an incidence of 0.16% of papillary carcinomas. Around 80% of patients were women and the average age was 47 years. Only two of their cases presented with extrathyroidal invasion and both of these patients had aggressive tumor behavior resulting in one disease-specific death and the other patient alive with pulmonary metastases at 9 years from diagnosis. Of the remaining patients, only two had evidence of persistent disease after an average of 5.8 years of follow-up. Because the clinical course appeared to correspond to the clinical stage of the disease, these authors suggest the absence of prognostic influence by the columnar cell variant morphology.

Diffuse sclerosing variant papillary carcinoma

This unusual variant is seen in 1.6 to 5.7% of papillary carcinomas (26-29). It is characterized by diffuse involvement of one or both thyroid lobes with dense sclerosis, abundant psammoma bodies, and frequently showing foci of squamous metaplasia. These tumors demonstrate a marked lymphocytic infiltration with numerous micropapillary formations within lymph vessels (30-33). There may be irregularly disposed thin bundles of smooth muscle within the fibrous stroma (33). Fine needle aspiration cytology may suggest this diagnosis (34). The biological behavior, in comparison to usual papillary carcinoma, is evidenced by a greater incidence of local lymph node metastases (28,31,35), a higher rate of pulmonary metastases (28,31,35), and a question of an increased likelihood of extrathyroidal invasion (27) or no difference in local invasive growth (28).

This pattern of metastatic behavior would suggest a less favorable prognosis than seen in usual papillary carcinoma. Although some clinicians report higher rates of mortality (30-32,35) others find this variant to have a good clinical outcome (26-29,33). A unique report of aggressive distant bone metastases despite a microscopic primary tumor further complicates this issue (36). It is possible that immunocytochemical staining for S-100 protein in associated dendritic/Langerhans cells may distinguish a good prognosis with this tumor variant (37).

Diffuse follicular variant papillary carcinoma

This suggested variant of papillary carcinoma has an uncertain status since it is described in a single report of eight such cases made by Sobrinho-Simões *et al* (38). These cases represented 1.6% of 503 papillary cancers evaluated by these investigators. It is characterized by diffuse involvement of the entire thyroid by papillary carcinoma in a follicular growth pattern, without fibrosis, lymphocytic infiltration, psammoma bodies, or discernible thyroidal nodules. Two of the cases were associated with Graves' disease. Most patients had locally metastatic disease and two patients had pulmonary metastases at presentation. After ten years, all patients had developed distant metastases to lung or bone; however, despite persistent tumor, the cancer remained responsive to radioiodine therapy.

Oxyphilic (Hürthle cell) variants of differentiated epithelial carcinoma

Hürthle cell variant follicular carcinoma. Follicular thyroid carcinomas in which the cells are predominantly oxyphilic, due to metaplastic changes with overexpression of large mitochondria, constitute a variant with unique clinical features (39). Just as for typical follicular neoplasms, in which carcinomas are distinguished from benign adenomas by the presence of vascular and/or tumor capsular invasion (40), the same criteria reliably distinguish benign Hürthle cell adenomas from the corresponding carcinomas (39). Since these adenomas share cytologic features, degrees of DNA aneuploidy, mitotic activity, and cellular atypia with carcinomas (41,42), it is likely that at least some of them are "carcinomas *in situ*" in which diagnosis by resection is curative.

Hürthle cell variant follicular carcinomas constitute 2.5 to 6.4% of thyroid carcinomas (43-46) and 20% of follicular carcinomas (43). Patients average 52 to 56 years of age with a female preponderance (1.3-7.3 to 1) (43-45). It differs in presentation from typical follicular carcinoma in that there is a higher risk of distant metastases (33% *vs* 22%) and a lower risk of local metastases (21% *vs* 30%) (47). Gross extrathyroidal invasion is seen in about 18% of patients (43, 44). Hürthle cell variant carcinoma patients have an appreciable disease-specific mortality of 13 to 35% (43-46) which may be greater than typical follicular cancer (47). One likely factor is that many of these tumors fail to concentrate sufficient radioiodine for effective therapy of recurrent or distantly metastatic disease (44).

Papotti *et al* (48) have recently described a significantly more lethal subtype constituting one third of Hürthle cell variant follicular thyroid carcinomas, with poorly differentiated features and a predominantly solid or trabecular growth pattern. Despite the absence of anaplastic carcinoma foci, 20% of cases over-expressed p53 protein and 50% expressed the *bcl-2* gene product. Mortality in this subset was positively associated with a small cell histologic pattern, p53 protein positivity, and absence of *bcl-2* gene product expression.

Hürthle cell variant papillary carcinoma. This variant of papillary thyroid carcinoma has a papillary architecture composed entirely of oxyphilic cells but does not show typical papillary nuclear changes (30), although one series reports that most cases had optically clear nuclei with variable expression of papillary nuclear features (49). Because of this, fine needle aspiration cytologies can be suggestive of an oxyphilic neoplasm, but are not reliably diagnostic of this tumor type (50-52). Surgical pathology reveals this variant in 2 to 4% of papillary carcinomas (49,53), with the female to male ratio at 1.8-3.9 to 1 (53,54), and average age at presentation of 44-57 years (49,54).

Hürthle cell variant is reported as having a more aggressive clinical course than typical papillary cancers with an 18 to 27% mortality at 10 years compared to 8-11% for typical papillary cancer (53,55). On the other hand, there was only one disease-specific mortality out of 39 cases described in two published reports, suggesting a less dangerous outcome (49,54). In the largest series of such patients, locoregional or distant recurrence was 28% at 10 years compared to 11% for typical papillary cancer and the presence of aneuploid DNA was 3-fold greater (53). One report (56) suggests that aggressive clinical behavior is seen with Hürthle cell variant papillary cancers which are invasive at presentation, while encapsulated primary lesions are less menacing.

A possible subtype of Hürthle cell variant papillary cancer was described by Apel et al (57) in 12 women and one man. This was suggested as a "Wartholin-like tumor", resembling a papillary cystadenoma lymphomatosum of the salivary gland, and appearing as Hürthle cells with a papillary tumor architecture bearing a lymphocytic stroma including lymphoid aggregates and germinal centers. All patients were free of disease at a short follow-up of 3 months to 9 years despite skeletal muscle invasion in one patient and local metastases in three patients.

Insular thyroid carcinoma

This thyroid epithelial carcinoma has been variously called: primordial cell carcinoma, solid variant of follicular cancer, poorly differentiated variant of papillary cancer, or "compact" subtype of anaplastic carcinoma (58,59). It is composed of nests of uniform cells and small follicles in an "insular" architectural pattern (60) representing 4 to 7% of thyroid carcinomas (61). Carcangiu et al (62) considered it a variant of papillary carcinoma which still retains papillary features, such as focal papilla formation and ground-glass nuclei, while featuring small tumor cells with scanty cytoplasm and microfollicles in a generally solid, lobular background. Thyroid capsular and vascular invasion are typical findings. Insular thyroid cancers may be misclassified as anaplastic cancer (63). Proper classification is critical since these cancers exhibit clinical behavior midway between papillary and anaplastic carcinomas (62,64,65) and may concentrate and respond to radioiodine therapy (63,65,66).

Cytological evaluation reveals both isolated cells and cellular clusters ranging from uniformly round to pleomorphic. There is often a necrotic background with poorly defined cytoplasm, without oxyphilia, and cytoplasmic vacuoles containing thyroglobulin. Nuclei are enlarged, hyperchromatic, and demonstrate features typical of papillary carcinoma with intranuclear inclusions and grooving (60, 61). This cancer may be seen in adolescents, as reported by Hassoun et al (65), with two female patients, aged 15 and 16 years, presenting with large and locally metastatic tumors which concentrated radioiodine and produced thyroglobulin; one patient dying of widely disseminated, distantly metastatic disease. An unusual presentation of an insular carcinoma featured a primary tumor appearing as an autonomously functioning thyroid nodule causing thyrotoxicosis, distant metastases, and revealing an activating mutation of the thyrotropin receptor on sequence analysis (66).

Insular carcinomas are typically aggressive with a 56% mortality in one series of 25 patients (64). In comparison to a similar number of poorly differentiated papillary carcinomas, 31 patients with insular carcinoma had a higher rate of recurrences and distant metastases (60% *vs* 19%), although mortality was similar (58). These tumors show a high rate of metastases to lung, bone, local lymph nodes, and show local recurrences (64,67). Isolated case reports may document variable clinical courses (68,69). Sometimes tumors have focal or varying portions of insular histology despite being predominantly papillary or follicular carcinomas. In a large series of such cases, Ashfaq *et al* (70) showed no correlation between the amount of insular component and the stage of disease, degree of aneuploidy, or mortality. This suggests that only predominant insular carcinomas have predictably aggressive clinical courses.

Mixed medullary and thyroid epithelial carcinoma

Carcinomas of follicular cell origin and parafollicular cell origin are thought to arise from separate embryologic origins. Rarely, primary tumors with features of both types of cancer are found, expressing both calcitonin and thyroglobulin, some with metastases of similar mixed phenotype. Many clinicians consider this to be an example of a "collision" tumor, in which the tumor is a coalescence of two independent primary cancers. Other possibilities include common expression of oncogenic mutations (such as those involving the RET proto-oncogene) resulting in simultaneous neoplastic transformation in two different precursor cells or development from multipotent stem cells. Some studies have suggested that rare examples of a common stem-cell origin can be inferred from immunohistochemical analyses and distinguished from collision tumors (71). The use of immunological staining of histological sections to verify co-expression of thyroglobulin and calcitonin in the same cells is of questionable reliability due to the detection of adsorbed thyroglobulin. Papotti *et al* (72) addressed this issue by using *in situ* hybridization to detect specific calcitonin and thyroglobulin mRNAs. In 2 of 11 cases, thyroglobulin and calcitonin messages were present in the same cells, while the remaining 9 cases showed distinct cell populations expressing each type of mRNA. This is the best evidence, to date, that the majority of these mixed tumors are collision tumors with a smaller number arising from a common stem-cell, as yet undefined. In this series, 45% of the patients died of their tumor by 8 years from diagnosis, suggesting this to be a clinically aggressive tumor. It is important to discriminate these tumors from metastases of other neuroendocrine tumors which may be mistaken for medullary carcinomas (73).

Anaplastic (dedifferentiated) thyroid carcinoma

Anaplastic thyroid carcinoma is the most aggressive solid tumor of any organ known. The incidence of this cancer has been variously reported to range from 5 to 20% of thyroid cancers; however its true incidence in the United States is best evidenced from the Surveillance, Epidemiology and End Results (SEER) Program which indicated that anaplastic cancer constituted 1.6% of thyroid cancers accumulated over the 18 years of the program (74). This is most commonly seen in older patients with a mean age of diagnosis at 57-67 years (74-78). The female to male patient ratio is 3.1-1.2 to 1 (74-76,78-80) which likely reflects the female preponderance of differentiated thyroid cancers, since anaplastic cancer represents a terminal dedifferentiation of pre-existing differentiated follicular epithelial cell carcinoma in most, if not all, cases (81-84). This feature places a burden upon clinicians to appropriately eliminate differentiated thyroid cancers in their early stages to lessen the opportunity for anaplastic transformation.

Most of these patients present with a rapidly growing thyroid mass, many of them with hoarseness and dyspnea, and some with dysphagia or cervical pain (77, 79). Fine needle aspiration cytology can permit a reliable diagnosis when properly performed and interpreted (85); however co-existent regions of differentiated carcinoma may contribute to diagnostic error (86). Pathologic assessment reveals a large, tan-white, fleshy, infiltrative tumor, with regions of necrosis and hemorrhage (39). There are three major histological patterns to this cancer, often coexisting in the same tumor: spindle cell (53%), giant cell (50%), and squamoid (19%) (59, 80). Common features include large foci of necrosis, marked invasiveness, and angiotropism. Tumor cells have a high mitotic rate (39) corresponding to their rapid rate of growth. An older designation of "small cell" anaplastic carcinoma is a misnomer and actually refers to misclassification of a lymphoma (87). This is a major problem in interpreting published therapeutic trials in this disease, since nearly all long term survivors or responders to chemotherapy were lymphomas or medullary cancers misdiagnosed as anaplastic cancer (88).

The clinical course is rapid and relentless despite most therapeutic interventions. Most patients die of local progression or distant metastases, sometimes within several weeks of diagnosis. The mean survival ranges from 2 to 7 months (78,80, 89,90), while the median survival is 4 to 12 months (76,77,91). Nearly all patients who survive their local disease will eventually reveal distant metastases. Those with distant metastases at initial presentation have shorter lengths of survival than patients presenting with only local tumor (74,78). Rare anaplastic carcinoma patients with longer term survival are younger, have small primary sites of localized tumor, and have received aggressive surgical resection, external radiotherapy, and systemic chemotherapy (although there have not been reliably effective agents) (76,78,90).

Therapeutic efforts may provide some prolongation of survival but have not been able to prevent mortality (see also Chapter 14). More extensive resection of the thyroid gland is associated with longer survival (92-94). Despite being relatively radioresistant, local external radiotherapy (sometimes with radiosensitizing chemotherapy (95)) has appeared to provide local disease control and prolong survival despite eventual death from distant disease (94,96). Many systemic chemotherapy agents have been tried, alone and in combination (particularly doxorubicin, cisplatin, bleomycin, and etoposide), but none of them are curative; although rare patients with partial responses have extension of survival. Initial investigations of mechanisms of chemotherapy resistance in anaplastic carcinoma have implicated over-expression of the multidrug resistance-associated protein (MRP1 gene product) which permits the cancer to survive chemotherapy agents by pumping them out of the cells (97,98). Since MRP is less able to expel paclitaxel (99), this may account for early evidence of significant antineoplastic activity of paclitaxel against anaplastic carcinoma cell lines (100).

Angiomatoid thyroid neoplasms (epithelioid angiosarcomas and hemangioendotheliomas)

Angiomatoid thyroid neoplasms are extremely rare cancers, particularly in the United States. By 1953, only 3 cases of malignant hemangioendothelioma had been reported in the United States despite an incidence of 16% of thyroid cancers in Switzerland at that time (101). Essentially, all of the literature reports only Alpine cases (or from the Andes in South America (102)), suggesting a remarkable geographic predilection. The incidence of malignant hemangioendothelioma in the Alpine goiter regions has progressively diminished coincident with the institution of iodine prophylaxis to prevent goiter (103). A recent report from Slovenia (Alpine country) shows only two cases of epithelioid angiosarcomas out of 327 thyroid carcinomas (0.6%) (104).

Angiomatoid thyroid neoplasms consist of epithelioid cells with prominent eosinophilic cytoplasm lining vascular-like spaces. Extensive immunohistochemical analysis of 8 angiomatoid thyroid neoplasms (105) demonstrated half of them to be angiosarcoma-like neoplasms with positive staining for: factor VIII-related antigen, CD31 (a vascular cell-to-cell adhesion molecule), CD34 (a hematopoietic progenitor cell antigen), and *Ulex europaeus* I lectin (an endothelial marker); while lacking immunostaining for epithelial markers other than cytokeratin. The other 4 tumors expressed one or more vascular markers as well as immunoactivity for cytokeratin, epithelial membrane antigen, and thyroglobulin; resulting in a designation of angiomatoid carcinoma. This demonstrates that angiomatoid thyroid neoplasms usually show some endothelial differentiation with "transitional" tumors having both epithelial and endothelial features, suggesting mesenchymal metaplasia (105). Additional reports of angiosarcomas reveal immunoactivity for factor VIII-related antigen (104,106) as well as *Ulex europaeus* I lectin, vimentin, cytokeratin, and laminin (104). Likewise, hemangioendotheliomas are positive for factor VIII-related antigen, suggesting a common endothelial origin (107-109).

These are aggressive tumors, usually presenting with sudden growth of a long-standing goiter in an older patient (mean age 67 years). Associated symptoms include radiating neck pain, dysphagia, dyspnea, emaciation, and fever. The tumors are locally invasive, causing asphyxia or bleeding (102,108). Most cases have hemorrhagic metastases to lung, pleura, lymph nodes, intestinal tract, bones, and heart (in order of frequency) (102,105,106,108). Survival is only a few months and the tumors appear unresponsive to surgery, radiotherapy, or chemotherapy (102,104-106,108).

Mucoepidermoid thyroid carcinoma

Mucoepidermoid thyroid carcinoma is exceedingly rare with just over 20 cases recorded in the literature. These tumors are solid, usually nonencapsulated, homogeneous masses; consisting of sheets of squamous cells with horny pearls and duct-like elements lined with mucous cells containing mucin cytoplasmic granules (110-112). Ultrastructural studies reveal aggregates of tonofilaments with well-developed desmosomal attachments (110). Immunocytochemistry demonstrates: positive staining for cytokeratin and carcinoembryonic antigen (CEA in mucous cells); negative staining for thyroglobulin, calcitonin, vimentin, chromogranin, and neuron-specific enolase; while vital stains are positive for mucicarmine and periodic acid-Schiff (110,111). On the other hand, Wenig *et al* (113) evaluated 6 cases described as mucoepidermoid carcinoma which had associated thyroiditis and a different immunocytochemistry pattern with positive staining for thyroglobulin, but negative staining for CEA, chromogranin, and calcitonin. The reason for this discrepancy is unclear; however their cases included only one tumor with extrathyroidal invasion and all were associated with thyroiditis. On the other hand, among the other cases in the literature, one third of the tumors were locally invasive, one third invaded vessels, and one third had nodal metastases (111).

These cancers are believed to originate from ultimobranchial-derived solid cell nests in the thyroid. To support this hypothesis, Harach *et al* (114) serially sectioned and stained the thyroid glands from 40 consecutive autopsies of fetuses (15-23 weeks of age), demonstrating solid cell nests in one third of the glands (usually in the middle to upper third of the lateral lobes) with 73% revealing the presence of mucosubstances. Harach's earlier study (115) had shown these solid cell nests to be composed of non-keratinizing epidermoid cells lacking intercellular bridges, surrounded by mucinous cells, and staining positively for cytokeratins and CEA. Half of these nests were positive for calcitonin. Additional support was provided by Pianzola *et al* (116), describing these solid cell nests in 21% of 100 consecutive autopsied thyroid glands; although a contemporary report analyzing 3,260 thyroidectomy specimens found solid cell nests in only 1.3% of the glands (117). To the contrary, Wenig *et al* (113) believe that mucoepidermoid thyroid carcinomas derive from thyroid follicular epithelial cells, reflecting the immunocytochemical staining pattern they described above.

With few clinical cases to evaluate, the prognosis of mucoepidermoid thyroid carcinoma remains unclear. Of 18 cases reported with some follow-up, only one patient had died of disease (13 months after diagnosis), despite three with local recurrences and half with distant metastases (110-113). Some patients received radiation therapy and some may have received various chemotherapies; however there is insufficient information to judge their therapeutic value, as well as likely insufficient follow-up time. An additional difficulty in assessing the clinical effects of this tumor results from cases in which the mucoepidermoid cancer co-exists with differentiated epithelial thyroid cancers (111) or anaplastic carcinoma (112), since the clinical effects of coexistent cancers may supersede those of the mucoepidermoid component. Further confusion results from cases with questionable classification (118) or potential thyroidal metastases from primary tumors of salivary, respiratory, or digestive sites (111).

Sclerosing mucoepidermoid carcinoma with eosinophilia (SMECE)

This is an apparent variant of mucoepidermoid thyroid carcinoma which is characterized by a dense fibrohyaline stroma infiltrated by numerous eosinophils. Approximately 10 cases have been described to date and the clinical reports suggest that this variant is more aggressive than "typical" mucoepidermoid carcinoma. Seven of 10 cases had extrathyroidal invasion with 4 cases involving the trachea or esophagus. Three cases were locally metastatic and one had distant metastases. Comparison of SMECE with "typical" mucoepidermoid thyroid carcinoma reveals involvement of older patients (mean 59 years *vs* 37 years), a greater predilection for women (100% *vs* 65%) and higher rates of extrathyroidal invasion (70% *vs* 13%). None of the SMECE patients were reported with disease-specific mortality for the period of follow-up (119,120).

Thyroid carcinomas with thymic differentiation

In human embryonic development, the thymus is derived from endoderm of the third pair of branchial pouches and descends in the neck, sometimes leaving behind "ectopic" thymus tissue in varied cervical locations, including the thyroid gland. This has been detected in around 20% of people (121,122). These thymic rests are the probable source of thymic neoplasms in and near the thyroid gland, as well as occasionally being misclassified as lymphomas (39). In order to clarify the nosology of cervical thymic neoplasms, Chan and Rosai (122) reviewed the literature and histologic material of reported cases to define four general categories: ectopic hamartomatous thymomas, ectopic cervical thymomas, spindle epithelial tumors with thymus-like differentiation (SETTLE), and carcinomas showing thymus-like differentiation (CASTLE).

In the Chan and Rosai schema (122), ectopic hamartomatous thymomas are found in supraclavicular or suprasternal locations as masses which may have been present for up to 30 years. These tumors consist of 20-95% spindle epithelial cells with 5-35% of the tumor having solid or cystic epithelial islands within fibrous stroma with entrapped mature fat cells. Resection is curative, suggesting a possibly non-malignant phenotype, with no metastases or recurrences noted in 15 reported cases. The category of ectopic cervical thymoma is characterized by anterolateral neck tumors which may be adjacent to the thyroid, rarely intrathyroidal, with histologic characteristics identical to those of mediastinal thymomas, featuring encapsulated lobular mixtures of plump or spindled epithelial cells and small lymphocytes in fibrous septa. In 16 reported cases, one was locally metastatic and two were locally invasive, all were treated with surgery (some with additional external radiotherapy), and no fatalities were recorded.

Spindle epithelial tumor with thymus-like differentiation (SETTLE)

This category from Chan and Rosai (122) is intended to include tumors known as thyroid spindle cell tumors with mucous cysts and some malignant teratomas. The tumors will be discussed in the following section on malignant teratomas.

Carcinomas showing thymus-like differentiation (CASTLE)

These cancers are also known as primary thyroid thymomas and are seen in adults at a mean age of 49 years with two thirds of patients being female. Approximately 40% have nodal metastases and nearly 30% of primary tumors are invasive (122). The tumor contains lobules and cords of squamoid cells separated by fibrous septa infiltrated with small lymphocytes and plasma cells; focal areas resemble Hassall's corpuscles (122). The tumor cells have vesicular nuclei and pale eosinophilic cytoplasm. Electron microscopy reveals numerous prominent desmosomes and intracytoplasmic bundles of tonofilaments. Immunocytochemistry is positive for cytokeratins and CEA, but negative for calcitonin, thyroglobulin, S-100 protein, chromogranin, somatostatin, and leukocyte common antigen (123). Some cases may be misdiagnosed as poorly differentiated squamous cell carcinomas (124). Since other lymphoepithelioma-like carcinomas, such as nasopharyngeal carcinoma, are associated with Epstein-Barr virus, Shek *et al* (125) used *in situ* mRNA hybridization to rule out evidence of viral influence in one such case. This tumor is clinically aggressive with a significant, but unquantified, mortality rate. There is suggestive evidence that external radiotherapy may enhance the therapeutic effectiveness of thyroidectomy and aid in the management of recurrent disease (122-124,126,127).

Malignant adult thyroid teratoma

These are extremely rare thyroid malignancies and extremely aggressive ones with unlikely survival more than one year after initial surgery. They are distinct from cervical teratomas of infancy, are presumed to arise from midline misplaced germ cells, and are histologically similar to immature teratomas or malignant germ cell neoplasms arising in teratomas (39). Patients with this tumor average 39 years of age and are typically female (70%) (128,129). Tumors are often locally invasive and nearly all locally metastatic as well as distantly metastatic (129,130). Patients have been typically treated with thyroidectomy, followed by external radiotherapy and/or systemic chemotherapy. Agents documented in case reports include: doxorubicin, cisplatin, etoposide (VP-16), bleomycin, vincristine, cyclophosphamide, and actinomycin-D (128-131). Mortality is nearly complete despite these therapeutic efforts.

Malignant adult thyroid teratoma appears to be distinct from the spindle epithelial tumors with thymus-like differentiation (SETTLE) delineated by Chan and Rosai (122). They describe cellular tumors, containing compact bundles of long spindle epithelial cells which merge with tubulopapillary structures or mucinous glands, which have been seen in patients with a mean age of 15 years (compared to 39 years for adult thyroid teratomas), with similar female predominance, but with a somewhat less aggressive clinical course. Only 38% presented with distant metastases and the mortality was only 25%, defined at a 6-7 year follow-up. Because of these differences, SETTLE patients should be classified as an aggressive subtype of thyroid carcinomas with thymic differentiation.

Paraganglioma of the thyroid

Paragangliomas typically develop in sites near the autonomic nervous system, but may rarely be found in unusual sites such as the thyroid, even though there is no evidence that normal paraganglions are found within thyroids (39). Livolsi (39) classifies thyroid paragangliomas as synonymous with hyalinizing trabecular adenomas and paraganglioma-like adenomas of the thyroid (PLAT). Both PLAT and hyalinizing trabecular adenomas may be more appropriately considered as variants of papillary carcinomas (1). LaGuette, Matias-Guiu, & Rosai (132) have recently reported 3 cases of paraganglioma of the thyroid, along with 11 additional cases gleaned from the literature, which are distinct from PLAT or medullary carcinomas.

The paragangliomas described by LaGuette et al (132) are thought to arise from the inferior laryngeal paraganglia. All of these patients were women between 40 and 60 years of age. Nearly 30% of them presented with their primary tumor invading the trachea or larynx and none had metastases. Immunohistochemistry revealed positive staining for neuron-specific enolase, synaptophysin, and chromogranin A; while there was no immunoreactivity for cytokeratin, epithelial membrane antigen, CEA, thyroglobulin, calcitonin, calcitonin gene-related peptide, serotonin, and vimentin. This is in contrast to PLAT tumors, which stain positively for thyroglobulin (133). Limited clinical experience suggests that thyroid paraganglioma patients respond well to surgical resection and have not shown any disease-specific mortality despite the absence of adjuvant treatments.

Primary thyroid lymphomas

Primary thyroid lymphomas are uncommon, representing 1 to 5% of thyroid malignancies (39,134,135) and less than 1% of all lymphomas (39). Although the majority of these tumors arise in glands with autoimmune thyroiditis (135), the high incidence of thyroid autoimmunity eliminates this from clinical consideration as a premalignant condition. Nearly all of these lymphomas are B-cell type with T-cell lymphomas distinctly rare (136). More than 80% have a diffuse histologic pattern and 70 to 80% are large cell lymphomas (histiocytic lymphomas), with 5-10%

intermediate grade (poorly differentiated), 10-12% low grade lymphoma (small cell; frequently mistaken for anaplastic or medullary carcinomas), and Hodgkin's disease exceedingly rare (39). The gross appearance is that of a large fleshy tan to gray mass with frequent extrathyroidal extension and vascular invasion (137). More than 70% of thyroid lymphomas have characteristic lymphoepithelial lesions (39,138) which suggest them to be mucosa-associated lymphoid tissue (MALT) malignancies. More than half of such patient fatalities, subjected to full autopsies, revealed tumors in the gastrointestinal tract, reflecting the tendency of MALT lymphomas to spread to other MALT sites (139).

Nearly all thyroid lymphoma patients present with a pre-existing goiter with 78% showing sudden rapid growth of the goiter, 13% with hoarseness, 7% with dysphagia, and 7% with fever (135). The finding of stridor on presentation has been highly associated with death from this disease (138). Patients average 60 to 68 years of age at presentation and 67 to 90% are women (134,135,139,140). Fine needle aspiration cytology has emerged as a preferred diagnostic technique (135, 141). In the largest published series of thyroid lymphoma patients (135), more than 78% were correctly diagnosed this way; with B-cell immunotyping by flow cytometry used to enhance diagnostic specificity. Other patients required open biopsy; and ultrasound examination produced characteristic findings of an asymmetrical pseudocystic pattern in the thyroid which was reputed to be seen in 93% of patients. These patients should be assigned a clinical stage based on assessments for distant disease using computerized axial tomographic scanning, magnetic resonance imaging, or gallium-67 nuclear scanning of the chest and abdomen. The majority of thyroid lymphoma patients are stage I-E (thyroid) or II-E (thyroid and local nodes) (140,142,143) with around 6% of patients presenting with distant metastases, usually of the stomach or abdominal cavity (135).

Disease-specific mortality following treatment with surgery and/or external radiotherapy, prior to the availability of chemotherapy, was 35 to 64% (134,135,140,143). This is related to a 30% incidence of distant relapses despite clinically localized disease (142). Use of combination chemotherapy (CHOP: cyclophosphamide, doxorubicin, vincristine, and prednisone) and external radiotherapy produces the best clinical results with close to complete survival in Stage I-E disease and moderately less in Stage II-E (135,138,142) (please see also Chapter 14). Due to frequent local bulky disease, more than 20% of patients treated with chemotherapy alone will have local recurrences (142). On the other hand, there is no difference in survival between patients treated with mere thyroid biopsy plus adjuvant therapy compared to those treated with thyroidectomy plus adjuvant therapy, suggesting that surgical resection offers no advantages over external radiotherapy (143). This is in contrast to a recent recommendation advocating total thyroidectomy rather than only biopsy (67). Lower external radiotherapy doses (140) and fewer courses of combination chemotherapy (135) produce worse clinical outcomes.

Strategies for therapeutic management

In consideration of the rare expression of these thyroid malignancies, there is a significant deficit of clinical experience on which to base choices of therapeutic approach. For this reason, the following recommendations of the author reflect his clinical judgment and limited experience with these rare thyroid cancers.

Variants of differentiated epithelial thyroid carcinoma

Treatment of differentiated thyroid epithelial carcinomas is predicated upon a total thyroidectomy with varying degrees of nodal resection, followed by adjuvant radioiodine ablation therapy. Apart from the question of additional local disease control with external radiotherapy, there is no doubt that radioiodine treatment remains the only effective systemic therapy. There is no convincing evidence that any currently available chemotherapy agents have significant activity in these cancers. For this reason, a general philosophy of enhancing and optimizing surgical and radioiodine treatments appears to be a rational approach.

Surgery. Surgical thyroidectomies should be as complete as an experienced thyroid surgeon can safely manage (144,145). Since radioiodine can more effectively destroy smaller metastases than larger ones, and the ability to concentrate radioiodine may be in question, it is important to do ipsilateral modified neck dissections at the initial surgery and later (if not previously performed), if local recurrence is noted. In practical terms, the diagnosis of a rare variant carcinoma is usually not immediately apparent at the time of the initial surgery, which may be less than a total resection. When the diagnosis is made, particularly if available clinical information suggests that the particular variant is associated with an aggressive disease course, there should be little hesitation to reoperate and complete the thyroidectomy and node dissection.

Radioiodine therapy. Some variants, particularly oxyphilic and tall cell carcinomas, are well known to lose iodine concentrating ability, rendering them resistant to radioiodine therapy (1,44). This may be a late phase of the disease with a narrow window of opportunity for effective radioiodine therapy early in the disease course. In such circumstances, as well as for other clinically aggressive variants or distantly metastatic disease, it is advisable to enhance I-131 treatment as much as possible. These enhancements include: increasing endogenous thyrotropin levels above 35 mU/L (treatment experience with recombinant human thyrotropin is not yet available) (146), use of an iodine-restricted diet (to reduce stable iodine excretion to less than 50 µg/day) (147), avoidance of tumor stunning by lowering or eliminating the radioiodine scanning dose prior to a therapy dose (148), use of maximal dosimetry-directed I-131 therapy doses to treat to the limits of marrow or lung tolerance (149,150), and enhancement of radioiodine retention in tumor tissue by adjuvant use of lithium carbonate (149,151,152).

Follow-up. Evaluation and clinical follow-up of patients must not rely solely upon I-131 scanning. The thyroglobulin level serves as an independent index for the presence of residual thyroid cancer, since there are no benign sources of thyroglobulin following total thyroidectomy and radioiodine ablation. Some patients, with micrometastatic disease, remain responsive to enhanced radioiodine therapy given on the basis of elevated thyroglobulin levels (above 5-8 ng/mL) (153). Functional diagnostic studies, based upon radioiodine uptake, may be supplemented with thallium-201 (154,155) or technetium-99m-sestamibi (hexakis 2-methoxy isobutyl isonitrile) nuclear body scans, which do not depend upon functional iodine transport. Tc-99m-sestamibi seems to have particular value in oxyphilic variants since it is mitochondria-avid (156,157). In a similar fashion, whole body positron emission tomographic imaging with fluorine-18 fluorodeoxyglucose appears to be able to detect thyroid carcinoma metastases (158,159). Likewise, anatomical imaging with gadolinium-enhanced magnetic resonance scans and high resolution non-contrast computerized tomographic radiologic scans (best for the lung) provide other opportunities to detect residual, recurrent, or metastatic thyroid cancer. In the absence of sufficient radioiodine uptake in tumor deposits, detection by these other modalities (as well as physical examination) denotes an intent for further surgical resection or treatment with external radiotherapy.

Mixed medullary and thyroid epithelial carcinoma

In view of the rarity of true mixed tumors, as opposed to collision tumors, all therapeutic suggestions remain highly hypothetical. Radioiodine therapy is of no value for medullary thyroid cancer since this tumor does not express the sodium-iodide symporter. Although Papotti et al (72) suggest the use of I-131 to treat mixed tumors, the effectiveness of this approach remains unproved. It is more reasonable to suppose that, despite such efforts, meticulous and extensive surgical resection remains the best available therapeutic option (160).

Anaplastic thyroid carcinoma

Current therapeutic options do not provide the opportunity for curative treatment of anaplastic thyroid carcinoma. Survival may be extended by careful management of local disease. If resectable, this should be the first step; however, hyperfractionated external beam radiotherapy can enhance local disease control, although patients will die of distant disease. Radiosensitization with concomitant low-dose doxorubicin has been claimed to enhance the response to external radiotherapy (95), but later experience suggests that there is significantly increased toxicity without enhancement of tumor response (161). Multimodality therapy, combining surgery, external radiotherapy, and systemic full-dose chemotherapy appears to delay (but not reduce) ultimate mortality (162). Preliminary results from our national phase II clinical trial suggests that paclitaxel is the most active available chemotherapy agent for this disease.

Angiomatoid thyroid neoplasm and malignant adult thyroid teratoma

Both of these categories of thyroid malignancies are extremely aggressive, do not appear likely to concentrate radioiodine, and have high rates of mortality. There are no clearly defined benefits to any particular therapeutic approach, suggesting that clinicians approach this tumor in a similar fashion as for anaplastic carcinoma (discussed above). The tendency for metastases from this tumor to be extremely vascular suggests the need to consider palliative surgery or angiographic embolectomy in situations of clinical hemorrhage.

Mucoepidermoid thyroid carcinoma and thyroid paraganglioma

The clinical courses of these cancers and their subtypes is uncertain; however they appear less aggressive than anaplastic, angiomatoid, or teratomatous malignancies. Local tumor control with complete surgical resection appears appropriate and reasonable. The role of external radiotherapy is not defined and should be considered on a case-by-case basis. In the absence of known active chemotherapy agents, as well as a lower rate of mortality in comparison with dedifferentiated thyroid neoplasms, empirical chemotherapy is not advised.

Thyroid carcinoma with thymic differentiation

The different categories of thymic-type thyroid malignancies vary widely in their disease course and mortality. Surgical resection is essential as initial treatment; however, the thymic differentiation suggests that external radiotherapy may have particularly important therapeutic effects.

Primary thyroid lymphoma

Matsuzuka *et al* (135) have demonstrated the best clinical outcome for thyroid lymphoma patients following their recommended approach. They suggest that, following diagnosis (using fine needle biopsy) and staging, patients undergo one course of full-dose CHOP chemotherapy, followed by 40 to 60 Gy of local external radiotherapy, then five additional courses of CHOP. This appears to be a reasonable plan with acceptably low morbidity.

References

1. Ain KB. Papillary thyroid carcinoma: etiology, assessment, and therapy. Endocrin Metab Clin N Amer. 1995; 24:711-60.
2. Fassina AS, Montesco MC, Ninfo V, Denti P, Masarotto G. Histological evaluation of thyroid carcinomas: reproducibility of the ÇWHOÈ classification. Tumori. 1993; 79:314-20.
3. Hawk WA, Hazard JB. The many appearances of papillary carcinoma of the thyroid. Clev Clin Quart. 1976; 43:207-16.
4. Merino MJ, Kennedy SM, Norton JA, Robbins J. Pleural involvement by metastatic thyroid carcinoma "tall cell variant": an unusual occurrence. Surg Pathol. 1990; 3:59-64.
5. Ozaki O, Ito K, Mimura T, Sugino K, Hosoda Y. Papillary carcinoma of the thyroid: tall-cell variant with extensive lymphocyte infiltration. Am J Surg Pathol. 1996; 20:695-698.

6. Egea AM, Gonzalez JMR, Perez JS, Cogollos TS, Paricio PP. Prognostic value of the tall cell variety of papillary cancer of the thyroid. Eur J Surg Oncol. 1993; 19:517-21.

7. Johnson TL, Lloyd RV, Thompson NW, Beierwaltes WH, Sisson JC. Prognostic implications of the tall cell variant of papillary thyroid carcinoma. Am J Surg Pathol. 1988; 12:22-7.

8. Rüter A, Nishiyama R, Lennquist S. Tall-cell variant of papillary thyroid cancer: disregarded entity? World J Surg. 1997; 21:15-21.

9. Terry JH, St. John SA, Karkowski FJ, et al. Tall cell papillary thyroid cancer: incidence and prognosis. Am J Surg. 1994; 168:459-61.

10. Gamboa-Domínguez A, Candanedo-González F, Uribe-Uribe NO, Angeles-Angeles A. Tall cell variant of papillary thyroid carcinoma: a cytohistologic correlation. Acta Cytologica. 1997; 41:672-676.

11. Ostrowski ML, Merino MJ. Tall cell variant of papillary thyroid carcinoma: a reassessment and immunohistochemical study with comparison to the usual type of papillary carcinoma of the thyroid. Am J Surg Path. 1996; 20:964-974.

12. LiVolsi VA. Papillary neoplasms of the thyroid: pathologic and prognostic features. Am J Clin Pathol. 1992; 97:426-34.

13. Harach HR, Zusman SB. Cytopathology of the tall cell variant of thyroid papillary carcinoma. Acta Cytolog. 1992; 36:895-9.

14. Leung C-S, Hartwick RWJ, Bédard YC. Correlation of cytologic and histologic features in variants of papillary carcinoma of the thyroid. Acta Cytolog. 1993; 37:645-50.

15. Rüter A, Dreifus J, Jones M, Nishiyama R, Lennquist S. Overexpression of p53 in tall cell variants of papillary thyroid carcinoma. Surgery. 1996; 120:1046-1050.

16. Flint A, Davenport RD, Lloyd RV. The tall cell variant of papillary carcinoma of the thyroid gland: comparison with the common form of papillary carcinoma by DNA and morphometric analysis. Arch Pathol Lab Med. 1991; 115:169-71.

17. Bronner MP, LiVolsi VA. Spindle cell squamous carcinoma of the thyroid: an unusual anaplastic tumor associated with tall cell papillary cancer. Mod Pathol. 1991; 4:637-43.

18. Sobrinho-Simões M, Nesland JM, Johannessen JV. 1988 Columnar-cell carcinoma. Another variant of poorly differentiated carcinoma of the thyroid. Am J Clin Pathol. 1988; 89:264-7.

19. Akslen LA, Varhaug JE. Thyroid carcinoma with mixed tall-cell and columnar-cell features. Am J Clin Pathol. 1990; 94:442-5.

20. Berends D, Mouthaan PJ. Columnar-cell carcinoma of the thyroid. Histopathol. 1992; 20:360-2.

21. Evans HL. Columnar-cell carcinoma of the thyroid: a report of two cases of an aggressive variant of thyroid carcinoma. Am J Clin Pathol. 1986; 85:77-80.

22. Ferreiro JA, Hay ID, Lloyd RV. Columnar cell carcinoma of the thyroid: report of three additional cases. Hum Pathol. 1996; 27:1156-1160.

23. Hui P-K, Chan JKC, Cheung PSY, Gwi E. Columnar cell carcinoma of the thyroid: fine needle aspiration findings in a case. Acta Cytolog. 1990; 34:355-8.

24. Mizukami Y, Nonomusra A, Michigishi T, Noguchi M, Nakamura S, Hashimoto T. Columnar cell carcinoma of the thyroid gland: a case report and review of the literature. Hum Pathol. 1994; 25:1098-1101.

25. Wenig BM, Thompson LDR, Adair CF, Shmookler B, Heffess CS. Thyroid papillary carcinoma of columnar cell type. Cancer. 1988; 82:740-763.

26. Fujimoto Y, Obara T, Ito Y, Kodama T, Aiba M, Yamaguchi K. Diffuse sclerosing variant of papillary carcinoma of the thyroid: clinical importance, surgical treatment, and follow-up study. Cancer. 1990; 66:2306-12.

27. Egea AM, Gonzalez JMR, Perez JS, Soria T, Paricio PP. Clinicopathological study of the diffuse sclerosing variety of papillary cancer of the thyroid. Presentation of 4 new cases and review of the literature. Eur J Surg Oncol. 1994; 20:7-11.

28. Soares J, Limbert E, Sobrinho-Simões. Diffuse sclerosing variant of papillary thyroid carcinoma: a clinicopathologic study of 10 cases. Path Res Pract. 1989; 185:200-6.

29. Macák J, Michal M. Diffuse sclerosing variant of papillary thyroid carcinoma. Ceskoslov Patol. 1993; 29:6-8.

30. Hedinger CE, Williams ED, Sobin LH. Histological Typing of Thyroid Tumours. (2nd ed.) Berlin: Springer-Verlag; 1988.

31. Carcangiu ML, Bianchi S. Diffuse sclerosing variant of papillary thyroid carcinoma: clinicopathologic study of 15 cases. Am J Surg Pathol. 1989; 13:1041-9.

32. Vickery Jr AL, Carcangiu ML, Johannessen JV, Sobrinho-Simoes M. Session I: papillary carcinoma. Sem Diag Pathol. 1985; 2:90-100.

33.   Chan JKC, Tsui MS, Tse CH. Diffuse sclerosing variant of papillary carcinoma of the thyroid: a histological and immunohistochemical study of three cases. Histopathol. 1987; 11:191-201.
34.   Caruso G, Tabarri B, Lucchi I, Tison V. Fine needle aspiration cytology in a case of diffuse sclerosing carcinoma of the thyroid. Acta Cytolog. 1990; 34:352-4.
35.   Rosai J. Papillary Carcinoma. Monographs in Pathology. 1993; 1993:138-65.
36.   Patchefsky AS, Keller IB, Mansfield CM. Solitary vertebral column metastasis from occult sclerosing carcinoma of the thyroid gland: report of a case. Am J Clin Pathol. 1970; 53:596-601.
37.   Schröder S, Bay V, Dumke K, et al. 1990 Diffuse sclerosing variant of papillary thyroid carcinoma: S-100 protein immunocytochemistry and prognosis. Virch Arch A Pathol Anat. 1990; 416:367-71.
38.   Sobrinho-Simões MA, Soares J, Carneiro F, Limbert E. Diffuse follicular variant of papillary carcinoma of the thyroid: report of eight cases of a distinct aggressive type of thyroid tumor. Surg Pathol. 1990; 3:189-203.
39.   LiVolsi VA. Surgical Pathology of the Thyroid. Philadelphia: W. B. Saunders Co. 1990.
40.   Franssila KO, Ackerman LV, Brown CL, Hedinger CE. Session II: follicular carcinoma. Sem Diag Pathol. 1985; 2:101-22.
41.   Schürmann G, Mattfeldt T, Feichter G, Koretz K, Möller P, Buhr H. Stereology, flow cytometry, and immunohistochemistry of follicular neoplasms of the thyroid gland. Hum Pathol. 1991; 22:179-84.
42.   Grebe SKG, Hay ID. Follicular thyroid cancer. Endocrinol Metab Clin N Amer. 1995; 24:761-801.
43.   Watson RG, Brennan MD, Goellner JR, van Heerden JA, McConahey WM, Taylor WF. Invasive Hürthle cell carcinoma of the thyroid: natural history and management. Mayo Clin Proc. 1984; 59:851-855.
44.   Har-El G, Hadar T, Segal K, Levy R, Sidi J. Hürthle cell carcinoma of the thyroid gland: a tumor of moderate malignancy. Cancer. 1986; 57:1613-1617.
45.   McDonald MP, Sanders LE, Silverman ML, Chan H-S, Buyske J. Hürthle cell carcinoma of the thyroid gland: prognostic factors and results of surgical treatment. Surg. 1996; 120:1000-1005.
46.   Tollefsen HR, Shah JP, Huvos AG. Hürthle cell carcinoma of the thyroid. Am J Surg. 1975; 130:390-394.
47.   Shaha AR, Shah JP, Loree TR. Patterns of nodal and distant metastasis based on histologic varieties in differentiated carcinoma of the thyroid. Am J Surg. 1996; 172:692-694.
48.   Papotti M, Torchio B, Grassi L, Favero A, Bussolati G. Poorly differentiated oxyphilic (Hürthle cell) carcinomas of the thyroid. Am J Surg Pathol. 1996; 20:686-694.
49.   Berho M, Suster S. The oncocytic variant of papillary carcinoma of the thyroid: a clinicopathologic study of 15 cases. Hum Pathol. 1997; 28:47-53.
50.   Chen KTK. Fine-needle aspiration cytology of papillary Hürthle-cell tumors of thyroid: a report of three cases. Diagn Cytopathol. 1991; 7:53-6.
51.   Doria Jr. MI, Attal H, Wang HH, Jensen JA, DeMay RM. Fine needle aspiration cytology of the oxyphil variant of papillary carcinoma of the thyroid: a report of three cases. Acta Cytolog. 1996; 40:1007-1011.
52.   Dzieciol J, Musiatowicz B, Zimnoch L, Kemona A, Sulkowski S. Papillary Hürthle cell tumor of thyroid: report of a case with a cytomorphologic approach to diagnosis. Acta Cytolog. 1996; 40:311-314.
53.   Herrera MF, Hay ID, Wu PS-C, et al. Hürthle cell (oxyphilic) papillary thyroid carcinoma: a variant with more aggressive biologic behavior. World J Surg. 1992; 16:669-75.
54.   Beckner ME, Heffess CS, Oertel JE. Oxyphilic papillary thyroid carcinomas. Am J Clin Pathol. 1995; 103:280-287.
55.   Sobrinho-Simões MA, Nesland JM, Holm R, Sambade MC, Johannessen JV. Hürthle cell and mitochondrion-rich papillary carcinomas of the thyroid gland: an ultrastructural and immunocytochemical study. Ultrastruct Pathol. 1985; 8:131-42.
56.   Barbuto D, Carcangiu ML, Rosai J. Papillary Hürthle cell neoplasms of the thyroid gland. A study of 20 cases. Lab Invest. 1990; 62:7A.
57.   Apel RL, Asa SL, LiVolsi VA. Papillary Hürthle cell carcinoma with lymphocytic stroma: "Wartholin-like tumor" of the thyroid. Am J Surg Pathol. 1995; 19:810-814.
58.   Papotti M, Micca FB, Favero A, Palestini N, Bussolati G. Poorly differentiated thyroid carcinomas with primordial cell component: a group of aggressive lesions sharing insular, trabecular, and solid patterns. Am J Surg Pathol. 1993; 17:291-301.

59. Rosai J, Saxén EA, Woolner L. Session III: Undifferentiated and poorly differentiated carcinoma. Sem Diag Pathol. 1985; 2:123-36.

60. Zakowski MF, Schlesinger K, Mizrachi HH. Cytologic features of poorly differentiated "insular" carcinoma of the thyroid: a case report. Acta Cytolog. 1992; 36:523-526.

61. Pietribiasi F, Sapino A, Papotti M, Bussolati G. Cytologic features of poorly differentiated 'insular' carcinoma of the thyroid, as revealed by fine-needle aspiration biopsy. Am J Clin Pathol. 1990; 94:687-692.

62. Carcangiu ML, Zampi G, Rosai J. Papillary thyroid carcinoma: a study of its many morphologic expressions and clinical correlates. Pathol Ann. 1985; 20:1-44.

63. Justin EP, Seabold JE, Robinson RA, Walker WP, Gurll NJ, Hawes DR. Insular carcinoma: a distinct thyroid carcinoma with associated iodine-131 localization. J Nucl Med. 1991; 32:1358-1363.

64. Carcangiu ML, Zampi G, Rosai J. Poorly differentiated ("insular") thyroid carcinoma: a reinterpretation of Langhans' "wucherende Struma". Am J Surg Pathol. 1984; 8:655-68.

65. Hassoun AAK, Hay ID, Goellner JR, Zimmerman D. Insular thyroid carcinoma in adolescents: a potentially lethal endocrine malignancy. Cancer. 1997; 79:1044-1048.

66. Russo D, Tumino S, Arturi F, et al. Detection of an activating mutation of the thyrotropin receptor in a case of an autonomously hyperfunctioning thyroid insular carcinoma. J Clin Endocrinol Metab. 1997; 82:735-738.

67. Burman KD, Ringel MD, Wartofsky L. Unusual types of thyroid neoplasms. Endocrinol Metab Clin N Amer. 1996; 25:49-68.

68. Bal C, Padhy AK, Panda S, Kumar L, Basu AK. "Insular" carcinoma of thyroid: a subset of anaplastic thyroid malignancy with a less aggressive clinical course. Clin Nucl Med. 1993; 18:1056-8.

69. Flynn SD, Forman BH, Stewart AF, Kinder BK. Poorly differentiated ("insular") carcinoma of the thyroid gland: an aggressive subset of differentiated thyroid neoplasms. Surg. 1988; 104:963-70.

70. Ashfaq R, Vuitch F, Delgado R, Albores-Saavedra J. Papillary and follicular thyroid carcinomas with an insular component. Cancer. 1994; 73:416-23.

71. Lax SF, Beham A, Kronberger-Schšnecker D, Langsteger W, Denk H. Coexistence of papillary and medullary carcinoma of the thyroid gland - mixed or collision tumour? Clinicopathological analysis of three cases. Virchows Archiv. 1994; 424:441-447.

72. Papotti M, Negro F, Carney JA, Bussolati G, Lloyd RV. Mixed medullary-follicular carcinoma of the thyroid: a morphological, immunohistochemical and in situ hybridization analysis of 11 cases. Virchows Arch. 1997; 430:397-405.

73. Matias-Guiu X, LaGuette J, Puras-Gil AM, Rosai J. Metastatic neuroendocrine tumors to the thyroid gland mimicking medullary carcinoma: a pathologic and immunohistochemistry study of six cases. Am J Surg Pathol. 1997; 21:754-762.

74. Gilliland FD, Hunt WC, Morris DM, Key CR. Prognostic factors for thyroid carcinoma: a population-based study of 15,698 cases from the Surveillance, Epidemiology and End Results (SEER) Program 1973-1991. Cancer. 1997; 79:564-573.

75. Agrawal S, Rao RS, Parikh EM, Parikh HK, Borges AM, Sampat MB. Histologic trends in thyroid cancer 1969-1993: a clinico-pathologic analysis of the relative proportion of anaplastic carcinoma of the thyroid. J Surg Oncol. 1996; 63:251-255.

76. Demeter JG, De Jong SA, Lawrence AM, Paloyan E. Anaplastic thyroid carcinoma: risk factors and outcome. Surgery. 1991; 110:956-963.

77. Nel CJC, van Heerden JA, Goellner JR, et al. Anaplastic carcinoma of the thyroid: a clinicopathologic study of 82 cases. Mayo Clin Proc. 1985; 60:51-8.

78. Venkatesh YS, Ordonez NG, Schultz PN, Hickey RC, Goepfert H, Samaan NA. Anaplastic carcinoma of the thyroid: a clinicopathologic study of 121 cases. Cancer. 1990; 66:321-330.

79. Hadar T, Mor C, Shvero J, Levy R, Segal K. Anaplastic carcinoma of the thyroid. Eur J Surg Oncol. 1993; 19:511-16.

80. Carcangiu ML, Steeper T, Zampi G, Rosai J. Anaplastic thyroid carcinoma: A study of 70 cases. Am J Clin Pathol. 1985; 83:135-58.

81. Aldinger KA, Samaan NA, Ibanez M, Hill Jr CS. Anaplastic carcinoma of the thyroid: a review of 84 cases of spindle and giant cell carcinoma of the thyroid. Cancer. 1978; 41:2267-2275.

82. Nishiyama RH, Dunn EL, Thompson NW. Anaplastic spindle-cell and giant-cell tumors of the thyroid gland. Cancer. 1972; 30:113-127.

83.   Harada T, Ito K, Shimaoka K, Hosoda Y, Yakumaru K. Fatal thyroid carcinoma: anaplastic transformation of adenocarcinoma. Cancer. 1977; 39:2588-96.

84.   Matias-Guiu X, Villanueva A, Cuatrecasas M, Capella G, De Leiva A, Prat J. p53 in a thyroid follicular carcinoma with foci of poorly differentiated and anaplastic carcinoma. Path Res Pract. 1996; 192:1242-1249.

85.   Us-Krasovec M, Golouh R, Auersperg M, Besic N, Ruparcic-Oblak L. Anaplastic thyroid carcinoma in fine needle aspirates. Acta Cytol. 1996; 40:953-958.

86.   Bauman ME, Tao L-C. Cytopathology of papillary carcinoma of the thyroid with anaplastic transformation: a case report. Acta Cytol. 1995; 39:525-529.

87.   Wolf BC, Sheahan K, DeCoste D, Variakojis D, Alpern HD, Haselow RE. Immunohistochemical analysis of small cell tumors of the thyroid gland: an Eastern Cooperative Oncology Group study. Hum Pathol. 1992; 23:1252-1261.

88.   Nusynowitz ML. Differentiating anaplastic thyroid carcinomas. J Nucl Med. 1991; 32:1363-1364.

89.   Lampertico P. Anaplastic (sarcomatoid) carcinoma of the thyroid gland. Sem Diag Pathol. 1993; 10:159-168.

90.   Jereb B, Stjernswärd J, Löwhagen T. Anaplastic giant-cell carcinoma of the thyroid: a study of treatment and prognosis. Cancer. 1975; 35:1293-1295.

91.   Spires JR, Schwartz MR, Miller RH. Anaplastic thyroid carcinoma: association with differentiated thyroid cancer. Arch Otolaryngol Head Neck Surg. 1988; 114:40-44.

92.   Tan RK, Finley III RK, Driscoll D, Bakamjian V, Hicks Jr WL, Shedd DP. Anaplastic carcinoma of the thyroid: a 24-year experience. Head & Neck. 1995; 17:41-48.

93.   Junor EJ, Paul J, Reed NS. Anaplastic thyroid carcinoma: 91 patients treated by surgery and radiotherapy. Eur J Surg Oncol. 1992; 18:83-88.

94.   Kobayashi T, Asakawa H, Umeshita K, et al. Treatment of 37 patients with anaplastic carcinoma of the thyroid. Head Neck. 1996; 18:36-41.

95.   Kim JH, Leeper RD. Treatment of locally advanced thyroid carcinoma with combination doxorubicin and radiation therapy. Cancer. 1987; 60:2372-75.

96.   Levendag PC, De Porre PMZR, van Putten WLJ. Anaplastic carcinoma of the thyroid gland treated by radiation therapy. Int J Radiation Oncology Biol Phys. 1993; 26:125-128.

97.   Satake S, Sugawara I, Watanabe M, Takami H. Lack of a point mutation of human DNA topoisomerase II in multidrug-resistant anaplastic thyroid carcinoma cell lines. Cancer Letters. 1997; 116:33-39.

98.   Venkataraman GM, Yatin M, Ain KB. MDR1 and MRP1 mRNA expression in primary thyroid cancers and cell lines. 79th Annual Meeting of the Endocrine Society. Minneapolis, MN. 248, 1997.

99.   Loe DW, Deeley RG, Cole SPC. Biology of the multidrug resistance-associated protein, MRP. Eur J Cancer. 1996 ; 32A:945-957.

100. Ain KB, Tofiq S, Taylor KD. Antineoplastic activity of taxol against human anaplastic thyroid carcinoma cell lines in vitro and in vivo. J Clin Endocrinol Metab. 1996; 81:3650-3653.

101. Chesky VE, Dreese WC, Hellwig CA. Hemangioendothelioma of the thyroid: review of the literature and report of a case. J Clin Endocrinol Metab. 1953; 13:801-808.

102. Egloff B. The hemangioendothelioma of the thyroid. Virchows Arch [Pathol Anat]. 1983; 1983; 400:119-142.

103. Hedinger C. Geographic pathology of thyroid diseases. Path Res Pract. 1981; 171:285-292.

104. Lamovec J, Zidar A, Zidanik B. Epithelioid angiosarcoma of the thyroid gland: report of two cases. Arch pathol Lab Med. 1994; 118:642-646.

105. Mills SE, Gaffey MJ, Watts JC, et al. Angiomatoid carcinoma and 'angiosarcoma' of the thyroid gland: a spectrum of endothelial differentiation. Am J Clin Pathol. 1994; 102:322-330.

106. Chan YF, Ma L, Boey JH, Yeung HY. Angiosarcoma of the thyroid: an immunohistochemical and ultrastructural study of a case in a Chinese patient. Cancer. 1986; 57:2381-2388.

107. **Ruchti C, Gerber HA, Schaffner T**. Factor VIII-related antigen in malignant hemangioendothelioma of the thyroid: additional evidence for the endothelial origin of this tumor. Am J Clin Pathol. 1984; 82:474-480.

108. Thaler W, Riccabona G, Riedler L, Schmid K. 1986 Zum malignen hämangioendotheliom der schilddrüse. Chirurg. 1986; 57:397-400.

109. Vollenweider I, Hedinger C, Saremaslani P, Pfaltz M. Malignant haemangioendothelioma of the thyroid, immunohistochemical evidence of heterogeneity. Path Res Pract. 1989; 184:376-381.

110.   Katoh R, Sugai T, Ono S, *et al*. Mucoepidermoid carcnoma of the thyroid gland. Cancer. 1990; 65:2020-2027.
111.   Miranda RN, Myint MA, Gnepp DR. Composite follicular variant of papillary carcinoma and mucoepidermoid carcinoma of the thyroid. Am J Surg Pathol. 1995; 19:1209-1215.
112.   Franssila KO, Harach HR, Wasenius V-M. 1984 Mucoepidermoid carcinoma of the thyroid. Histopathol. 1984; 8:847-860.
113.   Wenig BM, Adair CF, Heffess CS. Primary mucoepidermoid carcinoma of the thyroid gland: a report of six cases and a review of the literature of a follicular epithelial-derived tumor. Hum Pathol. 1995; 26:1099-1108.
114.   Harach HR, Vujanic GM, Jasani B. Ultimobranchial body nests in human fetal thyroid: an autopsy, histological, and immunohistochemical study in relation to solid cell nests and mucoepidermoid carcinoma of the thyroid. J Pathol. 1993; 169:465-469.
115.   Harach HR. Solid cell nests of the thyoid. J Pathol. 1988; 155:191-200.
116.   Pianzola HM, Ottino A, Castelletto RH. Solid cell nests of the thyroid gland: optic and immunohistochemical study at autopsies. Acta Anatomica. 1992; 143:79-83.
117.   Ozaki O, Ito K, Sugino K, Yasuda K, Yamashita T, Toshima K. Solid cell nests of the thyroid gland: precursor of mucoepidermoid carcinonma? World J Surg. 1992; 16:685-689.
118.   Mizukami Y, Nakajima H, Annen Y, Michigishi T, Nonomura A, Nakamura S. Mucin-producing poorly differentiated adenocarcinoma of the thyroid: a case report. Path Res Pract. 1993; 189:608-612.
119.   Chan KCJ, Albores-Saavedra J, Battifora H, Carcangiu ML, Rosai J. Sclerosing mucoepidermoid thyroid carcinoma with eosinophilia: a distinctive low-grade malignancy arising from the metaplastic follicles of Hashimoto's thyroiditis. Am J Surg Pathol. 1991; 15:438-448.
120.   Sim SJ, Ro JY, Ordonez NG, Cleary KR, Ayala AG. Sclerosing mucoepidermoid carcinoma with eosinophilia of the thyroid: report of two patients, one with distant metastasis, and review of the literature. Hum Pathol. 1997; 28:1091-1096.
121.   Martin JME, Sandhawa G, Temple WJ. Cervical thymoma. Arch Pathol Lab Med. 1986 ; 110:354-357.
122.   Chan JKC, Rosai J. Tumors of the neck showing thymic or related branchial pouch differentiation: a unifying concept. Hum Pathol. 1991; 22:349-367.
123.   Asa SL, Dardick I, Van Nostrand AWP, Bailey DJ, Gullane PJ. Primary thyroid thymoma: a distinct clinicopathologic entity. Hum Pathol. 1988; 19:1463-1467.
124.   Miyauchi A, Kuma K, Matsuzuka F, *et al*. Intrathyroidal epithelial thymoma: an entity distinct from squamous cell carcinoma of the thyroid. World J Surg. 1985 ; 9:128-135.
125.   Shek TWH, Luk ISC, Ng IOL, Lo CY. Lymphoepithelioma-like carcinoma of the thyroid gland: lack of evidence of association with Epstein-Barr virus. Hum Pathol. 1996; 27:851-853.
126.   Damiani S, Filotico M, Eusebi V. Carcinoma of the thyroid showing thymoma-like features. Virchows Archiv A Pathol Anat. 1991; 418:463-466.
127.   Mizukami Y, Kurumaya H, Yamada T, *et al*. Thymic carcinoma involving the thyroid gland: report of two cases. Hum Pathol. 1995; 26:576-579.
128.   Buckley NJ, Burch WM, Leight GS. Malignant teratoma in the thyroid gland of an adult: a case report and a review of the literature. Surg. 1986; 100:932-936.
129.   Kimler SC, Muth WF. Primary malignant teratoma of the thyroid: case report and literature review of cervical teratomas in adults. Cancer. 1978; 42:311--317.
130.   Ramadas K, Augustin J, Parameswaran S, Joseph F. Case report: malignant teratoma in the thyroid gland. Br J Radiol. 1996; 69:879-880.
131.   Bowker CM, Whittaker RS. Malignant teratoma of the thyroid: case report and literature review of thyroid teratoma in adults. Histopathol. 1992; 21:81-83.
132.   LaGuette J, Matias-Guiu X, Rosai J. Thyroid paraganglionoma: a clinicopathologic and immunohistochemical study of three cases. Am J Surg Pathol. 1997; 21:748-753.
133.   Bronner MP, LiVolsi VA, Jennings TA. Plat: paraganglioma-like adenomas of the thyroid. Surg Pathol. 1988; 1:383-389.
134.   Kapadia SB, Dekker A, Cheng VS, Desai U, Watson CG. Malignant lymphoma of the thyroid gland: a clinicopathologic study. Head & Neck Surg. 1982; 4:270-280.
135.   Matsuzuka F, Miyauchi A, Katayama S, *et al*. Clinical aspects of primary thyroid lymphoma: diagnosis and treatment based on our experience of 119 cases. Thyroid. 1993; 3:93-99.
136.   Abdul-Rahman ZH, Gogas HJ, Tooze JA, *et al*. T-cell lymphoma in Hashimoto's thyroiditis. Histopathol. 1996; 29:455-459.

137.   Oertel JE, Heffess CS. Lymphoma of the thyroid and related disorders. Semin Oncol. 1987; 14:333-342.
138.   Sasai K, Yamabe H, Haga H, et al. Non-Hodgkin's lymphoma of the thyroid. Acta Oncologica. 1996; 35:457-461.
139.   Anscombe AM, Wright DH. Primary malignant lymphoma of the thyroid — a tumour of mucosa-associated lymphoid tissue: review of seventy-six cases. Histopathol. 1985; 9:81-97.
140.   Logue JP, Hale RJ, Stewart AL, Duthie MB, Banerjee SS. Primary malignant lymphoma of the thyroid: a clinicopathological analysis. Int J Radiation Oncology Biol Phys. 1992; 22:929-933.
141.   Hamburger JI, Miller JM. Lymphoma of the thyroid. Ann Int Med. 1983; 99:685-693.
142.   Doria R, Jekel JF, Cooper DL. Thyroid lymphoma: The case for combined modality therapy. Cancer. 1994; 73:200-6.
143.   Pyke CM, Grant CS, Habermann TM, et al. Non-Hodgkin's lymphoma of the thyroid: Is more than biopsy necessary? World J Surg. 1992; 16:604-10.
144.   Clark OH, Levin K, Zeng Q-H, Greenspan FS, Siperstein A. Thyroid cancer: the case for total thyroidectomy. Eur J Cancer Clin Oncol. 1988; 24:305-13.
145.   Soh EY, Clark OH. Surgical considerations and approach to thyroid cancer. Endocrinol Metab Clin N Amer. 1996; 25:115-39.
146.   Goldman JM, Line BR, Aamodt RL, Robbins J. Influence of triiodothyronine withdrawal time on ^{131}I uptake postthyroidectomy for thyroid cancer. J Clin Endocrinol Metab. 1980; 50:734-39.
147.   Lakshmanan M, Schaffer A, Robbins J, Reynolds J, Norton J. A simplified low iodine diet in I-131 scanning and therapy of thyroid cancer. Clin Nucl Med. 1988; 13:866-68.
148.   Park H-M, Perkins OW, Edmondson JW, Schnute RB, Manatunga A. Influence of diagnostic radioiodines on the uptake of ablative dose of iodine-131. Thyroid. 1994; 4:49-54.
149.   Ain KB. Management of thyroid cancer. In: Braverman LE, ed. Diseases of the thyroid. Totowa, N.J.: Humana Press, Inc.; 1997; 287-317.
150.   Benua RS, Leeper RD. A method and rationale for treating metastatic thyroid carcinoma with the largest safe dose of ^{131}I. In: Medeiros-Neto G, Gaitan E, ed. Frontiers in Thyroidology. New York: Plenum Medical Book Co; 1986; 1317-1321.
151.   Gershengorn MC, Izumi M, Robbins J. Use of lithium as an adjunct to radioiodine therapy of thyroid carcinoma. J Clin Endocrinol Metab. 1976; 42:105-11.
152.   Pons F, Carrió I, Estorch M, Ginjaume M, Pons J, Milian R. Lithium as an adjuvant of iodine-131 uptake when treating patients with well-differentiated thyroid carcinoma. Clin Nucl Med. 1987; 25:644-7.
153.   Pineda JD, Lee T, Ain KB, Reynolds J, Robbins J. I-131 therapy for thyroid cancer with elevated thyroglobulin and negative diagnostic scan. Thyroid. 1992; 2:S16.
154.   Mallin WH, Elgazzar AH, Maxon HR. Imaging modalities in the follow-up of non-iodine avid thyroid carcinoma. Am J Otolaryngol. 1994; 15:417-422.
155.   Ramanna L, Waxman A, Braunstein G. Thallium-201 scintigraphy in differentiated thyroid cancer: comparison with radioiodine scintigraphy and serum thyroglobulin determinations. J Nucl Med. 1991; 32:441-46.
156.   Balon HR, Fink-Bennett D, Stoffer SS. Technetium-99m-sestamibi uptake by recurrent Hurthle cell carcinoma of the thyroid. J Nucl Med. 1992; 33:1393-95.
157.   Yen T-C, Lin H-D, Lee C-H, Chang SL, Yeh SH. The role of technetium-99m sestamibi whole-body scans in diagnosing metastatic Hürthle cell carcinoma of the thyroid gland after total thyroidectomy: A comparison with iodine-131 and thallium-201 whole-body scans. Eur J Nucl Med. 1994; 21:980-83.
158.   Grunwald F, Schomburg A, Bender H, et al. Fluorine-18 fluorodeoxyglucose positron emission tomography in the follow-up of differentiated thyroid cancer. Eur J Nucl Med. 1996; 23:312-9.
159.   Scott GC, Meier DA, Dickinson CZ. Cervical lymph node metastasis of thyroid papillary carcinoma imaged with fluorine-18-FDG, technetium-99m-pertechnetate and iodine-131-sodium iodide. J Nucl Med. 1995; 36:1843-5.
160.   Dralle H, Damm I, Scheumann GFW, Kotzerke J, Kupsch E. Frequency and significance of cervicomediastinal lymph node metastases in medullary thyroid carcinoma: Results of a compartment-oriented microdissection method. Henry Ford Hosp Med J. 1992; 40:264-67.
161.   Wong CS, Van Dyk J, Simpson WJ. Myelopathy following hyperfractionated accelerated radiotherapy for anaplastic thyroid carcinoma. Radiother Oncol. 1991; 20:3-9.
162.   Tallroth E, Wallin G, Lundell G, Löwhagen T, Einhorn J. Multimodality treatment in anaplastic giant cell thyroid carcinoma. Cancer. 1987; 60:1428-1431.

14 CHEMOTHERAPY AND BIOLOGICAL THERAPY OF THYROID CANCER

A.F. Cailleux
M.J. Schlumberger
Institut Gustave-Roussy
Villejuif, France

ANAPLASTIC THYROID CARCINOMA

Anaplastic carcinoma of the thyroid is one of the most aggressive cancers encountered in humans. It is a rare disease that occurs in elderly patients. In most cases, it represents the terminal stage in the dedifferentiation of a follicular or papillary carcinoma. In fact, anaplastic cells do not produce thyroglobulin, they are not able to transport iodine and thyrotropin (TSH) receptors are not found in their plasma cell membranes. Radioiodine treatment is useless in cases with an anaplastic component, even when it represents a small proportion of the tumor.

Most patients with anaplastic thyroid carcinoma present with a rapidly enlarging cervical mass. Pain and compressive symptoms are frequent. Lymph node metastases are frequent and distant metastases are observed initially in 20 % to 50 % of patients. The diagnosis of anaplastic carcinoma is established by biopsy or surgery.

Survival is not altered by treatment with surgery, radiotherapy or chemotherapy alone. In most patients, death is caused by local tumor invasion. The median survival is 2 to 6 months, and few patients survive for more than 12 months (1-3)

Some therapeutic trials have been carried out : more radical surgery was not more effective than less radical surgery ; radiotherapy failed to induce any significant regression. The most effective single cytotoxic agent against anaplastic carcinomas is doxorubicin, and a few responses have been reported with chemotherapy using doxorubicin and cisplatin (4). In fact, only combined multimodality therapy improved the local control rate, thus avoiding death from suffocation. Three types of therapeutic trials have been carried out.

Combination of Low-Dose Doxorubicin, Radiotherapy and Surgery

A combined regimen consisting of once weekly administration of doxorubicin (10 mg/m^2) during hyperfractionated radiotherapy (1.6 Gy (160 rads)) per treatment, twice a day for 3 days per week to a total dose of 57.6 Gy (5760 rads) in 40 days) was used in 19 patients (5). The rate of complete neck tumor response was 84 % initially and 68 % at the time of last follow-up or death. Four patients survived longer than 20 months and the median survival was 1 year, deaths being due to lung or brain metastases. Patients whose tumor volume exceeded more than 200 cm^3 at presentation did not respond and those patients who survived more than 1 year were those having radical surgery and minimal residual disease at the time of irradiation. There was no unexpected toxicity

A combination of hyperfractionated radiotherapy (1 Gy (100 rads) twice a day for 5 days per week to a total dose of 30 Gy (3000 rads)) and doxorubicin (20 mg per week) was followed by surgery after 2-3 weeks, when feasible. Then an additional dose of 16 Gy (1600 rads) was given with concomitant doxorubicin and was followed by additional doxorubicin (6). Among 16 patients, only 5 had complete local tumor control and 1 patient survived longer than 20 months. Six patients died from distant metastases and 6 from local growth. Despite the advanced age (> 70 yrs) of most patients, toxicity was moderate and no patients failed to complete the protocol because of treatment-related toxicity.

Multimodal Approach with an Aggressive Cytotoxic Regimen

A combination of hyperfractionated radiotherapy (1 Gy (100 rads) twice a day for 5 days per week to a total dose of 30 Gy (3000 rads) in 3 weeks) and chemotherapy (bleomycin 5 mg daily, cyclophosphamide 200 mg daily and 5-fluorouracil 500 mg every second day) was followed by surgery after 2 to 3 weeks, when feasible. Then radiotherapy was given with the same protocol to a total dose of 16 Gy (1600 rads) with concomitant chemotherapy and was followed by additional chemotherapy (7). Of 20 evaluable patients, 15 had an objective remission and three survived for more than a year ; 7 patients died of local tumor growth. Severe toxicity occurred in one third of the patients

A combination of chemotherapy (doxorubicin 60 mg/m^2 and cisplatin 90 mg/m^2 every 4 weeks) and radiotherapy was used in 19 patients aged less than 65 years (8). Radiotherapy was carried out in 3 courses between days 10 and 20 of the first four courses of chemotherapy and delivered 17.5 Gy (1750 rads) in 7 fractions to the neck and the upper mediastinum. Complete tumor control was obtained in 10 patients and 5 patients survived longer than 20 months, all of whom had undergone surgery. The median survival was 8 months. None of the patients not operated had complete local control of tumor. Death occurred in 15 patients, caused by distant metastases in 11 and by local growth in 2. Severe toxicity occurred in half the patients.

Hyperfractionated and Accelerated Radiotherapy

Accelerated and hyperfractionated radiotherapy enables the delivery of an efficient radiation dose in a limited period of time and prevents repopulation in rapidly growing tumors.

In a Swedish trial, the daily fraction was 1.3 Gy (130 rads) twice a day for 5 days per week to the same total dose pre and postoperatively as in previous Swedish trial, combined with doxorubicin (20 mg / week) and surgery (6). Among 17 patients, local control was obtained in 11 patients and death attributable to local failure occurred in 2 patients. These data suggested that acceleration and hyperfractionation of radiotherapy improve the effectiveness of the combined protocol .

A French trial, combining doxorubicin (60 mg/m2) and cisplatin (90 mg/m2) with hyperfractionated and accelerated radiotherapy (1.25 Gy (125 rads) twice a day for 5 days per week, to a total dose of 40 Gy (4000 rads)) between the second and third course was given to 17 patients. Local control was obtained in 14 patients (80 %) ; 4 patients survived longer than 20 months, of whom all had undergone surgery and did not have distant metastases at the initiation of the protocol (unpublished data). This protocol did not appear to be more efficient than the previous French protocol. Toxicity appeared to be similar or higher.

Conclusion

These treatment modalities are effective in some patients with anaplastic carcinoma. Acute toxicity is high and is the main factor limiting therapy in these elderly patients who are often in poor general condition. At the present time, we advocate a combination of surgery, accelerated and hyperfractionated radiotherapy with one of two protocols of chemotherapy : aggressive chemotherapy (doxorubicin-cisplatin) in patients less than 70 years and low dose doxorubicin in those over 70 years or in poor general condition.

In most protocols, only patients in whom surgery was feasible responded.

In these series, no response was observed in distant metastases. This underlines the need for treating these patients as soon as possible, before distant metastases appear. Even in patients with metastatic disease, these treatment modalities may be useful as they can avoid death by suffocation caused by local tumor growth. Debulking surgery should be performed whenever possible but should not delay the commencement of the combined protocol of chemotherapy and radiotherapy. In patients with distant metastases, further therapeutic trials using other cytotoxic agents are clearly needed. Preliminary data suggest that taxol (paclitaxel) is efficient in some patients with anaplastic carcinoma.

THYROID LYMPHOMA

Thyroid lymphoma is a rare disease that occurs in elderly patients. It almost invariably presents as a rapidly enlarging, painless neck mass. One third of patients have compressive symptoms (9,10). The mass is often fixed to surrounding tissues. Unilateral or bilateral lymph node enlargement is present in half of patients. Clinically evident distant disease is uncommon.

The majority of primary thyroid lymphomas arise in patients who have chronic autoimmune thyroiditis : most have serum anti-peroxidase and anti-thyroglobulin antibodies. When peritumor tissues can be examined, nearly all cases have histologic evidence of chronic autoimmune thyroiditis.

The diagnosis of thyroid lymphoma is established by biopsy or surgery. The majority of cases are of diffuse large cell type and of follicular center cell origin. A distinct subset of thyroid malignant lymphomas with small cells can be considered as « mucosa-associated lymphoid tissue » lymphomas (MALT-L). The differential diagnosis between MALT-lymphomas and autoimmune thyroiditis is difficult and can be made only on biopsies.

Accurate staging is very important for planning treatment. However, these patients are often elderly, in poor condition, or may require urgent therapy to relieve symptoms, making a full staging investigation before treatment impractical. Staging includes physical examination, complete blood count, serum lactate dehydrogenase and β_2-microglobulin measurements, liver function tests, bone marrow biopsy, CT scanning of the neck, thorax, abdomen and pelvis, and appropriate biopsies at other sites where tumor is suspected. Involvement of the Waldeyer's ring and of the gastrointestinal tract has been associated with thyroid lymphomas, and for this reason upper gastrointestinal radiographs or endoscopy should be performed.

Disseminated disease requires combined chemotherapy and external radiotherapy. In patients with disease apparently confined to the neck, three therapeutic modalities are available.

Small tumors are frequently treated initially as primary thyroid carcinomas. Aggressive surgery to debulk thyroid lymphomas is neither feasible nor necessary, and all patients should be treated with external radiotherapy and chemotherapy, whatever the extent of surgery.

External radiotherapy should be given in a total dose of 40 Gy (4000 rads) to the neck and mediastinum. In a third of patients with disease apparently confined to the neck and treated with external radiotherapy alone, a recurrence occurred at distant sites generally within the first year of treatment. It may be that patients having a relapse had disseminated disease at the time of diagnosis ; even with aggressive staging, distant disease may remain occult at the time of diagnosis. Chemotherapy should be an anthracycline-based regimen. It usually consists in 3 to 6 cycles of the

CHOP regimen (doxorubicin 50 mg/m^2 on day 1, cyclophosphamide 750 mg/m^2 on day 1, vincristine 1.4 mg/m2 on day 1 and prednisone 40 mg/m2/day on days 1-5) every 3 weeks. Most patients with thyroid lymphoma have bulky local disease, which is an adverse risk factor for local control with chemotherapy alone (10). Therefore, chemotherapy with an anthracycline-based regimen and radiotherapy should be given to all patients with stage I-II thyroid lymphoma, except those in poor general health or with advanced age, in whom only external radiotherapy is advised. In some series, the long term survival rate of combined chemo- and radiotherapy was nearly 100 % (9).

The therapy of MALT-lymphoma of the thyroid is not well defined, but can be derived from that used in MALT-lymphomas arising at other sites. In cases with localized disease after an accurate staging, treatment may consist in either external beam radiation alone or in chemotherapy with chlorambucil.

DIFFERENTIATED THYROID CARCINOMA

Differentiated thyroid carcinoma (DTC) has usually an indolent course. DTC patients with elevated serum thyroglobulin levels and no other evidence of disease and those with small distant metastases, even if not amenable to 131I radioiodine therapy, may survive for years or even decades. These patients are clearly not candidates for systemic treatment. In rare patients with a single or a few metastases that are slowly progressive, radical surgery may be beneficial. External radiotherapy on bone metastases may induce long term stabilization (3). However, some patients with multiple metastases have a rapidly evolutive course that may require systemic treatment.

Chemotherapy

Initially, doxorubicin alone was considered as the most effective regimen. However response rate is probably less than 20 % with most responses being transient (lasting only a few months) and partial, and side-effects being significant(4,11). Cisplatin alone was evaluated in a few studies, providing a low response rate (12,13). Combination of doxorubicin with cisplatin provided higher response rate, but toxicity was high (4,14). Combination of epirubicin and carboplatin was not more effective as compared to doxorubicin alone (13,15). In our series, no tumor response was observed with doxorubicin alone or in combination with cisplatin (13).

In 22 patients with neck relapse not suitable for surgery or radioactive iodine therapy, the combination of low dose doxorubicin (10 mg / m^2 once weekly) and external radiotherapy (200 cGy per treatment for 5 days per week) to a total dose of 56 Gy provided complete tumor response in 91 % initially, and 77 % at two years. Median survival was 4 years (5). This treatment modality may also be used in patients with poorly differentiated carcinoma confined to the neck in whom surgery is impossible.

Limited trials have used different drugs as single agents, such as bleomycin,, eliptinium acetate, cyclophosphamide, 5 fluorouracil, methotrexate, mitoxantrone or etoposide. No significant response was observed (12,13). Up to now there is no available data concerning the efficacy of taxanes and of the inhibitors of topoisomerase I.

In conclusion, chemotherapy is poorly effective in metastatic DTC patients. Further trials using other combination regimens are clearly needed and due to the rarity of this disease, preferably on a multicenter basis. Only metastatic patients with no radioiodine uptake and with evolutive disease should be included in such trials. Indeed, an informed consent should be obtained before inclusion.

Biotherapy

Interferon α2a alone or in combination with doxorubicin (15 mg/week) was ineffective in 10 patients. Similarly interleukin 2, alone or in combination with either doxorubicin or cisplatin did not provide any response in 6 patients (unpublished data).

Somatostatin analogs were ineffective in a limited trial (16).

Retinoic acid was reported to induce radioactive uptake, and to increase the expression of 5'deiodinase and of adhesion molecules in various thyroid carcinoma cell lines (17-19). A single clinical report showed stabilization of both tumor mass and thyroglobulin level during isotretinoin treatment (20).

Farnesyl-transferase inhibitors will be available in the near future for clinical trials. The ras proto-oncogene is activated in about 40 % of differentiated thyroid tumors (21). The farnesyl modification of ras protein is essential for the cellular transformation induced by ras, suggesting new targets for pharmacological research (22,23).

Due to the ineffectiveness of cytotoxic chemotherapy, there is a clear need for new trials, using either cytotoxic drugs that have not been already tested or other pharmacological agents.

MEDULLARY THYROID CARCINOMA

Medullary thyroid carcinoma (MTC) has usually an indolent course over decades. Patients with elevated circulating levels of calcitonin (CT) or carcino-embryonic antigen (CEA) after initial treatment and no other evidence of disease may survive for decades, and are not candidates for systemic treatment. Only MTC patients with evolutive distant metastases, may require systemic chemotherapy. In patients with metastatic MTC, metastases are multiple in each organ, and involve several organs (liver, lungs and bones). For these reasons, surgery for distant metastases is rarely indicated. Symptomatic treatments against diarrhea and pain are needed, when these symptoms are present.

Chemotherapy trials have been limited by the scarcity of these tumors.

Chemotherapy

Initially, doxorubicin was considered as the most effective single agent in MTC patients. However, response rate was only 15-20 %, and most responses were partial and transient lasting only a few month and with no beneficial effects on survival (4,11,14,24,25). Furthermore, toxicities were significant. Cisplatin was almost ineffective, with an overall response rate of only 13 % (12,26). Combination of doxorubicin with cisplatin or streptozocin (27), given during the early eighties, did not increase the response rate, as compared to doxorubicin alone (4,12,14).

Etoposide, given as a single agent appeared to be effective in limited trials, and among 9 patients, 5 tumor responses were observed (13,28), but this was not confirmed in a further study as no tumor response was observed with etoposide given as a second line of chemotherapy, among 16 evaluable patients (29).

In recent years, drugs that have been shown to be active in other neuroendocrine tumors have been used in MTC patients, such as 5-fluoro-uracil, dacarbazine and streptozocin. An anecdotal report suggested the efficacy of 5-fluoro-uracil and dacarbazine in one MTC patient (30). This was confirmed in a subsequent trial on 5 patients, of whom 3 had a tumor response (31). By alternating a combination of 5-fluoro-uracil and streptozocin with a combination of 5-fluoro-uracil and dacarbazine in 20 patients, we observed a partial response in 3 and a stabilization in 11, with an improvement of the performance status in 7 (29). A more recent trial has consisted in alternating a combination of doxorubicin and streptozocin with a combination of 5-fluoro-uracil and dacarbazine in 16 patients, and provided 3 partial responses (unpublished data) ; the response rate was therefore similar to that obtained with the previous combination despite the addition of doxorubicin. Another trial used a combination of cyclophosphamide, vincristine and dacarbazine in 7 patients, and provided 2 partial responses (32). The combination of doxorubicin, cyclophosphamide, vincristine and dacarbazine in 9 patients provided 3 responses (33). These regimens had an acceptable toxicity even in patients who had already been treated with other drug regimens. Response to therapy may be rapid or may occur after several courses of chemotherapy, in accordance with the slow growth rate of most of the MTC's.

Tumor responses with these combinations were observed in only 20 to 30 % of patients with metastatic MTC. Most tumor responses were partial, but some lasted more than one year. Toxicity, although acceptable, is significant. For these reasons, chemotherapy should be undertaken only in patients with distant metastases. In these patients, who may survive for years in the absence of systemic treatment, the initiation of chemotherapy should be decided only when a rapid progression of the metastases has been documented. Even in these cases an informed consent should be obtained from the patient. When chemotherapy is decided, the patient should be included in a controlled trial. Clearly, therapeutic trials are needed.

Biotherapy

Tamoxifen inhibits growth of a cell line of human MTC in vitro, as well as their xenographs in nude mice (34), but failed in 2 patients with metastatic MTC (35). Somatostatin analogs (Sandostatin®, 300-1000 µg per day) proved to be ineffective in metastatic MTC patients, even on diarrhea, flush or CT levels (36, 37).

Interferon α–2a, either alone or in combination with doxorubicin were ineffective in 9 patients with evolutive metastases from MTC (unpublished data)..

Combination of somatostatin analogs with interferon α–2b did not induce any tumor response in 8 patients (38).

Metabolic radiotherapy

A phase I trial has recently been conducted with bispecific monoclonal antibodies directed against CEA and labeled with ^{131}I radioiodine (39). Its efficacy has still to be demonstrated. Of note, iodine 131 metaiodobenzylguanidine has been used to treat MTC, but the response rate has been low (unpublished data).

Conclusion

Chemotherapy is effective in only a small proportion of patients with metastatic MTC. Further trials using other combination regimens are clearly needed, preferably on a multicenter basis.

Due to the low efficacy of chemotherapy, there is still some uncertainty to determine the optimal time to start systemic chemotherapy, even in patients with known metastases. Rapid tumor progression should dictate the initiation of chemotherapy, or any other systemic treatment. In any case, it should be given only after an informed consent has been signed by the patient.

REFERENCES

1. Nel C.J.C., Van Heerden J.A., Goellner J.R., Gharib H., Mc Conahey W.M., Taylor W.F., Grant C.S. Anaplastic carcinoma of the thyroid : a clinicopathologic study of 82 cases. Mayo Clin Proc 1985; 60:51-58.
2. Venkatesh Y.S.S., Ordonez N.G., Schultz P.N., Hickey R.C., Goepfert H., Samaan N.A. Anaplastic carcinoma of the thyroid A clinicopathologic study of 121 cases. Cancer 1990; 66: 321-330.
3. Tubiana M., Haddad E., Schlumberger M., Hill C., Rougier P., Sarrazin D. External radiotherapy in thyroid cancers. Cancer 1985; 55:2062-2071.
4. Shimaoka K., Schoenfeld D.A., De Wys W.D., Creech R.H., De Conti R. A randomized trial of Doxorubicin versus Doxorubicin plus Cisplatin in patients with advanced thyroid carcinoma. Cancer 1985; 56:2155-2160.

5. Kim J.H., Leeper R.D. Treatment of locally advanced thyroid carcinoma with combination Doxorubicin and radiation therapy. Cancer 1987; 60:2372-2375.
6. Tennvall J., Lundell G., Hallquist A., Wahlberg P., Wallin G., Tibblin S. and the Swedish Anaplastic Thyroid Cancer Group. Combined doxorubicin, hyperfractionated radiotherapy, and surgery in anaplastic thyroid carcinoma. Cancer 1994; 74:1348-1354.
7. Tallroth E., Wallin G., Lundell G, Löwhagen T., Einhorn J. Multimodality treatment in anaplastic giant cell thyroid carcinoma. Cancer 1987; 60:1428-1431.
8. Schlumberger M., Parmentier C., Delisle M.J., Couette J.E., Droz J.P., Sarrazin D. Combination therapy for anaplastic giant cell thyroid carcinoma. Cancer 1991; 67:564-566.
9. Matsuzuka F., Miyauchi A., Katayama S., Narabayashi I., Ikeda H., Kuma K., Sugawara M. Clinical aspects of primary thyroid lymphoma : diagnosis and treatment based on our experience of 119 cases. Thyroid 1993; 3:93-99.
10. Doria R., Jekel J.F., Cooper D.L. Thyroid lymphoma : the case for combined modality therapy. Cancer 1994; 73:200-206.
11. Gottlieb J.A., Hill C.S. Adriamycin (NSC - 123 127) therapy in thyroid carcinoma. Cancer Chemother, Rep 1975; 6:283-296.
12. Droz J.P., Schlumberger M., Rougier P., Ghosn M., Gardet P., Parmentier C. Chemotherapy in metastatic nonanaplastic thyroid cancer : experience at the Institut Gustave-Roussy. Tumori 1990; 76:480-483.
13. Hoskin P.J., Harmer C. Chemotherapy for thyroid cancer. Radiother Oncol 1987; 10:187-194.
14. Williams S.D., Birch R., Einhorn L.H.Phase II evaluation of doxorubicin plus cisplatin in advanced thyroid cancer : a Southeastern Cancer Study Group Trial. Cancer Treat. Rep. 1986; 70:405-407.
15. Magee M.J., Howard J., Bosl G.J., Wittes R.E. Phase II trial of 4'-epidoxorubicin in advanced carcinoma of head and neck origin. Cancer Treat. Rep. 1985; 69:125-126.
16. Zlock D.W., Greenspan F.S., Clark O.H., Higgins C.B. Octreotide therapy in advanced thyroid cancer. Thyroid 1994; 4: 427-431.
17. Van Herle A.J., Agatep M.L., Padua Iii D.N., Totanes T.L., Canlapan D.V., Van Herle H.M. Effects of 13 cis-retinoic acid on growth and differentiation of human follicular carcinoma cells (UCLA RO 82 W-1) in vitro. J Clin Endocrinol Metab 1990; 71:755-763.
18. Arai M., Tsushima T., Isozaki O., Shizume K., Emoto N., Demura H., et al. Effects of retinoids on iodine metabolism, thyroid peroxydase gene expression, and deoxyribonnucleic acid synthesis in porcine thyroid cells in culture. Endocrinology 1991; 129:2827-2833.
19. Schreck R., Schnieders F., Schmutzler C., Koehrle J. Retinoids stimulate type I iodothyronine 5'deiodinase activity in human follicular thyroid carcinoma cell lines. J Clin Endocrinol Metab 1994; 79:791-798.
20. Börner A.R., Simon D. Isotretinoin in metastatic thyroid cancer. Ann Int Med 1997; 127:246.
21. Challeton C, Bounacer A, Duvillard JA, Caillou B, De Vathaire F, Monier R, Schlumberger M, Suarez HG. Pattern of ras and gsp oncogene mutations in radiation-associated human thyroid tumors. Oncogene 1995; 11:601-603.
22. Jackson J.H., Cochrane C.G., Bourne J.R., Solski P.A., Buss J.E., Der C.J. Farnesyl modification of Kirsten-ras exon 4B protein is essential for transformation. Proc Natl Acad Sci. 1990; 87: 3042-3046.
23. Gibbs J.B., Oliff A., Kohl N.E. Farnesyltransferase inhibitors : ras research yields a potential cancer therapeutic. Cell. 1994; 77:175-178.
24. Husain M., Alsever R.N., Lock J.P., George W.F., Katz F.H. Failure of medullary carcinoma to respond to doxorubicin therapy. Hormone Res. 1978; 9:22-25.
25. Leight G.S., Farrel R.E., Wells S.A., Falletta J.M Effects of chemotherapy on calcitonin (CT) levels in patients with metastatic medullary thyroid carcinoma (MTC). Proc Ann Meet Am Assoc Cancer Res 1980; 21:622.
26. Kamalakar P., Freeman A.I., Higby D.J., Wallace H.J., Sinks L.F. Clinical response and toxicity with cisdichlorodiammineplatinum (II) in children. Cancer Treat Rep. 1977; 61:835-839.
27. Kelsen D.P., Cheng E., Kemeny N., Magill G.B., Yagoda N. Streptozotocin and adriamycin in the treatment of APUD tumors (carcinoid, islet cell and medullary carcinoma of the thyroid) (Abstr.). Proc Am Assoc Cancer Res. 1982; 111.
28. Kelsen D., Fiore J., Heelan E., Cheng E, Magill G. Phase II trial of Etoposide in APUD tumors. Cancer Treat Rep. 1987; 71:305-307.
29. Schlumberger M., Abdelmoumene N., Delisle M.J., Couette J.E. and the Groupe d'Etude des Tumeurs à Calcitonine (GETC). Treatment of advanced medullary thyroid cancer with an

alternating combination of 5 FU-streptozocin and 5 FU-dacarbazine. Br J Cancer. 1995; 71:363-365.

30. Petursson S.R. Metastatic medullary thyroid carcinoma. Complete response to combination chemotherapy with dacarbazine and 5-fluorouracil. Cancer. 1988; 62:1899-1903.

31. Orlandi F., Caraci P., Berruti A., Puligheddu B., Pivano G., Dogliotti L., Angeli A. Chemotherapy with dacarbazine and 5-fluorouracil in advanced medullary thyroid cancer. Ann Oncol. 1994; 5:763-765.

32 . Wu L.T., Averbuch S.D., Ball D.W., de Bustros A., Baylin S.B., McGuire W.P. Treatment of advanced medullary thyroid carcinoma with a combination of cyclophosphamide, vincristine and dacarbazine Cancer. 1994; 73:432-436.

33. Burgess MA, Sellin RV, Gagel RP. Chemotherapy for metastatic medullary carcinoma of the thyroid (MTC) with doxorubicin, imidazole carboxamide (DTIC), vincristine (VCR) and cyclophosphamide (CPA). ASCO, 1995.

34. Weber C.J., Marvin M., Krekun S., Koschitzky T., Karp F., Benson M., Feind C.R. Effects of tamoxifen and somatostatin on growth of human medullary, follicular and papillary thyroid carcinoma cell lines : tissue culture and nude mouse xenograft studies. Surgery. 1990; 109:1065-1071.

35. Garcia Pascual E.L., Millan M., Aglada J., Garau J. Tamoxifen failure in medullary thyroid carcinoma. Tumori. 1993; 79:357-358.

36. Mahler C., Verhelst J., de Longueville M., Harris A. Long term treatment of metastatic thyroid carcinoma with the somatostatin analog octreotide. Clin Endocrinol. 1990; 33:261-269.

37. Modigliani E., Cohen R., Joannidis S., Siame-Mourot C., Guliana J.M., Charpentier G., Cassuto D., Bentata-Pessayre M., Tabarin A., Roger P., Caron P., Guillausseau P.J., Lalau J.D., Tourniaire J., Bayard F., Aufevre P., James-Deidier A., Calmettes C. Result of long-term continuous subcutaneous octreotide administration in 14 patients with medullary thyroid carcinoma. Clin Endocrinol. 1992; 36:183-186.

38. Lupoli G., Cascone E., Arlotta F., Vitale G., Celentano L., Salvatore M., Lombardi G. Treatment of advanced medullary thyroid carcinima with a combination of recombinant interferon ?-2b and octreotide. Cancer. 1995; 78:1114-1118.

39. Bardiès M., Bardet S., Faivre-Chauvet A., Peltier P., Douillard J.Y., Mahé M., Fiche M., Lisbona A., Giacalone F., Meyer P., Gautherot F., Touvier E., Barbet J., Chatal J.-F. Bispecific antibody and iodine-131-labeled bivalent hapten dosimetry in patients with medullary thyroid or small-cell lung cancer. J Nucl Med. 1996; 37:1853-1859.

INDEX

Page numbers in *italics* indicate figures. Page numbers followed by "t" indicate tables.